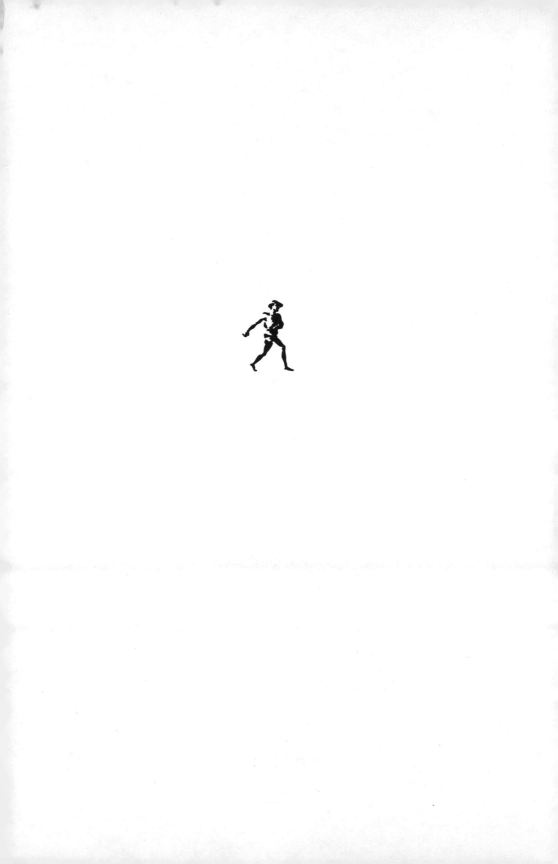

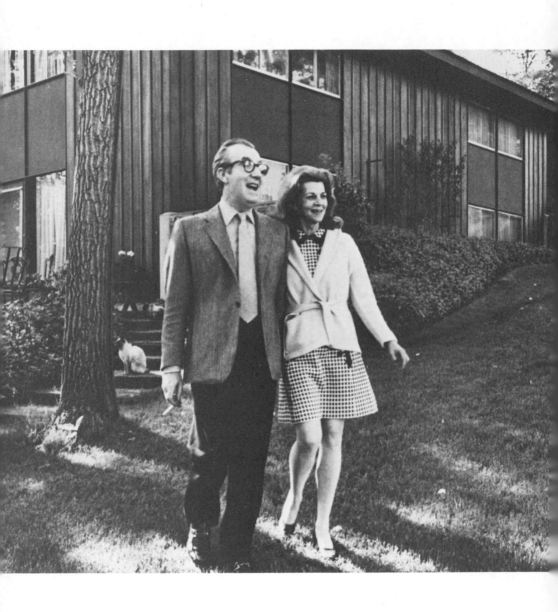

CORNELIUS RYAN
AND
KATHRYN MORGAN RYAN

A Private Battle

SIMON AND SCHUSTER · NEW YORK

DESIGNED BY EVE METZ
MANUFACTURED IN THE UNITED STATES OF AMERICA

1 2 3 4 5 6 7 8 9 10

LIBRARY OF CONGRESS CATALOGING IN PUBLICATION DATA

RYAN, CORNELIUS.
A PRIVATE BATTLE.

INCLUDES INDEX.
1. PROSTATE GLAND—CANCER—BIOGRAPHY.
2. RYAN, CORNELIUS.   3. JOURNALISTS—UNITED
STATES—BIOGRAPHY.   I. RYAN, KATHRYN MORGAN,
JOINT AUTHOR.   II. TITLE.
RC280.P7R93   362.1'9'699463 [B]   78-27037

ISBN 0–671–22594–4

CONTENTS

A PRIVATE BATTLE

ACKNOWLEDGMENTS
PAGE 445

ABOUT CORNELIUS

—

ON NOVEMBER 23, 1974, a bright, sunny Saturday more like spring than autumn, Cornelius Ryan died of cancer at 7:44 P.M. in New York's Memorial Sloan-Kettering Hospital. His last book, *A Bridge Too Far*, published two months earlier, was number two on nonfiction best-seller lists. He had other books planned. The book you are reading is one he had never mentioned. Yet until a month before his death he had worked on it in total secrecy for over four years while simultaneously writing *A Bridge Too Far*.

From July 24, 1970, until October 19, 1974, the Sunday before he entered the hospital for the last time, my husband had kept voluminous records of those four years and eighty-seven days. The material he accumulated is in the form of over 200 letters, more than 75 memoranda and medical reports, 8 bulging notebooks, and six 120-minute tapes.

Incredibly, neither his secretary, Anne Bardenhagen, nor I were aware of this hidden work. To Anne he had dictated an outline of events covering the two-week period immediately after he was told he had cancer. But that was all. The research for the book behind the book was entirely his own, seen and shared by no one.

He was able to build up his secret files by following a practice we were all accustomed to. He began work early in the mornings before Anne and I came in and remained long

9

after we left. Although confined to a wheelchair during much of the last four years of his life, he continued this work habit, going to the office across the driveway from our house seven days a week. His desk was sacrosanct, littered with interviews, war diaries, maps, pages of manuscript on *Bridge*. We had long ago learned never to disturb the seemingly random piles of material which cluttered it and the worktable behind him.

A week after his death, Anne and I began the task of putting away the files and books and work sheets he had used. In an unlocked file drawer in his desk, beneath a large manila folder containing a lengthy interview he had held with General Dwight D. Eisenhower, were the papers, jottings, journals, and tapes which form the substance of this book. A cursory glance showed that, with his tenacious ability to get at the facts, Connie had not only recorded his own case history of cancer but, in effect, he had written a miniautobiography as well. Only the tapes had not been transcribed. They were labeled with such headings as "Cancer I—1970" or "C—1974." It was several weeks before Anne and I could bring ourselves to listen to them and more weeks passed before she began transcribing the tapes.

As page after page was finished, we found countless references indicating that this, indeed, was prime research for a book Connie intended publishing—but not until others were finished, not until the cancer was killed or arrested. The tapes, products of many of the long hours he had spent in the office alone or in the confines of a hospital room, confirmed much of what I already knew about his illness. A cancer patient's innermost agony is quite apart from the physical torment he endures and it cannot be fully revealed or candidly shared. Connie obviously needed that time alone to examine his inner conflicts, to give way outside the presence of anxious friends and family to the incredible pain that racked his body, to renew again and again his adamant refusal to take drugs that would have eased his pain but might, he felt, have dulled his powers of reason. We were aware of the toll that *Bridge* had taken on his precarious health. Now we were discovering another, equally demanding chronicle whose existence had been the best kept secret of his life.

Anne and I, we very soon learned, had our secrets too. Without each other's knowledge or Connie's we had been keeping diaries of our own. Anne's recorded the page progress of *Bridge,* business and doctors' appointments, good days and bad. Mine was similar, but its references were to Connie's health, hospitalizations, and treatments. It was also a social calendar of those four years, a record of family life, lists of activities, speeches, trips, conferences, friends we saw, and, in the last three years of his life, notes on the progress of his disease. A sample entry reads:

No sleep again. Pain is unbelievable. Made tea around 4 A.M. C dictated outline for break-out of Horrocks' tanks. I'm to get out interviews of XXX Corps men, select best to use tomorrow.

A Bridge Too Far was the common denominator for all of us. Now we are sharing another book—the secret work that was to have been written in the better days Connie hoped would come.

I have depended on the tapes as a guideline for this book. Wherever they tend to abbreviate an episode, I have filled in with more descriptive material from my husband's written records or from the diaries Anne and I wrote. For example, the tapes mention the initial fear Connie had that his health was failing in April 1970, some three months before the cancer was actually discovered. I have amplified from his diary of that same April, which contains references both descriptive and reflective, relating to conversations he had, places he traveled to. It is the kind of minutiae the intrigued him all his professional life.

He had an insatiable curiosity about almost everything. The description of a place will occupy several pages in his diary, interspersed with detailed accounts of a particular day and particular conversations. Even in everyday life it was the Ryan way of making history human.

With his reporter's determination to get at the facts, Connie researched his cancer as completely as time and mobility would allow. He interrogated his doctors about his disease much as he would question soldiers about a military operation. He took copious notes, read position papers published in medical journals and available from cancer research centers; he learned to read some laboratory reports and to understand and recognize changes in his X rays. He trained himself to understand the gist of some clinical reports by querying his doctors and by hunting up references in medical books. He knew his way around the hospitals he was in and could come out a maze of turnings and corridors to end up at laboratories, radiology departments, and specialists' offices with the same ease as those who worked there. I remember one of his doctors once saying to him, "I may as well go over this report with you in detail. You'll find out about it somehow if I don't." The doctor then explained to me that he was once startled to see Connie appear in a hospital corridor, a medical coat open over his business suit. As the doctor watched in amazement, Connie nodded greetings to nurses and residents on his brisk trip down the hall, disappearing finally through a door marked Authorized Personnel Only.

The medical reports, his diary, my diary, Anne's diary, the tapes: together they tell, as accurately as it is possible to do so, the story of Cornelius Ryan's last four and a half years of life. They are the written record of how he was and what he did and how we worked and lived together. Since the material is basic, raw research—no single part able to stand alone—I have assembled and organized the whole into story form. I have augmented and developed notes and jottings, rewritten those portions of Connie's diaries and tapes (as he would have done himself) to meet the requirements of clarity and narration, and edited out irrelevancies.

Although the tapes run to less wordage than the written

material, it seemed fitting that the emphasis be placed on them. As they play, Connie's voice, vibrant and strong even in the last months, is compelling. If I had never found them, if I had never listened to them, I would have been forever without that extra dimension to his life and thoughts which the specter of cancer put between us.

After his death, hundreds of letters poured in over a period of nearly five months. They were from readers and admirers of his work, from fellow historians, heads of state, and the soldiers and civilians he wrote about. To paraphrase the dedication we used for *Bridge,* this book is for them all—from the two of us.

KATHRYN MORGAN RYAN

Throughout this book sections containing my work on the raw material Connie alone had gathered, written, or taped, is labeled, CORNELIUS. The remainder, expanded from my diaries and taken from memory, are identified by the heading, KATHRYN.

Part One
THE VERDICT
July 1970

$$\stackrel{=}{=} 1 \stackrel{=}{=}$$

Pathological Laboratory

Name: Ryan Cornelius   Age 50
Date: 7–23–70   Ward: D 612   Path No. K–3–1014

SPECIMEN LABELED (3) BIOPSY OF PROSTATE
CLINICAL—CARCINOMA OF PROSTATE

GROSS: Received in formalin are five elongated gray white soft tissues. Each fragment is attached on a separate piece of filter paper. The largest fragment measures 1.5 cm in length and 3 mm in maximum diameter. The smallest fragment measures 5 mm in length and 2 mm in average diameter. The entire specimen is submitted for microscopic study.

MICROSCOPIC: Prostatic tissue is heavily infiltrated by small irregular glands which frequently have a back-to-back configuration. One of the fragments contains a sympathetic ganglion and nerve and these are also extremely invaded by carcinoma.

DIAGNOSIS: Adenocarcinoma of prostate.

CORNELIUS

On this early summer morning my office is patched with sun and shade. Even the great stand of trees at the far edge of the lawn cannot bar the light that pours into the small hedged garden just outside my sliding windows and splashes into my workroom. As on so many other days, I have swiveled my chair to the landscape. Usually the view, stretching for miles to distant hills I have never yet identified, simply exists. But today, everyday sights take on uncommon importance. The bronze marigolds in the little garden are lush and thick and just now a bird swept down intent, I suppose, on an insect or worm in the still-damp grass. Farther back in the forest other birds are on the wing. The world hums with life outside the office. Inside, I am not so sure. On this soft morning I think I must begin to acknowledge the distinct possibility that I am dying.

The replay of my voice speaking such words into the tape recorder is uncanny in this silent room. I started this tape with the thought that it might serve a therapeutic use. To record unsettling thoughts and feelings here alone, away from the presence of others may, in time, ease the awful feeling that I am under a sentence of death. I may even learn to grow accustomed to the knowledge although, at the moment, the probability seems very far away.

I am self-conscious, almost embarrassed, to sit here and speak aloud on such a subject. I notice how quiet the office is, a silence as heavy and mournful as my mood permeates the building. I miss the absence of workaday noises—the jangling phones, the hum of the copying machine, the sounds of my secretary at work in the next room. More than any of these, the sight of my wife's tidy desk and empty chair across the way from where I sit makes me unbearably lonely. I am apprehensive and frankly afraid.

On this Saturday, July 25, 1970, only the big synchronous clock on the wall across the room from my desk makes its customary noise. It has just flapped over another minute. The time is 6:13 A.M. Just under twelve hours ago—at precisely 6:35 P.M. yesterday—my wife and I were told by a prominent New York urologist that I have a primary carcinoma of the prostate. He meant that I've got cancer. In these tormented hours this is the first time I've said that word out loud.

18

The diagnosis changes everything. Familiar objects conjure up their histories. Here in the office the memorabilia of my life are all around me. On the desk near the tape recorder a young Kathryn—now my wife for twenty years—smiles out from a small silver frame. Sitting possessively beside her is our first dog, Sean, a parti-colored cocker spaniel. I am reminded that he never liked men and allowed me to live in our first apartment under his constant scrutiny and abiding suspicion.

Opposite Katie's picture is one of the children, Geoff and Vicki, baby fat not gone then, mugging for my camera. Time doesn't fly. It hurtles. I took that picture nine years ago when they were seven and four. That little lad with face and ears and almost noble brow has disappeared beneath a hirsute avalanche and I almost feel like that father in a comic strip: I can't be sure Geoff's facing me unless I see the zipper on his jeans. Vicki, on the other hand, has not changed her hairstyle in all these years. It sweeps back from her forehead, straw colored as mine once was, and only slightly longer than her brother's. The plump little oval face has thinned in adolescence, disclosing cheekbones and, a father's thought, a growing beauty. There is also temper, so her mother says, but I prefer to think of it as spirit because it's in me, too.

On the same wall where the clock is constantly reminding me of time are my favorite photographs—heads of state, friends I love, journalists so renowned in their profession the very word was lustrous because of them. And on the table facing my desk are awards, plaques, and medals, each one less an honor than a challenge to make my work better. Nearby are my helmet, musette bag, and map case from World War II, conjuring up memories both good and bad, tempered and diluted by the years. Before today these objects were the trappings of my office. This morning they are the essence of my life.

Now cancer will be my closest possession, going with me from office to house, to conferences and dinner parties, as I go myself. I have got to get used to having it always here. I have got to think about what influence it may assume in time, not only over me but on my family, friends, and work. This seems as good a time as any to start to talk it out on tape. I want to spare Kathryn and the children as much as possible. I will only be able to deal candidly with this subject through the tape recorder or in notebooks I will have to hide somewhere among the research material only I delve into. For now, the space behind the Russian atlas seems as safe a place as any. The book is within arm's reach on the shelf where I keep translations and no one ever looks at them but me.

What comes to mind immediately is how fast cancer alienates one from the usual routines and behavior. I suppose I'm less alive than I was yesterday and by tomorrow I'll be dying more than I am today. Not in the manner of the old cliché that you began to die the minute you are born. That is not much consolation. There's not a time limit inherent in that old bromide. My time as of now is most definitely limited, predetermined by cancer survival statistics and the absence of real progress against the disease.

I feel such a terrible sense of injustice. What did I do to deserve this? Yet, that's just the kind of question I've got to eliminate from my mind. I do not exactly trust my ability to maintain objectivity publicly unless I can release the body quakes and shocks in private. And how can you make people who haven't got cancer understand what's happened to you without having to endure their pity as well? I'm damned if I want pity. Self-pity is bad enough.

In the long hours since we got the news I've tried to rationalize the verdict. But all the pat, logical, arguments—like, "You're good for at least fifteen years," or, "Look, you might be run over by a truck this afternoon"—work for only a second. Then I hear the doctor's voice again and there is no logic or reason that helps me. It is odd that apart from a slight aching of the prostate after a series of tests and examinations this week, there is no pain, no dramatic change, caused by this malignancy. Except in my mind.

Does this cancer really exist? Did some harassed technician mix my biopsy slides with those of some other poor bastard's? How can I accept the proposition that maybe I won't be around much longer when the only evidence I've been shown was a couple of slides that appear to have a few thin red streaks on them?

Those last few sentences are illogical. The slides weren't mixed. The biopsy report is most certainly mine. I know I'm attempting to grasp at straws.

I suspect that is not uncommon in these first few hours. There is simply no way to maintain a precise progression of thoughts and actions after such an emotional shock. My mind swings from disbelief to fatalism. I am vacillating between a surging belief that all will be well and a maudlin conviction that nothing will ever be right again.

The diagnosis is causing me not just anguish, but anger as well. Why has cancer invaded *my* body? Why did *I* acquire these virulent deadly cells? Those are selfish, arrogant questions but objective thought seems to have deserted me for the moment. I can only think "Why me?"

I haven't even reached the halfway mark in the histories I am writing. If I have to get cancer, why can't it show up later, say twenty years from now?

Why couldn't I have had heart disease instead? The medical profession appears to have acquired a fund of sophisticated knowledge in that field. Every day one reads of complicated, successful surgery, of diets, medicines, and exercise to help mend an ailing heart.

Who mends cancer? The New York urologist tells me that a radical prostatectomy is my one hope of "cure." His definition of being "cured" is to survive cancer-free for five years following the surgery. I find such a standard ludicrous!

Will I die within months instead of lasting out the "cure"

if I don't have this operation? The doctor wants me to have the prostatectomy next week. Such urgency appalls me. I cannot make that crucial decision without more time. Professionally, I have never accepted a single piece of historical data without researching it to the fullest, collecting all the opinions and interviews I could.

With my books I have had the time to do the research and determine the accuracy of a fact. This doctor has so frightened me that I don't know if I have time to get other medical opinions. Perhaps he is painting the grimmest picture possible in order to goad me into action. But I am not at all sure that the operation he wants to perform *is* the right course of action.

For all I know the cancer may be firmly entrenched and radical surgery may not be the answer. Just how far *has* this disease progressed? The doctor believes it is confined to the prostate. Suppose it's not? Then what good would the operation do? Wouldn't it all be for nothing? Doesn't cancer kill you anyway?

Even if the urologist is correct I have to try to resolve this dilemma by methods that I know best. I must get other views. Somewhere out there in the medical world, a profession as foreign to me as the theoretical physicist's domain, are the sources, statistics, and terminology I will need in order to assess my chances of survival, to find precisely the course of action that will work best in my particular case. I cannot unequivocably accept one lone medical opinion. I simply cannot do it.

Just now I thought of something that is probably the closest comparison to my present predicament I have ever experienced. During World War II I found myself caught up with a patrol in a minefield. My reaction, and I remember it so very well, had two distinct plateaus: how did I get myself into this situation? and, now, let's get out of it!

Curiously, back then, I cannot remember experiencing

fear. Neither do I recall any great surge of courage. I think my reaction was almost mechanical. There was no point in dwelling on the fact that we were in the minefield. The sole objective was to get through it safely—and somehow we all did. Luck would appear to play a rather large factor in life. At the moment mine seems to be running out. Now, as in those wartime days, I don't know what steps will bring me through this grave ordeal, but I can't stay rooted to one spot forever.

Unless, unwittingly, I have already stayed too long. It may be too late to extricate myself, for, if one uses the approximate time of the pathological expert's diagnosis, I began dying forty-two hours ago.

No, let me correct that. The first indication I had that something was wrong occurred about four months back. So presumably I have been dying for the better part of this, my fiftieth, year.

I've just played those last few sentences back. Presumably at this early stage, the mathematics of self-pity can be raised to infinity. It must be due to the shock. Without scientific knowledge to back me up, I would guess that the worst time emotionally is in these first few hours after you get the bad news.

There's a mosquito in here buzzing around the desk. If it stings me I hope the damn thing gets cancer.

I'm reasonably certain that no one in my family ever had this particular illness. Being Irish, we've had our share of tuberculosis, heart problems, poverty, the odd famine now and then, and in recent years a couple of uncles went a little queer in the head, but all that reflects our Irishness more than any medical predisposition. To be Irish is to be a little mad to begin with. Otherwise our whole mystique would crumble.

On the fireplace wall opposite my desk is a tapestry of the Ryan family arms. It shows a writing pen and sword in base *in saltire proper*, which means they are X-shaped or crossed and belong correctly to our particular family tree. I don't know who the first Ryan scribes or soldiers were, but sitting here I think back on the two who shaped my life. My grandfather, Cornelius the First, was a journalist; my father, John, was a soldier. Both their vocations rubbed off on me. As did their names—Cornelius John Ryan.

Even now, I remember him well. Cornelius the First, arrogant and wise, possessor of the renowned Ryan nose— long, formidable, but extremely subject to breakage. Our family's prominent, fragile proboscises have been damaged frequently on rugby or soccer fields and once, in my case, by a piece of shrapnel which honed in on my large facial adornment like one of today's guided missiles. But just as often that distinctive Ryan feature has been flattened during a burst of careless talk in a Dublin pub. Still, I like to think we gave as good as we got.

Cornelius the First acquired three or four fractures in his lifetime, about evenly divided as to cause. To him the pen was certainly as mighty as the sword, and just as deadly. It got both him and his nose into a number of irretrievable positions. Grandfather was a pamphleteer whose political writings caused ire, exasperation, and danger to his spectacular profile in some circles in Ireland. Still, he was not deterred by opposing opinions or the authority that often went with them. He was taken off fairly regularly to jail, where he not only set about converting his keepers to his philosophy but scribbled ever more damaging prose from his cell which, strangely, was always ready for his arrival.

As a very young lad, I, often accompanied by my brother Joe, was sent daily during Grandfather's temporal retreats to get his copy which he lowered to me by rope-tied basket in plain view of the constabulary and passersby. Those who noticed our little byplay seemed to regard the procedure as quite unremarkable—a rather sensible Irish view given the nature of our people.

As soon as the basket reached me, I would pocket Grandfather's article, free the little copy container, and tie the rope to the handle of a large, heavy bucket that I had brought by pull cart over precarious cobblestones to the prison. When Grandfather was in jail, I was never to appear below his cell without it. With two light jerks on the rope to alert him that help was on the way, I would laboriously lift the bucket and Cornelius the First would begin carefully to haul the weighty pail up the front of the prison wall, deftly avoiding any protruding masonry that might threaten the delicate balance of the load. Then, with consummate skill he would empty the bucket's contents through the bars of his cell into a washbasin he had conveniently set on a table just inside his open window. By this taxing procedure Grandfather's daily supply of porter would arrive safely to his cell. He seldom lost a drop during the hazardous journey up the wall or in the still more finicky decanting into the washbasin. That risky operation completed, he'd send the empty can back down and I'd tie the copy basket on again and watch the rope whiz up to his cell where he hitched it fast against the bars. With the porter to fortify him against the damp and the demons, Grandfather would begin his next incendiary writing while I hurried off to his printer with his latest communique.

In the Irish Free State, as it was then called (we did not become a sovereign nation until 1937), Cornelius the First scourged in his writings the bitter divisions among our people north and south, ridiculed our ancient fears and superstitions, ranted against our Irish shortsightedness—one thunderous piece began "How long shall we content ourselves with the knowledge that Ireland is but a bee sting on the backside of Europe?"—and, in general, flailed away at the mentality of politicians, from the lowest clerk to whichever parliamentary representative had most recently happened to incur his ire. He was totally objective in the matter. Sinn

Feiners, Labourites, Independents, and De Valera's then new Fianna Fail party—all received nearly equal time from his abrasive pen.

It always seemed an exercise in futility for the authorities to persist in locking up Cornelius the First, particularly as he never minded much unless the sentence was longer than the usual few days and he could not get at scissors and a mirror to trim his beard. His writings continued to circulate whether he was in jail or out, and to this day I have never understood how his underground printer eluded detection. But at the age of eight or thereabouts I didn't give much thought to the political reasons that caused him to "board out" so often. I simply admired him and wanted to be like him. In time, his influence was stronger on me than my father's soldierly traits although I have spent my life within the borders of their two professions.

Now, I wonder, is my life, the extension of theirs, to be soon ended and all I learned from them snuffed out with it?

Grandfather and Father never lived to enjoy the best part of my life: Katie, the children, the success of my books. Grandfather died when I was ten, and I would guess death took him totally by surprise, not giving him the time for one more argument. My father, in many ways, had simply given up. He died some eighteen months after Katie and I were married, his honors all behind him, leaving Mother with meager funds and three young children, of a total of six, still in the process of struggling for an education.

That job fell heavily on Katie and me because a widow's pension from the British army is never enough to keep body and soul together, excluding the necessity of taking care of others. My father's brothers could have helped, but our branch of the Ryan family tree was rather spectacularly lopped off when Mother's Irish nationalism became locked in battle with the pro-British views of Father's older brothers. After Cornelius the First died, his elder sons, lacking the humanity of that irascible but generous old man, severed my father's allowance which, in the years he served abroad in the British army, had sustained us at home quite handsomely with servants, nannies, and the little luxuries one too often takes for granted until they disappear.

Father was invalided out of the army when I was still a boy. He came home to us a pensioner, trying to deal with our reduced circumstances and the family rift between Mother and his brothers which neither side had warned him of. Too poor to resort to lawyers and the courts to recover his rightful monies, too loyal to Mother to do so if he could, Father barely managed food for the table. He was trained for nothing but soldiering. He ended up bicycling to a bakery shop each morning where he worked as a menial until he died of bronchial pneumonia and, quite possibly, of a psyche made ragged by his attempts to conciliate the warring attitudes of Mother and his brothers. Yet in all those years I never heard him complain. He stubbornly clung to his loyalties to the British army and the Crown as he tried to pacify Mother, her justified anger against his family, and his total failure to effect any amnesty between the sides. As the firstborn, I grew up in a household torn between their opposite allegiances. To this day I have never totally resolved the problem, but at eighteen the need to choose sides was taken out of my hands.

In the one positive action he had taken since he had left the army, Father sent me to England, where he had secured a position for me as junior secretary to Garfield Weston, the biscuit magnate and M.P. He spirited me out of the house and onto the ferry that carries Ireland's sons and daughters over the furies of the Irish Sea (which is maddened, our people say, because the young are being taken from our shores). "There's nothing for you here, Con," my father said. "I can't give you a university education. All I can do is supply you with the chance to make opportunities for yourself. There's a world beyond this little island. Find it as I once did."

With my education from the Christian Brothers acquired at some cost to my knuckles and head from leather straps wielded by a few choleric teachers, plus a stint at the Irish Academy of Music (where my nose was first broken by false friends who didn't understand my affinity for the violin), I was sent out to make my place in the world. In my best suit of rough tweeds, wearing a cloth cap and carrying a cardboard suitcase whose undependable fastenings constantly threatened to expose my linens to the public eye, I arrived in Great Britain.*

Within a year I had moved from Weston's employ to what I knew by then I had always wanted: to be a journalist like Cornelius the First. I was hired by Reuter's at a much lower salary than Weston had paid me and I continued to learn my trade on the job. There was no meteoric rise to my career. It was damn difficult. I wrote most nights, training myself, producing reams of stuff that embarrasses me now but eventually I managed to talk my way into Fleet Street and onto the prestigious *London Daily Telegraph* as a reporter, eventually assigned to cover the U.S. forces in Europe.

The late Lord Camrose, then owner of the paper, called me into his office one day and said, "Ryan, we've got to have someone reporting the doings of these American chaps. Since you're Irish, would you mind?" My impression was that I was being picked not because he thought the Irish had any particular affinity with Americans but simply because my nationality made me expendable. I very nearly was. American MPs who had not heard that I was the *Telegraph*'s gift to their nation were constantly carting me off, certain that my new American uniform and weird accent were the most inept kind of cover for an enemy agent. I always failed their basic test questions: I hadn't a clue who won the World Series in 1943—I had never even heard of the World Series—and worse, much worse, I didn't know that Betty Grable was married to Harry James, probably the man U.S. forces the world

---

* I have never been without good luggage or well-cut clothes since that time. I would go without food or a single cent, but fine leather and impeccable tailoring are absolute essentials. The Irish in me demands them.

over envied most. It is a wonder that I ever got down eventually to "the doings of these American chaps." Among those brash, irreverent, confident soldiers I found my spiritual home and, covering the war in Europe, I furthered my training as a reporter by working with some of the finest correspondents the United States had in that theater. Young, dumb, brash, and Irish, I learned more from them than any school could ever have taught me.

At least Father lived to see that part of my success—if dodging fire while reporting from the front, being constantly afraid, and bulldozing my way to equal by-lines with my English counterparts covering the British armies could be called success. Years later, on a trip back to Dublin, Mother showed me scrapbooks my father had kept. In them was every story I had ever written for the *Telegraph,* neatly cut and pasted on the pages, the dates of each piece running in order. All during the war I sent almost all my salary home so that my sister and younger brothers could have the education we three older sons had missed. And in 1952 when Father died, Katie and I managed, by some rather spectacular deprivations to ourselves, to complete their education and to help out in the renovation of a respectable old house I had put up most of the money for my father to buy for the family.

Even today, especially today, I miss that black-haired, dark-eyed, courtly gentleman who was my father. He had taught me to fish, to ride, to hunt, had forced me out into the world to carry, I hope, his honor and to remember his staid, old-worldly codes. Neither he nor Cornelius the First will know how fervently I have tried to uphold their values, how much of my career and, vicariously through me, theirs, I thought still lay ahead.

Now comes news of this illness. This incredible pronouncement. How on God's earth will I handle it? Will I live with it—or die from it—with all the grace and impeccable manners I can muster from my father, or will I fight and argue and rebel like my grandfather? I think that much as I loved my father, my inclinations and personality are more closely allied to those of Cornelius the First.

Yet, unlike that grand old man who always knew the reasons for his jail sentences, I feel as though I've been condemned in some court for a crime of which I'm totally innocent and no one has told me when I'm going to be led out to the hangman.

≚ 2 ≚

KATHRYN

Throughout the next four years the events of our lives would be governed by cancer. It would change not only Connie but our entire family. A day would come when I would order my only son from home and in so doing lose both my children. I would find myself wondering how other wives coped with such an illness and if they found release through extramarital experiences and how they felt about it afterward. Little did I know that my own mental and physical exhaustion would turn me into a semi-invalid at the exact time when Connie was struggling against becoming one. Nor could I even anticipate the agonies of body and mind that would haunt each of us to the end.

We would come to discover the highs and lows of character, ambition, and personality in the foreign world of medicine which was about to engulf us. Cancer would force my husband to battle narcotics and to discover a talent he had not believed he possessed. There would come a time in the middle of all this when accolades and honors we had only dreamed of would come his way.

Cancer would threaten our sanity, our family's morals, and rip our lives apart. And finally, its awful work done, cancer's survivors would try to put their lives back together. But like a priceless smashed vase, the vital part that had been Connie would be forever missing.

On Friday night, July 24, 1970, the evening before Connie began his secret tapes, he and I had come home from the city hours later than we had planned. Connie had spent two and a half days in the hospital undergoing tests that I had assumed naively were routine and would produce a solution to a persistent prostatitis that had plagued him for some months. Instead, the findings had revealed the grim invasion of cancer.

We did not talk as we drove through the soft dark night toward Connecticut. For the moment we were out of words. Connie sat rigidly behind the wheel, remote and, to me, somehow unreal. I did not think of him as Connie. He was simply someone steering through the night.

Emotionally exhausted, our thoughts on cancer rather than the road, we passed our regular turnoff from the throughway and continued up the highway, moving farther away from home. It was Connie who discovered the mistake.

"Katie, where the hell are we?" he asked.

From the darkness of the car I stared out at the greater darkness of unfamiliar country and said dully, "I don't know."

Connie drove on until we came to a sign. He swung off the road to get his bearings. Then he said, "It's a good half hour back to our turn and another forty-five minutes home from there. What a damn-fool thing to do, but it's been a damn-fool day all around."

Normally, being detained in town, missing our throughway exit, would have been trivial irritants. On that Friday they were two more setbacks in a day already full of anguish. I threw my arms around Connie, crying bitterly. I had always found it difficult to cry. That night I could not seem to stop. "CJ, it isn't true. The doctor's wrong. It isn't happening."

Connie shook me gently. "Hey, little girl, stop this," he said. "Nothing's happened to me yet."

In the dashboard lights his face was shadowed but his voice was controlled and even. His composure made me fleetingly optimistic and then the grief washed back. "Connie, I wish with all my heart that this was happening to me instead of to you."

I saw a faint smile. "Promise me you won't be jealous," Connie said. "I'll give you almost anything else I've got."

"We have to share this," I insisted. "If it's happening to you, it's happening to me. You've always said that we're a team."

"That we are," Connie said, "but like it or not, Katie, there's been a change in the team rules." He kissed my forehead, gave me his handkerchief to dry my eyes, and lit a cigarette. Then he got us headed home. One thing was certain and didn't need discussion, then or in the days to follow. Grief had come to join our team. We would be able to push it away from time to time, although never for long—and the crucible was still to come, somewhere ahead, awaiting us.

We are called "the immediate family," we close relatives of the sick. It is a term used often by hospital personnel and by morticians. It implies a solidarity (however temporary), bound by blood and marriage, and summoned up by tragedy. For the first time in nearly seventeen years, three generations of our family were under one roof: Connie's mother, Emily, vacationing with us from Dublin; my father, Eldon Morgan, visiting from Iowa; and the four of us—these were our immediate family. Tragedy was, indeed, our common denominator. In spite of hope, prayer, or rebellion, Connie's cancer now would dominate our lives.

It had already begun to do so. My father was the first of the family to realize that disaster, not relief, would be in store. As we entered the house shortly after 10:00 P.M. that Friday, he stood at the bottom of the steps leading to the living room awaiting us. His face, I thought, reflected what he must have seen in ours.

My gentle, quiet parent had experienced much in his then-eighty years of life, including, the previous November, my mother's death. They had been married fifty-two years and I was their only child, the lone survivor, following three stillborns. My own first friends and closest companions, my parents had assimilated Connie into our little circle from the day they first met him. Perhaps they trusted my judgment; more likely, Connie's charisma, his queries regarding Iowa— a state he had known nothing about—beguiled them. The first time I took him home to meet my parents he asked in mock seriousness if he should take his Winchester "in case of Indian attack or your father's disapproval of our marriage plans." He did not need the rifle for either contingency. Father regaled him with tales of U.S. Western history and the life of pioneer families. Mother, early on, enlisted his help in her indefatigable researches into her family's history. Together, those two tracked down some missing genealogical links—an accomplishment that pleased them equally. When Mother died suddenly in November 1969, my father's love and interests became more bound than ever with Connie, me, and his grandchildren. His long life, his experiences with both happiness and tragedy, may have alerted him to our mood. Certainly he felt the presence of impending trouble that July evening when we walked silently into the house.

In an agitated attempt to stave off the inevitable moment

when the question about the outcome of Connie's tests would be asked, I moved down the stairs and past Father with all the short-lived sputter of a sparkler firework. I went from room to room, tossing out apologies for our late arrival home. Encountering the children, Geoff and Vicki, I asked them about their day without waiting for their answers.

Finally, in the kitchen, I snatched up pots and pans to start a dinner long since over. My frenzied actions had drawn our parents and Connie to this room. I saw them staring at me and the growing piles of cookware on the counters, enough utensils to fix food for fifty.

My father reached out and drew me to him, holding me still. And then he asked the question all my erratic actions could no longer delay.

"What is it, Connie?" Father asked, holding on to me. "What's wrong?"

"It's malignant," Connie said.

Emily, Connie's mother, rushed to him and threw her arms around his waist. She began to moan. Slowly she knelt to the floor and started a litany of prayers. Connie had often spoken jokingly of his mother "storming heaven" for her children, but that was something I, not Catholic, had only heard about. I stared at her uncomprehendingly.

Emily seemed oblivious to us all. She prayed aloud, her words racing, their clarity obscured by tears. Connie's face was ashen. He reached down and touched her head and then walked past her and out of the room, leaving my father and me with Emily.

"Help me with her," Father said, and we got Emily to her feet and walked her between us into the living room and onto a sofa. Shaken and wan, she drank the brandy my father handed her, staring sightlessly out into the room. The children and Connie were nowhere in sight. I tried to think if Geoff and Vicki had overheard and if the word "malignant" had any meaning for our young. If not then, it would—and all too soon.

At some point I went up to our rooms. Connie was on the phone to Dr. Patrick Neligan, only short months earlier more Connie's friend than doctor. I sat down, watching Connie as he spoke with Pat. Sick? How could anyone who looked like Connie be sick? His blond hair was just then beginning to gray a bit at the temples. His wide shoulders, the strength and leanness of his body, his hands—long-fingered with square, broad nails—the crisp, organized manner in which he spoke, all these were Connie traits. He was not bowed or drawn or less vital than before. He couldn't have cancer. The frightening diagnosis of that day was wrong. It made no sense.

Leaving Connie still on the phone to Pat, I went back to the main foyer and across the hall to the children's wing. I had been aware of Vicki's face peering in from time to time, but I hadn't seen Geoff since I passed him in the hall.

Thirteen-year-old Vicki was sitting on her bed, a tray with a smattering of jigsaw puzzle pieces fitted together on her lap. Nearby, Geoff's door was closed as usual. For some time now we had been asked to knock and wait until we were invited in—a proper enough request for privacy. Still, it was disquieting.

I sat beside Vicki, blond like her father, and with his temperament and will. We chatted aimlessly. She'd been upstairs twice, she told me, but Connie—on the phone—had motioned her back down. She wondered why. Until I talked with Connie, I thought it best to tell her only that Daddy had been in the hospital and might have to go back at some point, but we weren't sure. She nodded, apparently satisfied, and went back to the puzzle. "Tell him to kiss me good night," she said as I left her room.

In the hallway outside Geoff's door, I knocked, waited, then knocked again. He asked what I wanted. "To see you," I said to the door. After a few minutes it opened. Only one bulb was lit, making his room almost as dark as if there was no light at all. His rock albums were scattered across the room; the montage of psychedelic posters on his walls looked menacingly iridescent in the dim glow. Impulsively, I sat down in a chair and told him everything. At sixteen, he had a right to know, I felt, and to learn in future everything that we would. I wanted him to be prepared for that future—whatever it was—and in this sharing with him to reestablish a rapport that seemed to have vaporized.

Perhaps I was wrong to give him the crushing news so quickly. I could not come to terms with it myself as yet, and age sixteen is a nether world between youth and maturity. Geoff seemed almost too placid, I thought. Yet I remembered my mother's death eight months earlier and the strength with which he had supported us all, his own anguish subordinated to ours. He had loved her dearly all his young life. At her grave he stood longest by the bier, his single yellow rose laid last on the blanket of flowers that covered her casket.

He never shared that grief with anyone as far as I know. Nor did he when I told him about his father's illness. Whatever he was feeling was lost to any sight or sound or touch of mine. He simply sat and listened. When I'd finished, he seemed remote and distant. I don't know when the barrier between us had been built. But it was there, undoubtedly as much my fault as his. I felt a rush of remorse and sorrow for us both. I had exposed him to my pain. His, if it was there that night, was guarded and private, not mine to share. I left him in the shadows of his cluttered room, feeling we were further apart than ever, longing for the boy I used to know and seemed to have lost without remembering when.

The pressures of the books were always bad enough on all the family when Connie and I were working long hours in the office, guilty about not spending enough time with our young. This dreadful news would change our lives still more. It would not be easy to maintain even the tenuous contact we had with Geoff when, obviously, it should be strengthened— and soon. But he would have to help a little, too. We all would have to help each other.

Later, the older members of the household mercifully re-tired. I sat with Emily until she fell asleep. My father had sensibly locked up and turned out lights and, after good nights to the children, had taken himself off to his own room.

Connie was in his dressing room when I came back to our bedroom. I went into my own and stared into the mirror. It seemed to me I looked the same as always but that seemed incredible. I was not the same woman who had driven to the city that morning to pick up her husband in a hospital. A change had taken place whether it showed or not, and it would cause ever deepening tracks in body and mind until the horror that hung over us was ended—one way or the other.

I filled my tub and soaked, hearing Connie's shower run-ning on the other side of my bathroom wall. He finished first and the bedroom was dark when I came in. In bed, I turned to him, putting my head against his chest, hearing the strong beat of his heart, feeling the intense body warmth that Con-nie and Vicki share in common. The bleak news we had been given was despicable, grossly unfair. We were committed to *A Bridge Too Far*, the new book; we had Geoff and Vicki to love and care for. We had a marriage, mutual interests, the fun of the rare times we played hooky from work to golf, to spend a day or two in town, to fly suddenly off, short-term truants, to London, Paris, or Dublin. Such news should not have come in a lovely July month, our grounds bright with summer sunshine, warm and dusky in the evenings when, after a day's hard work, we sat and savored silence on the terrace. Especially this news should not menace our private lives, setting us apart, dividing us in health, affecting our relationship as husband and wife. As we lay in silence I knew, as Connie had said in the car, that the rules had changed, the doctor's findings had already begun to make a difference. Cancer had separated us. In spite of physical closeness a barrier, invisible but everlasting, had come be-tween us.

It was close on dawn when Connie said, "You haven't slept at all." "Neither have you." Then he said, "Katie, you remember when we went to Saint Martin in April? Remember how I felt? Katie, I think I had it then."

≟ *3* ≟

CORNELIUS

I've just made myself a cup of coffee. As I sit here sipping it, I believe that the best way to pull myself out of shock, away from the feeling that the world has gone mad, is to try and put the events of this illness in some sort of order. The coffee is hot and soothing. I don't feel quite so empty, so close to tears. I must try to regain perspective, to produce on these tapes a rationale. Somehow I have to pass through that World War II minefield once again, alert and hopefully intact.

The peculiar lassitude I've been feeling for several months is now far too easy to understand. I have put it down to the rigors of research trips and to the fact that, at forty-nine or fifty, after years of traveling around the world, I might, indeed, be aging if only a bit. The energy I've always taken for granted has lessened more than I like to admit and, not for the first time, I have experienced a severe mental block about coming to grips with writing.

I've always experienced cold fear when the research for a book was finished. The subject material has always seemed greater than my ability to handle it. But in the past I've been able to settle down to the job, only occasionally muttering that the book couldn't be done, it had been an unworkable idea to begin with, and I'd never get to the final sentence. On this book "writer's block" has persisted for so long that I've been panicked. Now, at least, I understand some of the cause. The prolonged fatigue has to be due to cancer. Despite all talk of surgery and "cure," right at this moment I believe it will kill me. All the more reason to drive myself to work. I can't die with *A Bridge Too Far* unwritten. But how do I start with this sword of Damocles hanging over my head?

The ways I've found to avoid work have certainly come back to plague me now. Still, I did think one postponement— a brief trip to see our friends, Mel and Margery Thompson, at their Caribbean home on Saint Martin some four months back—would stoke up the fires again. The little trip was supposed to be good for both Katie and me. Instead, as I see it now, it produced the first ominous warnings that my inability to begin work would turn into a battle to survive long enough to get any work done at all.

We'd planned the trip for April 11. I've just gone through my diary and notebooks for this first quarter of 1970. I think I had some idea of writing a piece eventually about the place we were visiting. In any case, I'd made some initial notes while we were there: journalists' shorthand describing Saint Martin, the differences in Dutch and French handling of the thirty-seven-square-mile territory which is roughly divided between their two countries, the problems of water, electrification, and road building, some data on early Saint Martin Dutch settlers and the probable origins of the native population. Thinking back now, I'm amazed I took as many notes as I did.

It was to the Thompson's Shangri-la, a pink villa overlooking the water and reached by tortuous roads thick with volcanic ash, that Kathryn and I were heading in April four months ago. There was no warning that anything unusual was about to happen as I walked into the bathroom about 5:30 A.M. on Saturday, April 11, the day we left. There was

39

nothing unusual about the time, either. I've always been an early riser no matter how little sleep I've had previously. During World War II, correspondents, like soldiers, learned to grab their rest whenever they could, and this ability to fall asleep for fifteen minutes or six hours has stayed with me ever since. I felt fit and refreshed. My morning humor is very good, my wife tells me. She has also remarked from time to time that I might conserve a little of it for later in the day.

Within seconds whatever good humor I had that morning was shattered with devastating suddenness. As I started to urinate, a burning, scalding pain unlike anything I've ever experienced hit me with the force of a small electric charge. A sudden intense pressure in the bladder area almost doubled me over. My plumbing seemed blocked, paralyzed by some tremendous weight.

At the time, I think I was more stupefied than afraid. Whatever it was would disappear. I figured my body had rebelled against something I'd eaten or drunk the day before. I went through the other customary ablutions, resisting an almost unbearable urge to try to relieve myself again, but the searing pain had slackened and I didn't want to aggravate it further. Besides, I had no intention of letting anything keep us from flying to Saint Martin.

I dressed and woke Katie, whose morning mood differs from mine in every respect. I have to cajole her out of bed, speaking softly but continuously until the penny drops and she surfaces. But once she sits up and adjusts to the idea of leaving her bed, she moves into action with an efficiency I've never been able to match.

While Katie began her morning, I got a suitcase from the closet and began to pack for both of us. With her usual thoroughness, my wife had laid out her clothes the night before. The sight of them amused me as always. She'd collected much more apparel than she'd need for our short trip. To Katie, a weekend visit with friends would be unthinkable without at least a third of her wardrobe along, while I can live in Europe during a three-month research trip with one suit and a couple of pairs of slacks and jackets. As usual, my own packing took only minutes before I began the longer task of filling one side of the case with as many of Katie's clothes as possible. The rest went in on top of mine.

Yet even as I worked, the inexplicable experience in the bathroom continued to haunt me. On that morning I was the silent one, not Kathryn. It was difficult to concentrate on mundane procedures I had followed hundreds of times before. Traveler's checks, passports, airline tickets, usually inspected once and put into a folder in my inside jacket pocket, were brought out again and again. I simply couldn't remember that I'd already gone through them before. At one point I even remember thinking, somewhat wildly, that the children would be home alone. But Geoff, sixteen, was in boarding school and Victoria, thirteen, was staying with the family of a school friend. The animals were gone, too. Only the evening before Katie had taken our German shepherd and the four Siamese cats to be boarded.

So why was my mind so muddled? And, more important, how soon would this malady disappear? I could only wait and hope the problem was temporary. It had to be a good day.

But it may well turn out that by last April 11 I had already used all the good days up.

Katie and I took an 11:00 A.M. flight to Saint Martin from JFK. I have that notation in my diary and next to it I had written:

Urinary problem continuing. Feel like hell! Am wearing a path to the lavatory. Never had this before!

I had told Katie about my distress but, on the threshold of a holiday, we both tried to minimize it. Yet I remember how acutely uncomfortable I was. I fly hundreds of air miles every year in connection with my books and usually I get on the plane, settle in, read up on my notes, check the list of countries and people where I have interviews, and sleep a little. This trip was different. My earlier mood of cautious optimism that the problem would end as quickly as it had begun was giving way to a darker outlook. A feeling I couldn't suppress was growing stronger all the time. I was beginning to have the distinct impression that someplace inside me something was going very wrong.

Margery and Mel were at the airport to meet us. I'm never totally prepared for tropical heat. My Irish blood is too thick, I guess. Between the heat and this constant urge to void, I felt terrible. It was all I could do to get our passports stamped and follow Katie through the mob of tourists. Mel took our baggage ticket and the girls and I went outside. Away from the crowds, I felt a little better.

At the house, after a kidney-wrenching ride over the rutted island roads, Katie started to unpack while I headed for our bathroom. This time I noticed a kind of yellowish discharge, a staining, which had not been there before.

I told Katie about this new development. We still tried not to place any particular importance on it. There was nothing we could do there anyway. Going to one of the small island hospitals for some kind of medicine or relief for this unknown disorder didn't appeal to me. Besides, I kept rationalizing that whatever I had was temporary. I never get sick. Maybe that's why Katie and I played this down. Probably our attitude was foolish and we should have taken the first plane home. I think now that the cancer was already present and had been for a longer time than we will ever know.

We stayed on. I would have felt like a bloody idiot to go all the way home for treatment of an infection that would surely clear up unattended in a matter of days. And under the circumstances our stay with the Thompsons was almost all we could have wished. Despite discomfort, I did that little research about the island and got in some fishing—something I do wherever I can. The four of us swam, drove all over the island, ate at a couple of good restaurants, and imbibed some hefty rum punches at breezy, lattice-shaded bars where we could look out past bathers and native boats to the blue-green sea beyond. But the burning, excruciating need never to be far from a bathroom was getting worse, no question about it. I thought maybe the local brand of liquor was stronger than at home and that it had accelerated the pain and pressure. I cut out juices and booze and drank a lot of water, hoping to flush whatever I had out of my system. It didn't work. Each hour seemed worse than the last.

We didn't mention my problem to Margery and Mel, but my sudden bolts for a bathroom must have caused them some puzzlement. Yet, I couldn't explain. This distress was to personal. I was embarrassed by what was happening in a way that's difficult to describe. Perhaps being fastidious about that part of the body, one can't help having a feeling that what was happening was repulsive. I felt that I was dirty. I didn't put my underwear in with the house laundry and I couldn't let Katie wash it. It was something I had to do myself. I didn't want anyone, not even Katie, to witness the evidence of my disgust and humiliation.

It was increasingly obvious to me that whatever I had did, indeed, need medical attention. My home remedies weren't working and I didn't think I could keep control much longer. On Wednesday, April 15, we came home and on the sixteenth I saw my friend and physician, Dr. Patrick Neligan.

⹋ 4 ⹋

NELIGAN'S OFFICE is like the man himself—neat, sparse, un-
pretentious. I'd come in early that April Thursday nearly four
months ago. I had no appointment and the waiting room was
already filled. I didn't want to push past all the people who
had appointments but neither was I sure I could maintain the
control I'd need for a long wait. I went inside the receptionists' cubicle and got Mary Chapin, Pat's nurse, to come there.
I didn't tell Mary much but it was enough for her to lead me
to an examining room with a bathroom adjoining. She said
Pat would be in shortly.

Pacing the room I remember feeling suddenly embarrassed, foolish about taking up Pat's time. There was going to
be some simple explanation for all this and knowing Neligan
I'd never hear the end of it. Yet I didn't leave. My eyes kept
coming back to a little Irish figurine Pat has on a bookshelf in
that room. It's a badly cast impression of a leprechaun, incon-
gruous in the office of a man whose tastes run to classical
music and fine antiques. But it has been there on that shelf
like a talisman as long as I can remember, a little piece of
Irish legend that maybe binds Pat to the past.

Neligan and his wife, Veronica, are former Dubliners like
me. Some years back I met Pat and Vera for the first time at a
local party. Discovering our origins, the people and places
we had in common, we three were quickly engrossed in talk.
Katie, who had been across the room, left another group to

44

join us, but because she stood a little behind me, I didn't see her, and the Neligans and I continued comparing schools, friends, families, the mucked-up state of Irish life, and the idiosyncrasies of the Irish character which, of course, had not tainted the three of us at all.

"Who did you marry anyway?" Pat suddenly asked.

"Kathryn Morgan."

Pat mulled it over. "Where's she from? Dublin city? Rathmines? Rathgar?"

"Iowa."

Neligan was totally baffled. He said later he thought maybe I was referring to some small island in the Nile Delta. "How in God's name did you marry somebody from Iowa?"

"And what, exactly, is wrong with Iowa?" The familiar voice was just over my left shoulder. "Strange as it may seem, there *are* native-born Americans and they aren't all Irish. I do hope that's all right with you?"

I turned and sure enough there was my good wife, eyes blazing. I made hasty introductions, but the damage was done. Katie stalked off to another part of the room and the Ryans and the Neligans didn't speak for the next three years. As Pat remarked some time later, "built on this solid foundation, our four-way friendship has since grown and even flourished."

I was thinking about that when the door opened silently and Pat walked in. After we had exchanged a few insults, one of the more common Irish ways of showing affection, I told him somewhat offhandedly what had been happening to me. Immediately his face and manner changed. The banter stopped. To Pat illness is an affront to his patients and a personal challenge to him. He began to throw questions at me, and trying to respond, to get it all out in the open, made me feel a little better. Whatever I had, Neligan would come up with the answer. He called in Mary, who led me to a cubicle to undress and don one of those paper garments surely designed to make even the best of figures a subject of mirth. Neither a shirt nor a robe, "it barely covers the high-water mark," as an elderly lady once said about the mini.

In that abbreviated wrap, I got on the examining table and Pat went over me thoroughly, pressing here and there, asking if this hurt or that was tender, raising question after question. My answers were all negative. I'd already told him all I could. He began a prostatic massage which filled me with less than enthusiasm since, apart from its other aspects, it prohibits any semblance of dignified or comfortable posture. As Pat began to expel the urethral discharge, he said I was certainly exhibiting clear signs of prostatitis. Curiously, although I'd heard about it on and off, I didn't really know what prostatitis was. Pat's explanation was brief. Put simply, prostatitis is an inflammation of the prostate gland. A kind of tube or canal, the urethra, extends about an inch into the prostate. This duct carries urine from the bladder to the penis. If the prostate becomes inflamed, the urethra can't expel secretion at a normal rate. The stream slows and becomes sluggish, somewhat like the clogged top of a sauce bottle. The side effects are similar to those I was experiencing: the feeling of a need to void frequently without much success and a painful, burning sensation when one tried. I asked a few more questions and found the problem could show up in almost any age group, from postpubertal to elderly men. It wasn't all that uncommon. I felt a little better, even a little foolish about the way I'd raced back from Saint Martin.

Because of the swollen condition of the prostate, Pat could not tell whether anything was suspicious there. He put me on an antibacterial pill called NegGram and told me I would need prostatic massages for some time to come to expel all the urethral secretion.

The NegGram did help some, I remember. The burning pain and the constant urgency to void diminished. For the first time in over a week I could walk into the bathroom without having to steel myself for the ordeal, which was fortunate, since my diary indicates the following week was fairly active but not productive at all as far as writing was concerned. I note that Kathryn and I went to a couple of parties, I had meetings in New York, a couple of lunches with old friends like Ben Grauer and Walter Cronkite and a two-day stay—on April 23–24—in Boston with General and Mrs. James Gavin to talk with Jim about *A Bridge Too Far*. While the painful symptoms lessened, the draining and staining continued, and on Sunday, April 26, I called Pat and told him the medication didn't seem to be functioning in those departments. He told me to meet him at the office.

One incident made that Sunday's treatment different from the first. Pat gave me another prostatic massage and during it I remember he asked if I could notice any particular pain on the right lobe of the prostate. The question seemed anything but significant, yet it stuck in my mind. I told him the whole area felt so inflamed that I couldn't determine any localized pain. Pat didn't ask anything more about it. He took me off the NegGram and gave me a medication called Furadantin. I didn't ask what it was or why the NegGram was being changed.* I just wanted the damned thing to work. I was becoming more and more annoyed by the staining. Perhaps the Furadantin would clear that up, just as the NegGram had presumably been responsible for relieving the voiding problem. Still, it was taking a long time to get rid of the infection or whatever it was. Maybe I was just impatient with a problem that was stubbornly defying even Pat.

---

* Like NegGram, Furadantin is an antibacterial tablet given for urinary tract infections.

= 5 =

TEN DAYS AGO, July 15, the visible signs of prostatitis had been present for ninety-one days. In all that time I had become increasingly concerned by what was happening to me. By the fifteenth that concern had reached the proportions of an obsession. It was critical that something positive be done to end my problem. On that Wednesday I called Neligan and, shouting into the phone, told him I had just about reached my limits; I was becoming desperate for a cure.

In contrast to my explosiveness Pat's voice was warm and reassuring. He told me to come in and he would fit me into his appointments. It was cold comfort but I agreed. I hoped to God there was something he could do that would finally work for me. I had reached the stage where anything would be better than what I was going through. Since the discharge first appeared in April I have been changing my underclothes and showering three or four times a day. Kathryn, overriding my objections, daily washes my linen. And weekly I buy more, for in spite of the ads one sees on television that this liquid or that powder produces spanking clean garments, there comes a time when it just isn't so. No matter how thoroughly soaked, rubbed, and churned in the washer, I see the faint trace outlines of discoloration. I find them repellent.

Far more crucial, this physical disorder has been affecting my behavior toward Katie and the children. I have been irritable and on edge and they have had no way of knowing that my anger is directed at my own body. Ever since April 26 when Neligan put me on the Furadantin, I believed the medication would work, the drainage would stop. Even the four or five prostatic massages Pat has given me during all this time have been incapable of bettering the situation. I could hardly wait to see Neligan on July 15. I wanted him to get me back to normal. I needed to get to work on the book.

The fact is I may never get started again. Since that fateful April 11, three and a half months ago, when the first visible symptoms of this illness surfaced, I have been totally preoccupied with ridding myself of prostatitis. Now I am faced with something far more sinister and its implications can't help but affect the book and all our lives.

For weeks Katie has been after me about my "procrastination." I know she believed the work would divert my mind but all that has changed now. Even if I start up again, can I do the material justice? This will be the most difficult writing I've ever attempted. And this book is the greatest challenge I've ever faced. I've got to do it well or not do it at all. No matter what happens to me, I want my books to stand the test of time.

Here in the office everything to do with A *Bridge Too Far* is organized and ready. Kathryn has filed every military interview from division headquarters' personnel down to soldiers at company level, with metal tabs affixed to those whose experiences will probably be the heart of the book. Five large black folders—one each for the Dutch, Germans, Americans, British, and Poles—lie here on my desk. In each she's included the best individual accounts of action with cross-references to people who witnessed or experienced the same event.

Anne Bardenhagen, my secretary, has checked and rechecked the name spellings of all the men and women who have been interviewed or who sent in information, so that the entire list of contributors which we always include at the back of the books under a section entitled "What They Do Today" is completed. The bibliography is nearly finished and the photographic files are bulging with pictures of people, places, bridges, parachute drops, landing fields—all labeled, thanks to Annie, and awaiting captions.

Street maps of the Dutch towns of Eindhoven, Nijmegen, and Arnhem as they were in 1944 are ready to be pinned on our big bulletin board, which takes up half of one wall of the office. On the maps Dutch underground locations, principal buildings, homes which lay in the battle areas are marked in with colored inks. The war diaries and messages are in order by day and hour. Along with reference books, telephone logs, weather forecasts, and newspapers for September 1944, the research is all at hand in the bookcases alongside my desk.

Looking around this room I feel more than a little frightened. Everything's ready to go but me. The word "cancer" has completely changed my world. Why didn't I force myself to start on the book sooner? After all these months, I have yet to write even an acceptable opening sentence.

KATHRYN

The files and back-of-the-book material for *A Bridge Too Far* had long been cataloged and typed by Anne and me. Throughout 1969 and early 1970 we found ourselves doing odd jobs in the office, putting correspondence files in order, moving the material belonging to Connie's previous World War II histories—*The Longest Day* and *The Last Battle*— into a room in the office specially designed to filter the air and prevent the aging process of these invaluable documents, so many of which are handwritten by participants in those battles. The work was tedious and less than fulfilling. Anne and I wanted to get on with the intense activity for which there seemed never enough time when Connie was actually writing.

But he avoided the new book. Inexplicably he began a search for a private public relations person, a move that was totally unlike Connie. He was and had always been his own best publicist. My frustration built up through 1969 as month after month rolled by while Connie gave his time to articles projects, speeches, lectures and interviews, dinners with foreign publishers, lunches at the various clubs to which he belonged, a twenty-fifth D-Day anniversary trip to the Normandy beaches with other correspondents, an article for the *Reader's Digest* on the lunar landing of Apollo 11—anything, it seemed, that would keep him from getting started on the book. He even helped on the production of a school play in which Victoria was involved.* Anne and I were puzzled by the constant swings and shifts in Connie's moods. His diary for 1969 reads like that of a man harassed by demands on his time. But most of those demands were manufactured or self-created.

In November 1969, M-G-M, which had acquired the motion-picture rights to *The Last Battle* and for which Connie had already written the screenplay, decided not to make the picture. Connie was downcast and bitter. I was less so. I thought he had no more excuses not to begin the new book and every reason, including income, to get going. He did not appear to see it that way.

Anne and I had no insight into the physical factors which, I believe, were beginning to affect his state of mind sixteen months before he knew he had cancer. Yet disquieting things were occurring, although at the time they seemed of little consequence. I do not know if they were the forerunners of his final illness, but they seem worth mentioning.

On March 6, 1969, I wrote in my diary, "Connie ill at dinner at '21' with Tom and Mary Lenk." In fact, he had not eaten dinner at all. We had met the Lenks, who had driven into New York City from New Jersey as we had driven down from Connecticut, for a long-overdue reunion. Good friends, they traveled as much as Connie, if not more, and for the four of us a quiet evening together was a rare treat. We were barely seated

* It was to be the first of several such collaborations between father and daughter. The last and most ambitious would take place only three months before his death.

at the table when Connie excused himself, went to the men's room, and lost consciousness just as he went through the lavatory door. Thanks to the ministrations of the restaurant staff and to Connie's close friend and part owner of the club, Peter Kriendler, he was brought around, rested a few minutes in Pete's office, and came back to the table.

He was unable to eat and his face was very pale. Usually loquacious, bounding with vitality, Connie seemed drained and uncharacteristically silent as he sat while Tom, Mary, and I tried to carry on normally. We were not successful. Connie had not even ordered his favorite bourbon prior to dinner. Although many of his correspondent friends loved to write or speak about his drinking prowess, I think those references owed more to a trait the Irish are expected to possess than to any actual proclivity. In truth, two bourbons were his limit. He always said that he had no tolerance for alcohol, and after a time he developed a kind of sleight of hand in spiriting away unwanted drinks without companions being the wiser. Still, I think many of his journalism friends would dispute that fact; they could all recite the many instances in which he had drunk them under the table. If he ever did that it was because he had fortified himself some way in advance. To the men he had worked with and admired, that ability was a part of Connie's charisma. I am glad he ranked so high with them that they considered Herculean drinking another of his virtues. I am glad they cherished him.

On Sunday, March 9, 1969, Dr. Neligan put Connie in the hospital. He had complained of vague aches and pains, and after the blackout he had suffered in New York three days earlier, Pat wanted him in for tests and a complete physical. On that Sunday, as time neared for him to enter the hospital, his mood, gray in the morning, grew black. He had a horror of hospitals and was uneasy around sickness. If an illness demanded hospitalization, something within him snapped. To mask his apprehension, he could become truculent, belligerent to nurses, antagonistic in his refusal to comply with ordinary hospital rules. Whenever I had had to go to the hospital, Connie objected to nearly everything from the admittance forms to his banishment from my room during the visits of interns and technicians doing routine work-ups.

Much as he wanted to protect and be with me, he was an appalling sickroom visitor. He was uncommunicative, pacing the room as though caged, peering into drawers and cabinets, and eyeing members of the staff who came into the room with ill-concealed suspicion.

He knew and understood these changes in his personality when he went to a hospital. "It's dehumanizing," he once told me. "You take off your clothes and you're in their hands, defenseless, unable to decide when you come and go or to plan the next day yourself. You aren't a person any longer. You're a patient—without dignity or a sense of self. There's no way to keep your guard up."

"But why should you need to if you're sick?"

"When I was seven I was put into hospital in Dublin with a high fever," Connie told me. "My mother left and I was never so alone or frightened in my life. Everything was cold and white and foreign. A doctor took out my appendix and there wasn't a damn thing wrong with it. I had diphtheria, which they got around to discovering later. I remember crying and calling for my mother. Someone came in and told me to knock it off. I was a big boy and men don't cry. Not even when it hurts and when they took out a healthy appendix. I've been afraid of hospitals ever since. Few nurses have time to care if you're lonely or apprehensive. Whenever I walk through the doors of a hospital I become sick with anxiety. Suppose something is done there that was totally unnecessary, the real problem not treated? You won't be able to protest or demand more time to think things out or be comforted by your own people. Because, in hospital, you don't make the decisions governing your own life. You've got to trust the doctors to be right. And if they're not, you've gone through it all for nothing—the pain and the fear and the unfamiliarity of a world where sickness, not health, is normal."

Yet, strangely, his spirits depressed, his anxiety all too apparent, Connie had gone into the hospital that March in 1969. Perhaps he did so because Pat was on the hospital staff and he trusted Pat to be with him, Pat's face to be the familiar one he had been kept from seeing when he was a boy. Perhaps he believed that if Pat was there, he, Connie, would be able to maintain his own dignity. He would still be Connie.

But even with Pat nearby, he was nervous about his confinement. He went irritably through the schedule of tests Pat ordered. He did not want me to come to see him and on the telephone his voice was grim. He came home on Friday, March 14, after six days in an institution he feared and detested and, in a frenzy of activity, went to a dinner party in Ridgefield that evening, and gave a speech to the National University of Ireland Club at the St. Regis Hotel in New York the following night.

I watched him as he worked on the speech in a large room at the Plaza Hotel almost up to the time the benefit dinner began, polishing his address, surrounded by the opulent fittings of the most expensive suite he was able to acquire. He was easing himself away from the hospital. The rich appointments of the rooms, the ministrations there of his barber and my hairdresser, the constant scurry of waiters bringing trays of hors d'oeuvres and champagne—all were buffers to help him forget one small, white room where he felt helpless and without dignity.

He told me Pat had discovered some little-known parasite that Connie might have picked up during the early postwar years when he was assigned to General Douglas MacArthur's headquarters in Tokyo, and which had lain dormant until then.*

---

* Only recently did I think to ask Pat about it. He told me that Connie had complained of diarrhea and weakness. In the hospital, after numerous stool cultures, Pat found an intestinal parasitic infection, giardiasis. With medication the stool cultures cleared up and, other than praising Pat's detective work, Connie appeared to put the incident out of his mind. It was too closely associated with his dislike of hospitals.

Until April 1970, Connie made only one further entry concerning illness in his diary. On March 17, 1969, three days out of the hospital, he wrote "very sick again." On March 18 and 19, among other appointments, Anne's diary reads:

"Dr. Neligan."

Connie's diary of those dates gives no mention of Pat's name. The frantic pace he had initiated early in the year continued until the fateful events of July 1970.

It was in 1969 also that Connie and I had the most serious argument of our married life. Angry at what I considered his total lack of concern about starting on *Bridge* while he was giving time to a variety of outside activities, I told him that perhaps I could begin the book and he could put a double by-line on it. I have never seen him so outraged. He challenged me to do a book on my own and ordered me to leave his work completely alone. I retaliated by saying that he couldn't do his own book without me and that I was tired of his overextended ego trip. He said very quietly, "I never needed you in the past and I don't now. If you want to write, get yourself an idea and do your own book. If," he added, "you ever can."

With equal sarcasm, I asked, "You mean the way you do yours?"

Connie stared at me. "I was writing a long time before I ever met you," he said. "I'll do it again. On my terms. When I'm ready."

"And so will I," I said. "I want just one promise from you, Cornelius. Don't intrude your work on mine. Don't ask me to look up something or edit a page. I'll write a book of my own and you know something? You won't be asked for any help because you'll never see a line of it until it's in print."

"You don't even have the nerve," Connie said. "You wouldn't know where to begin."

I didn't answer. I spent that night alone in our bedroom, sleepless, wondering what I'd got myself into. I knew I would have to accept his challenge. But did I have the ability for the job? It was too late for either of us to undo the bitter words we had spoken. That night Connie did not come up to bed at all. Neither, as time passed, did he start to work on *Bridge*.

Over the next three weeks we were polite and distant. I never went near our office. For a long time I had been thinking of trying to write a novel based on the real-life experiences of four teenage girls growing up during World War II whose personalities and actions I might be able to incorporate into that of a single character. In part, the idea was a nostalgic trip. In part, it was a means of conveying my belief that the herd instincts and peer pressures of young people had not changed very much over the decades, despite each new generation's insistence that it is unique in its individualism. And, finally, I had felt that the slow disintegration of family life and parental control—which existed even in my own household—had its beginnings on the home front during World War II. These notions were to become central to the theme of the book.

Working in the house I did produce a story outline and I did get a publisher. I also got an advance for the book. I didn't tell Connie about any of it. I opened a new bank account and put the book advance into it. Then I went to work on my first novel, *The Betty Tree*.

Connie had never worked in solitude and I think he had become unable to work without having me nearby. Even Anne's presence, the routine daily work, and the constant telephone calls into and out of the office, did not, according to Anne, substitute for my being at my own desk across from his. One evening he came into the kitchen where I was preparing dinner and Victoria was doing homework. He winked at Vicki. "Your mother's mad at me," he told her.

"Oh? How come?"

"She's been mad at me for weeks because I hurt her by something I said and she knows how to hurt back."

He came over and put his arms around me for the first time

in weeks. "Katie, there's an old Irish saying which I just made up. You stick out your tongue behind my back and all the anger between us will go away."

"It's not that simple."

"Try it."

I did. And suddenly I kissed his cheek and we were laughing. Vicki left her homework and Connie caught her up in one arm, his other arm around my waist. Slowly we three revolved in a tight little circle.

"Stick out your tongues, girls," Connie said. "If my women don't adore me, I'm lost."

Giggling, Vicki complied. "You've got the longest tongue I've ever seen," Connie told her. "That's a lot of anger passing out of one little girl."

He kissed her face and leaned across her to kiss me. "Come back, Katie," he said. "I'm lost without you. I always will be."

The next day I went back to the office. I worked on *The Betty Tree* while Connie continued his phone conversations, his dictation, his arrangements for future activities. None of them included any mention of *A Bridge Too Far*. Still, I was happy to be back in the fold. Connie didn't ask about my book, nor did I talk about it. Occasionally he would stroll over to my desk and I would quickly cover the work with papers or a book. When I had enough material written, I handed it over to Anne for clean typing. A manuscript folder, such as she always made up for Connie, now held my work and began to thicken a little more each week. It sat on my desk, a constant reminder of our argument, not nine feet from Connie's work area. He seemed totally indifferent to whatever I was doing at my own desk, but Anne told me only recently that every evening when I left to begin some household chores, he would take the little manuscript and read it carefully. Then he would put it back precisely as I had left it.

In November 1969 my mother died suddenly. The shock and the countless details that follow a death, including the arrangement of my parents' big house in Iowa for my father's easier convenience, delayed my work on the book considerably. Still, by early March of 1970 I had written enough to earn another advance and this one, too, I deposited in the new bank account. I had great hopes for that book and, even so long after the serious rift between us, I savored the thought of showing Connie the money I had earned on a book he had never believed I would or could do. *The Betty Tree* was published finally in 1972. It was a flawed first novel but I thought there was merit to it—and still do. Moreover, I had had a compelling reason to write it—Connie's dare that I could never do it. But my book was finished by sandwiching it in during the hours I began to work once again with Connie. By the time he got around to asking me to help as I had done in the past, the importance of getting *Bridge* written far outweighed the pride I felt in writing my own book. And, even before *The Betty Tree* was finished, I drew on its advances and put those monies to a far different use than the spiteful purposes which had caused me originally to deposit them in a new account.

It is strange that in his diaries, tapes, and notebooks Connie never mentions the party I gave him at "21" on June 5, 1970. It was in honor of his fiftieth birthday. I wanted his friends from all over the world to come and help him celebrate—and I would not use the money for his party from our joint account. So *The Betty Tree* paid for the biggest party I had ever given, a surprise for Connie on his birthday.

Anne and I worked for weeks drawing up lists of people, sending out invitations, telegrams, and letters. Peter Kriendler, Ben Wright, Paul Gitlin, Tom Lenk, Paul Slade—all friends of Connie's—were first sworn to secrecy and then took over some of the work entailed to make this a memorable party. It was. People came from France, from Britain, and from Holland. They arrived from the West Coast and from all the states in between where Connie's friends could be found. Ben Wright, Mary Hemingway, Walter Cronkite, Pierre Salinger, Art Buchwald, and Jack Thompson roasted him unmercifully on that evening, after I'd propelled Connie, not unwillingly, into "21" for dinner.

In an upstairs private room, the guests were all assembled. As Connie walked in, General Omar Bradley embraced him and Kitty Bradley led eighty guests in one earsplitting shout of "Happy Birthday." Paul Slade, then chief North American photographer for *Paris Match,* had supplied large blowups of Connie with cartoon blurbs. The photographs hung on the walls of the still-larger banquet room we occupied after the first toasts and festivities were over. Tom Lenk had engaged an Irish singer and a group of correspondents and friends had worked on a fiftieth-anniversary booklet of pictures and text which went to every guest. For once, Connie was almost at a loss for words, but he rallied quickly and we had difficulty getting him away from the microphone where he had gone to protest Art Buchwald's comments on him. I have never seen him so happy as he was that night and I was glad I'd taken up Connie's challenge. The novel, then in the process of completion, had provided me the opportunity to give him the party entirely out of funds I'd made on my own. I felt both satisfied and vindicated.

By the time of that fiftieth birthday Connie had been plagued with prostatitis for two months. I believed it was temporary, certainly not serious, and I had great hopes that the party, bringing together tried and true friends who knew about the new book and were expecting its publication shortly, would be the impetus that would set him on the road to work once again.

Even as late as July 24, I thought a cure would be found for his difficulty. Connie had seldom mentioned it since the onset in April and then only to imply that he was on the mend. And if he was on the mend, surely his reluctance to begin the book would disappear as well. Even now I cannot believe the blithe unconcern with which I viewed his "little problem."

CORNELIUS

Can it really be only ten days since my world started to collapse around me? At the outset there was nothing to distinguish my July 15 visit to Neligan's office from any previous appointments. The paper gown, the examining table, the questions, the uncomfortable, inevitable prostatic massage were by now familiar. Then, unexpectedly, the customary routine snapped. Probing the inflamed area, Pat suddenly seemed to tense and stop. The room went very still. I started to say something but Neligan said, "Shush," and the strange, brooding quiet continued even as he resumed the massage. It seemed a longer time than usual before Pat peeled off his glove, dropped it in the disposal can and turned to the washbasin.

"Get dressed, Concubhair, and then we'll talk," he said over his shoulder. I should mention that Neligan is a fair Gaelic scholar and that Concubhair is Gaelic for Cornelius. If one was to write it the way it sounds, it would look something like "C-u-h-o-o-r." Pat, like Katie, usually calls me Connie or CJ. Only once or twice before has he ever used the Gaelic pronunciation of my name.

I remember looking over at him as I got off the table, but his back was to me, his face turned away. He was scrubbing up very thoroughly, but in spite of the sound of the running water and the hard whish of the brush on his hands and nails, I still felt an uneasy silence in the room. I wondered what was troubling him. Curiously, even though I had become aware of the change in mood during the massage, I didn't associate it with myself just then. Pat's mind is very often on another problem, even as he deals with the one before him. Whatever that problem was, Pat's concern was clearly showing.

He was on the phone when I came out of the dressing room.

"Can you hold a minute until I find out?" he asked. Covering the mouthpiece he glanced up at me. "What's your schedule look like for the rest of this week?"

I sat down and got out my notebook. "I've got a hectic week right up to Wednesday, the twenty-second," I told him. "Why?"

"Not 'til the twenty-second," Pat said into the phone and waited. "At nine." He nodded, looking at me.

"Nine, what?"

Impatiently he gestured for me to be still.

"All right, Doctor, thank you." He hung up and sat watching me light a cigarette. "Oh, hell," he said and took out one of his cigars. "We might as well pollute the atmosphere."

"Who were you talking to, Neligan?"

"A urologist. I want you to see him. On the twenty-second. At 9:00 A.M." He scribbled a name and address on a piece of paper and shoved it across the desk."

"For Christ's sake, Pat. I suggested we do something new on the medication angle. I'm not doubting you. Why should I see some other doc?"

"Because I want you to."

"Why?"

Pat assumed his professional manner: squared shoulders, narrowed eyes, a totally misleading sternness. "Because I want another opinion, you silly bastard. All right?"

"An opinion about what?"

He hesitated, drawing on the cigar. "Today, during the massage, I thought I could feel a small hardening along the base and lateral border of the right lobe of the prostate. I want to find out if somebody else thinks it's there and I want to know more about it. You've had that damn prostatitis for so long that it's been hard to detect anything. Maybe this hardening, if it is there, is the result of the prostatitis. In any case, we want to find out. O.K.?"

"How can this doc tell me more than you can?"

Neligan was becoming exasperated. "Because he's a urologist, understand? And I'm an internist. It's his specialty."

"O.K. If that's all you've got to suggest. Can he come up with anything new to stop this staining? It's driving me up the wall."

Pat nodded. "I know. Two heads are better than one. That's why I want you to see this man."

I glanced at the address on the paper. "Good thing he's in New York," I told Pat. "Katie and I have to be in town almost all the rest of this week and again the early part of next week. While we're gone, Eldon and my mother will have to cope with the house plus Geoff and Victoria."

I should mention that my mother had recently arrived from Dublin for a visit and Kathryn's father, Eldon Morgan, had come from Iowa to stay for a couple of weeks. His birthday was last Sunday, July 19, and we gave him a small party before heading back into New York and a string of appointments on Monday. I had to be on the Barry Gray radio show last Tuesday night, the twenty-first. Since the show aired late, I figured that Katie and I would simply stay over another night at the Plaza and I would see the urologist at nine on Wednesday morning, July 22. Incredibly, that was just three days ago.

Before Wednesday's appointment I hardly gave my forthcoming meeting with Neligan's urologist friend any thought at all, except to hope that he would come up with something to stop the staining. If anybody could clear up that problem and end the mental stress the prostatitis was causing, I was all for it. I was sick of the strain I've put on Katie and the kids, ashamed of my bad temper and its effect on them. To cherish my wife and to enjoy Geoff and Vicki were vitally important to me, more important even than to have the freedom from the physical worries that, I kept telling myself, were all that hindered me from getting back to work.

That last bit is pretty ironic. As a result of Wednesday's appointment and its aftermath I will never again have a trouble-free thought. Or be a normal husband to my wife or the father my children would want and will need. I don't even think I can protect their future. Quite frankly, the more I dwell on it, I doubt if I have either the time or the ability now to write the book.

$$= 6 =$$

SO MUCH HAS HAPPENED in these three short days that I am somewhat disoriented. My mind refuses to accept the almost certain termination of my future in this short time span. I've interviewed men involved in sudden, sharp skirmishes who have sworn that the battle went on for hours when the fact was that the action was over in ten or fifteen minutes. Fear, and the extent to which one is involved, tend to make an ordeal endless, and I suppose that this is what is happening to me.

Yet it is less than seventy hours since I set out from the Plaza in New York for the appointment that began to bring my world down around me.

Katie was still sleeping when I left the hotel. Since we'd had to stay over another night, she'd made a hair appointment for later in the morning and we'd arranged to meet at "21" for lunch before driving home.

The doctor's address was a few blocks uptown on Park Avenue, a short walk from the hotel. I remember feeling extremely fit, in spite of the persistent discharge. I know I was much calmer emotionally than I had been for some days. I had come around to Pat's point of view that a second opinion by a specialist was the right course of action. It would surely move us closer and more positively to a solution. As I look back it is curious that I felt no uneasiness at all about the hard area Pat had found in the prostate exactly a week before. If anything, I think I was relieved. To me it was an indication that the swelling had gone down enough, thanks to Neligan's ministrations, to reveal the remaining problem. I believed that Pat wanted to find out if the prostatic infection had triggered this thickening in the lining of the gland. We had come to the last bit of the trouble. Now, I thought it, too, could be treated. So, on Wednesday morning I really had no worries about it at all. I walked leisurely to the doctor's office, absorbing the sights and sounds of the city I like as well as any in the world except Paris.

It was about ten past nine when I got to the urologist's office and gave the receptionist my name. Surprisingly, there was no wait. I was shown immediately into an examining room where I filled out the usual medical history form for a nurse and then the doctor came in. A rather remote type but quite impressive—Dunhill suit, Church's shoes undoubtedly (I had on a pair myself), and the shirt and tie looked like Tripler's. We chatted briefly. He said he'd had a letter from Pat and he asked me most of the same questions about the prostatitis that Neligan already had.

Then came the procedure to which I had become uncomfortably accustomed: I stripped to the buff, got into the crackling paper horror, and climbed on the table. The poking and prodding began and then the digital manipulation of the prostate. I attempted some small talk. But this man lacked Pat's ability to put me at ease. Intent and aloof, he answered either in monosyllables or not at all.

The examination seemed longer somehow than those with Pat. Finally the doctor asked me to get dressed and said that the nurse would show me to his office. Before I could get to the dressing room, he disappeared through the door.

The urologist's private office was an awesome departure from the conventional paneled or painted rooms of the doctors, dentists, or optometrists I'd been in before: heavily stuccoed white walls, a couple of decorator-type seating areas that looked as though no one had ever sat there, and a bloody great desk at the far end of the room. The doctor was already seated at it, shadowy against the brittle light surrounding him. Behind his desk fluorescent tubes concealed in a curtained window recess shone down on a variety of plants arranged on rows of glass shelves. I was motioned to a leather chair in front of the desk, where I faced directly into the cold light. This unsocial chamber seemed more like the setting for an inquisition than the relaxed surroundings one would expect for a conference with patients.

The doctor spoke with no preamble. "Dr. Neligan is to be congratulated. I'm frankly amazed that he found the firm area in the prostate, Mr. Ryan. I had some difficulty locating it myself."

"But it's there?"

"Oh, yes. It's there. Until we do a complete urological check, I can't tell you whether it's fibrous or neoplastic. You've had long-standing prostatitis and this may well be the result. We'll see. But if I had to make a pronouncement right now, my bet would be one thousand to one that it is benign."

I must have stared at the man. I remember a feeling of utter bewilderment. My mind was so jumbled with questions that I couldn't think which to put first.

But two words he'd said were uppermost in my thoughts: benign, neoplastic. I knew the meaning of the first; the other—contrast it with fibrous, I told myself. Contrast it with benign. The opposite of benign would be malignant. My God! What was the man talking about?

I remember feeling a sudden, violent nausea. The face of the man across the desk was impassive. He seemed unaware of the effect his words were having on me. I could understand that in his profession words like "benign" and "neoplastic" were as commonplace as any I might use to describe a military plan. Still, I think one should lead into a subject. You don't jolt a reader or a patient until rapport has been established. The doctor and I seemed to have none. I attempted to bring that about.

"Doctor, let me try to understand. My view is that Dr. Neligan wanted an expert's opinion about this continuing discharge and how we proceed in stopping it and clearing up the problem. He mentioned a hardening but I'm under the impression it's come about because of the duration of the prostatitis."

"That may be so." He was not giving me much help. He reminded me of some of the people I've interviewed over the years. There are the arrogant ones, sometimes hostile, their responses reluctant, revealing little. And then there are any reporter's favorites—the outgoing people, wanting you to understand their actions, keen on setting the record straight, delving into notes and papers in order to add their own little footnotes to history. This man could be one of the difficult ones. Our compatibility was tenuous at best. I had to take the risk of severing it completely. I had to know more of what was in his mind.

"What I'm trying to understand is your terminology," I told him. "You said you'd bet this hardening is benign. It never occurred to me to think along the terms you've used. Have you the slightest reason to think it may not be benign?"

"There's always that possibility. That's why Dr. Neligan asked me to see you."

Pat had not put it that way. I was feeling more confused

and alarmed by the minute. By then, too, I was certain that my questions were not going to produce the kind of forthrightness I had hoped for. The doctor may have sensed my bewilderment. His next words were less harsh.

"Mr. Ryan, we want to clear up this problem. You've had it too long." Then, to my astonishment, he reached for the phone and dialed a number. Waiting while it rang, he said, "I'm going to put you in the hospital this afternoon. We'll do a laboratory workup and tomorrow I'll do a cystoscopy and biopsy the area."

I was stunned by his words. I cannot remember anything of his telephone conversation except hearing him spell my name carefully. He had not asked my permission or told me the reasons behind his decision. Audaciously, I thought, he had proceeded, setting strange gears into motion without the courtesy of consulting me. For a moment I felt like a small lad, lost and defenseless in unfamiliar territory. I experienced a moment of blinding panic.

"Look," I recall saying, "you're moving too fast for me to even understand what's to happen. I haven't agreed to any of this. I'd like to talk with Dr. Neligan before any further decisions are made."

"I already have. While you were dressing. He agrees we should go ahead."

"Doctor, Pat is my friend as well as my physician. I'd like to speak with him."

Wordlessly, he pushed the phone toward me. Pat wasn't in his office. Mary Chapin told me he was on his way to the hospital but, yes, he had spoken with the New York doctor shortly before he left and, no, she didn't know what they had discussed.

If Pat had, in fact, agreed then I probably ought to go along with this unexpected development. However, since I was unable to reach him and find out for myself, I tried another tack.

"My wife and I are due to leave for Connecticut this afternoon," I told the doctor. "I would much prefer that this be postponed until I can speak with Dr. Neligan."

"Mr. Ryan, I strongly advise you to stay over. What we're going to do is quite simple and it will reveal the problem. Let's take this one step at a time. Now," as Pat had done he wrote on a paper and handed it over to me. The hospital name was familiar. "I've asked them to expect you before four P.M. today. I probably won't see you myself until tomorrow morning since I want the laboratory work done first. This is a very simple, routine procedure. You'll be able to leave probably by midafternoon tomorrow."

I realized he was standing. My appointment was at an end. We parted without any exchange of pleasantries. In minutes I was out in the warm summer noise of Park Avenue. Although the urologist had made the hospital confinement sound, as he put it, "simple and routine," I felt as if I was in a suddenly frightening dream, alarmed and full of foreboding.

I discovered myself at Sulka's. There, I wandered around the men's store, chatting about God knows what with salesmen I knew, idly flipping through shirt swatches, looking at ties. I don't remember anything I saw.

I did try to reach Kathryn from the store. I got Hans Schroeder—the young German who does Katie's hair and has become almost a member of our family—on the phone. She'd already left and Hans didn't know where she was going next, only that she was meeting "Father"—me—for lunch.

After calling Hans, I walked over to Mark Cross and then to Cartier's to chat with Ken Van Atten. Then, finally, far too early to meet Katie, I went to "21". The restaurant was not yet officially open for lunch but it is my home away from home and, as always, Chuck was there to unlock the door and let me in. I needed the banter, the easy camaraderie, which the staff and its owners unfailingly supply. I found Pete Kriendler in his private quarters where he ordered coffee for me and his customary cup of tea and for a while everything was all right.

Jerry Berns and Bob Kriendler came in to give Pete and me their habitual razzing about our fishing trips. We always share a room together and we always swear that we will never do so again. Pete insists he developed chronic insomnia from my snoring. I claim even the fish are stunned by the stentorian utterances which emanate from his side of the room.

The familiar byplay relaxed me. I switched to a bourbon and put my feet up on Peter's paper-strewn desk, which drew snarls about my manners and speculation on the kind of building in which I had been raised. Listening to Kriendler complain always makes me feel better. I didn't tell Bob or Jerry or Peter about my morning. Once about six weeks back I had casually mentioned to Pete that I had "a touch" of prostatitis. "So what else is new?" he demanded. "Get something that half the guys in this world haven't had and then maybe I'll feel sorry."

Remembering, I wondered what had happened to "half the guys"? How many of them had been told there was a hardening in the prostate that only tests could define? What odds did they get from *their* doctors? And what happens if the specialists' bets are wrong? I didn't want to know the answers. I wasn't ready in case Pete's face took on a look of sudden concern.

Somebody telephoned to say that Mrs. Ryan had arrived and Pete and I went out to meet her. Katie was looking pretty and high-spirited, chatting with the lobby staff. She saw us and got kissed soundly by Pete, who announced that "since the class in the Ryan family" had arrived, it would be all right for me to lunch there. How happy she looked! Those dark blue eyes, which Geoff inherited, swung to me and something changed in her face. She reached up and kissed me and suddenly put both hands around my arm. I had the damnedest feeling there were tears in my eyes.

I told her at the table over drinks. She traced a pattern over the back of my hand with one finger, a habit she has.

"I'll call home after lunch and tell them we've been delayed until tomorrow. You've got to see somebody about the book. I'll think of something."

"No," I told her. "After lunch we're going back to the hotel to pack and you're going home. I hate to ask you to drive back in to pick me up tomorrow but I think the grandparents will have had it by now. Besides, you'll worry about being away from home another day. We told the kids we'd be back."

"What do I tell them at home?"

"The truth."

She looked at me. "What is the truth?"

"I've got to have some routine tests. That's all."

Katie played with the silverware. "Routine tests. O.K. You'll call me tonight and tell me what room you're in?"

"Of course."

"And I'll call you tomorrow to find out what time to pick you up."

"Better not. I'll call you. He's got to do his stuff in the morning. I'll call when I get back in the room."

"Can I have another drink?"

"Sure."

"Sometimes I forget to tell you," Katie said. "I love you."

꞊ 7 ꞊

I WAS TOO DISTRACTED to read. There are few things more unreal than sitting in a dressing gown on the edge of a hospital bed when you don't feel sick, when only a few hours earlier you have been in the hustle-bustle of the city chatting with friends. Several times I was strongly tempted to simply dress and get out of there, only to tell myself that I had come this far and I might as well see this brief stay through.

Since lunch with Katie, I'd tried to reach Neligan several times without success. Surely he'd ring back, if only to confirm that he had indeed agreed with the urologist that I should go into hospital for tests. I couldn't concentrate on the magazines and papers I'd brought with me. Instead, I brought my diary up to date.

I wrote:

July 22 cont'd. Now 6:30 p.m.: Two interns have been in. More examinations. More questions. Getting sick of repeating myself for each new visitor. Lab girl came for blood; somebody else for a urine specimen. Still no word from Pat. 8 p.m.: Just called Katie, gave her room number, asked her to try to track down Neligan. Everything at home all right. Vicki wanted to know where I was. Katie said another night in town on business. Mother apparently calm; Eldon, too. Both agreed best to get to the root of my problems. I am not so sure, I don't want these tests.

Shortly after 7:00 A.M. Thursday, July 23—only the day before yesterday I was taken down to an operating room. In a group of look-alikes—capped, gowned, and with masks in place—the urologist was difficult to pick out. Then one of the men came over to me. As he began to speak, I recognized the specialist's voice, muffled by his mask.

"How are you feeling?" he asked.

"All right, Doctor, but I would like the drill on what you're planning to do."

There was such a long silence that I thought he did not intend to answer. Finally, he said, "Suppose you let me worry about that. It's an innocuous procedure, as I explained yesterday."

It is my belief that every patient has a right to know as much as he wants about the medication or medical services that are prescribed for him. To be fair, I suppose that comprehension, intelligence, and the capability to absorb a doctor's information without developing grave misgivings or morbidity should be taken into account. But I think if a patient questions something, it is a doctor's obligation to explain within those limits. It was clear that this doctor felt no such compulsion. It was equally clear to me that I was going to press for the information. I think I had fairly taken his own profession into account, the amount of knowledge and expertise he surely possessed to bring him to his standing in his field. But it is *my* profession to ask questions, to probe, to get at reasons, more so now than ever when my unreliable body must function in spite of what ails it.

"What you propose to do may be innocuous, doctor. I would still like some idea of what this procedure entails."

"You ask a great many questions."

"I would never be able to write if I didn't."

"Oh, yes," he said. "You write. But these are technical matters."

"So is much of the material I deal with in my own work."

He hesitated and then said, "I am going to take a visual look inside the bladder by means of an instrument called a cystoscope. I shall also take a small amount of tissue from the hard area in the base of the right lobe of the prostate. That process is called a Silverman needle biopsy, Franklin modification, with one finger in the rectum. You will be anesthetized. There will be no pain." He moved a step back from the table. "Now, Mr. Ryan, have I enlightened you? We are ready to begin."

He turned from the table and walked out of my sight. I remember the last thing I thought of before they put me under: I couldn't understand why Pat Neligan hadn't called me. It simply wasn't like him.

My watch was strapped back on when I woke up on Thursday, but I couldn't seem to focus on the dial. I was quite alone in my room. As my mind cleared, I realized there was a catheter in me. The pain it induced brought me to full consciousness as constant bladder spasms made me want to alternately retch or yell. No one had told me to expect anything like this.

I have a hazy recollection of later talking to a nurse. I think I was both angry and tearful because no one had told me what would be done or how I would feel after the time on the table. Surely I could have been told to expect both the catheter and the bladder spasms that racked my body? The knowledge would have helped me anticipate the pain and be prepared to deal with it. The nurse just listened. I don't recall her saying anything.

Later still, the phone rang. I felt a wave of relief to hear Pat's voice. I told him about the catheter and the spasms. His was the first soothing voice I'd heard since before I'd gone down to the OR. He tried to calm me. He'd been in touch with the specialist and the catheter would be removed any time now. Then, almost offhandedly, he said they'd be keeping me in overnight again. That meant I had to stay in hospital until midmorning Friday, yesterday. In spite of his reassuring tone, Pat didn't sound like himself. There was an element of worry or emotion, some nuance in his words that triggered an alarm in me. Obviously, something was not right.

After Pat rang off, I got Katie on the phone and told her it appeared I wouldn't get out until the morning. I explained my discomfort, but I didn't mention my talk with Pat or the haunting feeling I had of something he had left unsaid. That was devious. There has always been honesty between Katie and me. It was devious, too, to ask casually if Pat had called her with any news—perhaps she knew something I had not been told. He hadn't. Katie sensed my pain and tried to cheer me up; the medicos would now know how to proceed in clearing up the prostatitis. Within a week, she said, this would all seem like a bad dream and I'd be working on the book. I said I'd see her in the morning. "And tomorrow night we'll celebrate," she said. "Let's all go out to dinner and put this thing behind us." It was obvious that she expected the outcome to be a good one, the persistent prostatitis all but over.

Late Thursday afternoon the urologist telephoned. I told him about the bladder spasms and that the unexpected catheter, which still had not been removed, was driving me up the wall.

"Just how severe are the spasms, Mr. Ryan?"

"I feel like I'm peeing barbed wire," I said baldly. As a joke the statement left much to be desired but it accurately described the pain.

"I've ordered the catheter removed," the doctor told me. "You'll be given something for your discomfort."

"When will you be in, Doctor?"

"I'll see you in the morning."

"I am going home tomorrow?"

"You'll be free to leave before noon."

There was one more question I had to ask—the most vital of all. "Doctor, did you win your bet?"

He rang off. I couldn't be absolutely certain he had even heard my query. But neither could I shake the feeling that the odds had changed on his 1000 to 1 bet. That strangeness in Pat's voice, the urologist's haste to end the telephone call, were sending fear signals all along my body. I didn't believe the tissue removed by biopsy was benign.

Katie had not arrived when the doctor came by yesterday morning. He inquired if I'd had a good night and, before I could answer, told me he'd signed my hospital release. I was free to go whenever Katie got there. He said he'd be talking to Pat about the future handling "of your case." Before I could ask anything, he was striding out the door. He had not even mentioned the biopsy, yet he surely knew that the results of it were the first information I wanted. Any patient would. I got out of bed as quickly as I could manage and went to the door. I looked up and down the hall but the specialist was nowhere to be seen. I went back and began to dress.

Kathryn and I were passing the nurses' station on my floor when one of the women behind the desk spoke to me.

"Mr. Ryan, the doctor left word for you to telephone his office before you leave. You're to ask for his nurse. Here's the number. You may use the white phone over there."

She handed me a slip, neatly printed—the nurse's name, the doctor's number. Katie and I exchanged glances. I tried to joke about it. "He didn't tell me good-bye this morning. One must observe the formalities."

The receptionist at his office was expecting the call. I was put through to the nurse immediately.

"Oh, yes, Mr. Ryan. Are you all ready to go?" Her voice was pleasant. Yet, as with Pat and the urologist, there was something about her tone that disturbed me—a brightness that somehow didn't ring true.

"We're leaving now," I told her.

"Is Mrs. Ryan with you?"

"Yes. May I ask what this is all about?"

"Doctor wanted me to say that he's sorry to have to detain you. I'm sure you're anxious to get home. However, he does want to see you again today. Here in the office at six. Please bring Mrs. Ryan with you." She rang off.

I stood by the telephone, stunned. I was afraid that Katie might see my fear. Without turning around, I called over to the nurses' station. "Nurse, can I call Connecticut from here?"

"I'm sorry," someone said. "It isn't permitted. There are pay phones in the lobby."

"I've got a telephone credit card. I'd like to call from here."

"We have our rules, Mr. Ryan."

Wordlessly I shook my head. I seemed to be frustrated at every turn.

Kathryn took my arm and we walked to the elevators. Waiting for a car, she asked me, "Who do you want to call?"

"Pat."

"Why?"

I jabbed the Down button again.

"He wants to see us at six tonight."

"Who does?"

"The urologist."

"Is that what the call was about?"

I nodded. I didn't want to talk about it just then.

All along, I'd found the doctor's behavior disturbingly similar to that of the reluctant subjects often encountered by reporters and correspondents trying to track down a story. The evasive routine seldom varies: questions are tabled or ignored, appointments are canceled, new meetings are set up—all to buy time for the interviewee to collect thoughts, review papers or notes, or decide how much or how little he's willing to put on the record. I was familiar with such practices. What was unfamiliar was that this was happening in a situation where my right to know the specialist's information should not be subject to debate. What knowledge he possessed about the outcome of my tests concerned me more vitally than it could ever matter to him. I didn't tell Kathryn any of this, but the doctor's behavior and a desperate fear that the 6:00 P.M. meeting was going to turn out badly were destroying the control I had been trying to hang on to.

In the main lobby, Katie asked, "CJ, why call Pat?"

"Why not?"

"What time did you say you have to see the doctor?"

"At six. Don't you listen? It isn't just me. He wants you to come along."

"Why shouldn't he see us both? He probably wants to explain where we go from here."

"That's how *you* interpret it."

Katie was annoyed. "Why are you making so much of this? You might recall that I've had two benign cysts removed from my breasts. In each case the surgeon asked you to be there when he explained what he'd done and what he found."

"Kathryn, I can't explain it, but this is different."

"I think it's senseless to worry. They kept you an extra day because of your discomfort. I'm sure the doctor wants to explain your future course of treatment. He wouldn't have released you if anything was wrong."

"Then why insist on seeing us today?"

"I should think to get the pressure off as soon as possible and start you on whatever medication is finally going to clear this up."

"Look, if he wanted to take the pressure off and write prescriptions, he surely could have done it this morning."

"Surgeons always have tight schedules. He was probably rushed and wants the leisure to go over it with enough time to fully explain everything—what he's done and what he'll recommend to Pat for the future."

Katie's reasoning annoyed me. My fear had been building far too long for my mind to accept a sensible explanation. "All right," I told her angrily. "I won't call Pat. We'll just muck around town and waste time waiting for six o'clock. We'll do it your way."

I headed toward the entrance doors and went through them, letting them swing back without waiting for her. Behind me, I could hear them being pushed open again and Kathryn came up alongside me. We walked up the street side by side. I had never felt so totally apart from her.

$$\overset{=}{\underset{=}{8}}$$

KATHRYN

We had come a block or more from the hospital without speaking. Connie was setting a punishing pace, his face grim and tight. He did not once glance at me and I had no breath to speak. It took all my effort to keep up with him. Then, abruptly, he slowed, the tension left his face. He reached out and caught my hand. I locked my fingers tightly into his. We went on at an easy walk.

Connie's wrath never lasted long. He could forget anger as quickly as if it had never surfaced. Victims of one of his stormy moods had longer memories and he was often baffled by a cold encounter with someone he had unsettled weeks before. Still, his tempers that spring and early summer had been all too frequent and they worried me. He blamed them on the stubborn continuance of the prostatitis. I thought they stemmed from a sense of guilt about his procrastination on the book. The problem of beginning *Bridge* was a great deal different from the problems he'd experienced in past writings. He was approaching this new book with health problems much more critical than his habitual search for the perfect lead.

Connie's tapes and diary notes go far toward clarifying other occurrences that troubled me during those midyear months of 1970. His account of the onset of the prostatitis and its persistence makes me feel ashamed of my selfish optimism that his problems were not only of a passing nature but of little importance, rather like a cold that would run its course and disappear. He never admitted how acutely he worried about the problem. He minimized even the pain he experienced in April and the consequent lingering discharge which he relates so irritated and obsessed him. At the time I never knew the extent to which these troubles occupied his mind.

What was important to me was Connie's withdrawal from physical love. The zest and joy and gentleness of that side of our marriage was slipping away and becoming, rather quickly, nonexistent. In all else the bond between us seemed strong as ever. But this missing dimension of our lives worried and confused me. Now I know that his love had not diminished as I feared, it was beginning a subtle, delicate change. In time, our lives together would become more intensely entwined than they had ever been before in marriage.

In retrospect, my ignorance of the many times Connie was in touch with Pat, either by phone or at his office, astonishes me. My own diary of those months contains commonplace social, family, and business engagements. We spent evenings with Pat and Vera alone or at someone's dinner party, but neither Pat nor Connie spoke of other meetings. Connie mentions that Pat had changed the original medication—Neg-Gram—ten days after he first went to Pat for professional help. My diary has a note that the Neligans were here for dinner on that same Sunday, April 26. Connie had never mentioned the afternoon medical visit.

I wonder now if on that fateful Friday after his release from the hospital, he might have been better left on his own. We could have gone our separate ways until 6:00 P.M. and met at the doctor's office. Connie might have relieved some tensions in the company of our friend and lawyer Paul Gitlin, whom Connie always referred to as "my brother," just as Vera Neligan and his French literary agent, Marie Schebeko, were always his "sisters." He could have spent time with Jerry Korn, his former editor in the *Collier's* days, whom he invariably used as confidant and sounding board throughout the writing of each of his books. Or Ben Wright, Connie's longtime friend from World War II days, would have been only too glad to concoct with him some new plan for fishing or travel.

Surely, a talk with Paul, a discussion with Jerry about the problems of *Bridge,* or an embryo plan for still another trip with Ben would have eased him on that day. But I believe by Friday afternoon, July 24, 1970, Connie knew he was upon the threshold of a new journey on which none of us who loved him would be along.

The day dragged. Connie wasn't hungry; neither was I. We window-shopped aimlessly and browsed in bookstores, growing gradually more comfortable with each other. It was nearly five when Connie suggested we have a drink at the Plaza's Oak Room bar before our appointment with the doctor. My husband's mood during that hour was uncharacteristic. He would be strangely apathetic one minute, only to talk nonstop the next. His anger seemed to have dissolved. As usual, I thought, he had forgotten it. But his pensive moments made me search for topics that would stir his imagination and start him expounding again. I have always found Connie's views more entertaining and stimulating than those of anyone else I knew. And so, in valleys and peaks of musings and talk, we passed what seemed to me an unimportant hour. In fact, it was to be the last carefree one of my marriage. We would never again share the future brightly as we had done the past.

The day had been warm and still bright outside. In the doctor's empty outer office it was night. The air-conditioned room had a wintery chill and lamps were lit, shining on the glossy covers of current, expensive magazines—*Country Life, Realities, Art in America.* No one was in the receptionist's glassed-in office. I stared into it at rows of plum-colored metal files along the room's far wall. A desk to match the cabinets' color held a steel basket of folders; and a message spindle, papers jutting at all angles, was alongside a sensible black phone. The most jarring note in the little room was the typewriter, a bright red, on still another plum-colored piece. I remember wondering who had devised the color scheme.

Connie seemed not to notice the clashing decor. He was pensive again, mentally far away. We both lit cigarettes and flicked the ashes into pristine heavy glass trays. I sat down and leafed through *Country Life.* Connie paced. Except for his footsteps and the slight hum of the air conditioner, everything seemed almost too still. I glanced up at my husband on one of his turns about the room. His face was pale; his fine, taut, Irish skin seemed almost luminescent.

"Do you think they've forgotten us?" I asked. "It would seem everyone's gone home."

Connie looked at his watch, shrugged, and continued pacing. My own watch showed 6:15. I thought of going to the hall and ringing the bell once again. There was no telling how long we might wait or how long the conference would last. After it, we still had more than an hour's drive home.

I was beginning to feel the irritability common to many of us when we sit in a doctor's office, waiting our turn long past the appointment time. Yet it had only been fifteen minutes. Still, putting aside the usual nervous annoyance this kind of wait can produce, I began to feel my own first nudgings of fear. If I was now becoming uneasy, what had it been like for Connie over these three days, his loathing of hospitals heightened by a series of tests given to a man totally at odds with sickness?

A door beside the files opened and a woman in white pushed back glass panels at the reception desk and smiled out at us. "I am so sorry, Mr. Ryan. Doctor is running a little late. He'll be with you in just a few minutes."

Connie stared vacantly at the woman. Her smile faded and she closed the glass panes between us softly. We seemed frozen in a tableau: Connie rooted to the carpet, my hands folded on the expensive stock paper of the open magazine, the uniformed woman framed in the glassed-in cubicle.

Then the door leading into the inner offices opened soundlessly. The doctor looked out at us. Silent as we three, he stood viewing Connie and me, our cigarettes, and his used ashtrays. I felt guilty about those ashtrays because the doctor had a look I recognized and had often employed: that of a parent disappointed by small children's stunts.

"Will you come in now?" He pushed the door farther back and stood against it.

I looked at Connie, tense and silent.

"Both of us?" I finally asked the doctor.

"Yes, Mrs. Ryan."

We were directed down the corridor to his private office. Two leather chairs were drawn up before the desk. The urologist motioned us to sit and took his own place opposite us. He opened a single folder on the desk and began to study it. His aloofness, the uncomfortable silence, were unnerving. My mouth felt dry. Our posthospital visits to my doctors had never begun like this.

$$= 9 =$$

CORNELIUS

Very often in the hours before dawn I've come awake with a solution to a problem that had tied up my writing all the previous day. In those minutes I could see clearly the direction a particular section had to take in order to maintain the drive and accuracy of the book. The organization, dormant during the waking hours, had surfaced only in sleep.

So it has been with hunches and intuitions. Sometimes I've acted without knowing why, almost always to discover later that what I had done was right, the impulse that had driven me correct. More than once, I would have lost an opportunity, a story, even a job, without that blind urgency that set everything else in motion.

Now intuition was working in a far more personal way. Even without clear-cut evidence, I knew my worst fears had been realized. But I was unable to act, to turn that inner knowledge to an advantage. The summons directing Katie and me to see the urologist at six had induced an incubus I could not get free of. I moved numbly through the hours until the appointment with the doctor, feeling as if I had been given a massive shot of Novocain, unable to steel myself for what I was now certain the outcome would be.

And then, with absolute clarity of mind, I found myself once again in the doctor's private consulting room, Kathryn by my side. The uninviting setting, the harsh lights, brought me to my senses. I could think again.

Perhaps there is some protocol involved in similar consultations between doctor and patient or relatives, but I wanted desperately to get to the point. Besides, as I well knew, this doctor was not given to exchanges of meaningless pleasantries.

"Doctor," I began, "I doubt that you have asked us both here if you have good news. I assume the biopsy was positive."

He was obviously astonished that I had taken the initiative and, possibly, annoyed by my bluntness. His attitude seemed to imply that the patient is expected to be mute and wait to be told his fate, rather in the manner of a courtroom, silent until judge or jury speaks. The air seemed charged with his disapproval. For seconds he was silent.

Then, "Yes," the doctor said finally, "that is correct."

Katie made some small sound but I didn't look at her. For three days no one had given me any information. Now the facts had to come out.

"Please tell me exactly what you have found," I said.

"I think, Mr. Ryan, much of the findings are too technical to go into. I would prefer to explain this in my own way."

I was baffled by his continuing brusqueness, but at the risk of increasing it I had to know the answer to the question uppermost in my mind: did I have a chance to go on living?

"Doctor," I began, "the technical findings concern me and my future. I'd very much appreciate your telling me what they are."

He did not unbend.

"You are a difficult man, Mr. Ryan, in your persistence in groping for details you could not possibly understand. I have my way of handling these talks. I should have preferred that you accept that. However, this problem has been with us from the start. You are not medically trained, yet you insist on medical language."

"No, not precisely. I simply want to know what you have found, and I want permission to question what I don't understand. Doctor, I am not trying to be either difficult or unreasonable."

He shrugged. I remember he picked up a sheet from the folder on his desk and referred to it from time to time as he talked.

"The diagnosis, to proceed, is early carcinoma of the prostate, confirmed by Silverman needle biopsy. Since you are just fifty and have no other disease of which we are now cognizant, I strongly recommend that you have a total radical prostatectomy. It is the only cure, and I stress the word, that medical science knows of today."

He seemed to be speaking to something or someone at a point above my head. The calm, crisp evenness of his voice made the report even harder to bear than I had imagined.

"You can probably live fifteen years, following surgical procedures and setting aside other health problems which could surface," he continued. "You will be impotent and there is about a twenty percent chance that you will have some incontinence, varying from slight to total. If it occurs, you will require a rubber bag device which would be strapped on to catch the urine.

"You could, of course, take Stilbestrol. It is a hormone. And have orchidectomy. However, the hormones will make you impotent in any case and the percentage chance of some degree of incontinency would remain the same. But your only real hope lies only in the prostatectomy. We will perform a metastatic series prior to the operation but, as of now, my examination indicates that the malignant change is confined to the base of the right lobe of the prostate."

Well, I had asked for it.

After a moment Kathryn spoke in a voice that I would have been hard put to recognize. "What is an orchi— Whatever you said?"

"The excision of the testes, Mrs. Ryan."

"Oh," Katie said in a small voice.

I expect my voice was as strange as Katie's seemed to me.

I asked about the recovery time for a radical prostatectomy and was told that I'd be in hospital at least three weeks, bladder spasms would be quite painful, and postoperative time would be difficult but within the normal limits of the procedure. I did not think to ask what "normal limits" meant. All I did think of, like the intuitions so often helpful in my work, was that I must not do anything immediately. One doctor's opinion was just not enough. I could not agree to such a procedure until I knew more about cancer of the prostate and what other avenues might be open to treat the disease. Surely, there had to be other choices.

Kathryn was obviously thinking the same thing. She asked about the hormones the urologist had mentioned. Would that treatment be preferable, she inquired, if the malignancy was confined to just one place? Instead of answering, the urologist began an oversimplified explanation of hormones. There were male hormones and female hormones. The first produced characteristics common to men, the second— Katie interrupted.

"We do understand the difference," she said. "I'm asking if hormonal treatment might be the first step before resorting to a drastic operation."

"I've said, Mrs. Ryan, that the radical prostatectomy is the only known cure." His words were flat and final.

"Now," he turned to me, "I'd planned to be on vacation but of course I will postpone it. I will schedule you back into the hospital Monday morning, July twenty-seventh."

"Doctor, this is all too sudden," I said. "I must have time to think it over."

The doctor looked directly at me. "I find your attitude almost impossible to understand. Why would you postpone what must be done if you're to be cured?"

I took a minute or two to assemble my thoughts as logically as possible under the circumstances.

"First, I don't know if there is a 'cure' for something like this, Doctor. You say so. Another doctor might not agree.

Second, if I'm not precisely at death's door I need time to think about an operation as total and final as this. I need to know much more background, statistics, survival records, and the steps that would have to be taken if you're wrong and the malignancy, God forbid, is not confined to the right lobe."

"I am not wrong. There is nothing to indicate that I am. I have already told you we will do a metastatic series prior to the operation but you need worry about nothing concerning those tests. I am convinced there is no spread."

"You also bet one thousand to one that the biopsy would prove benign."

He did not answer. His face was totally devoid of expression.

"In either course of treatment—hormones or the operation—you say I'll be impotent," I continued. "That destroys whatever sexual attributes I have. But what will happen to my mental drive? It's of utmost importance to me as well."

The urologist shook his head. "I can't predict," he told me. "That depends on you, and your desire to work. You may not work as well as in the past. Your thought processes, your 'drive,' as you call it, may be slower. Only time can tell."

Katie spoke up quickly. "I don't think any of us would want to commit my husband to a particular course of treatment without obtaining more opinions. Unless time is vital." She paused. "Is time vital, Doctor?"

He ignored the question. Instead, annoyance, a sudden anger with both of us, surfaced quickly. His tolerance for such attitudes as ours seemed very short. He launched into a curious monologue in which he referred to other urologists as "my opponents." His "opponents" would tell us to opt for hormone treatments; for radiation therapy, a treatment he contemptuously dismissed; and some "opponents," he warned, might advise us to do nothing at all, thus giving the malignancy time to spread. Surgery was the only course. "There is no alternative," he said flatly.

"Must it be done immediately?" Katie asked again.

"Since it must be done, what reason could you possibly have to postpone it?" he asked me. Yet he had still not answered Katie's question. Was this operation in any way elective? Was there time for other opinions? He had not helped us understand his decision. He had simply decreed that it had to be.

He seemed unaware of my necessity to make plans, impossible to complete over the weekend, between last evening, Friday, July 24, and Monday morning, July 27, when he wanted me back. His seeming indifference to our home situation and to the psychological effect his words were having on Kathryn and me were inexplicable. I understand them less today than yesterday.

I stood up and pulled Katie to her feet. I could feel her body trembling and I put my arm around her shoulders. She looked up at me and, startlingly, she smiled.

"Mr. Ryan," the doctor said, "I must insist that you telephone me tomorrow if I am to postpone my vacation. There is a great deal to do and I must let the hospital know. Private rooms are at a premium but I shall try and get you one."

I honestly do not think the man had heard a word either of us had said.

"Doctor, please hear me out," I told him. "I have your opinion that a radical prostatectomy must be done. I want to get other points of view in case there is a less drastic option open to me. I want to discuss our conversation with Dr. Neligan. I am not disputing you; I simply need more time, if in your view, I need not have an operation immediately."

"Why not now?" he asked. "You are illogical. If you were a black man and I told you I intended to perform a radical prostatectomy, I could cope with your attitude. In my experience I've found that a black will do anything to keep his sexual organs intact—even die from the disease although the cure is there. But you're an educated man. I'm sure you can adjust to the trauma of the sex part of this. After all, you and your wife are surely not expecting any more children."

Kathryn reacted as if someone had hit her violently across the face. She walked straight to his desk. "Never have I heard a doctor speak this way." She was on the verge of tears. "I can't believe what I've heard in this room. And you still haven't answered me. Has he time or hasn't he?"

"That," said the doctor, "is now up to the two of you. Isn't it?"

Wordlessly, Katie turned to stare at me and now there were tears—in her eyes and coursing down her face. I put my arm around her and together we walked out of his office. This time the absence of good-bye pleasantries did not seem strange. Among the three of us there was nothing further to be said.

Talking out this problem to myself has begun to help. I think I know what I must do. I've got to research this cancer as I do my books. I just can't take the word of one doctor or two—or even three—unless the opinions are the same. If it turns out that I must have a radical prostatectomy, then I'll have to go about it quickly. But I want some other surgeon to perform the operation. I'll need access to medical sources and to the whereabouts of every top urologist in the world. I'll have to discover and see for myself where the most advanced work on cancer is being done. I'll also have to do my book. I'll never be able to pay for this research if I don't, and now, somehow, I feel the strongest urge I've ever known to settle down to the writing of A Bridge Too Far. I can't let cancer kill me until both my knowledge of it and my work on the new book is done. I have to keep going, even if all the odds are against me. Somehow, someway, I will win. I will.

KATHRYN

It was close to 1:00 P.M. on Saturday, July 25, 1970, when Connie came up to the house from our office. For more than

six hours he had been alone with his thoughts and I had felt
a strong reluctance to intrude on him. It was impossible to
guess what his mood might be. If his spirits were low then I
would have to make my own appear far brighter and more
optimistic than indeed they were. If he was as composed as
he had been the previous evening, I, too, must once again
summon courage, even hope. Emotionally I was fluctuating
erratically. All morning I had felt tears welling up unexpectedly as I went through routine chores. Only by seeing Connie when he chose to appear could I be given the cue for my
own reactions in this now haunted world we had suddenly
entered.

Emily and I were having coffee on the terrace when we
heard the outer door of the office slam. Then Connie walked
past the garages, skirting the back entrance of the house, and
up the grassy hill to the big, semicircular terrace where we
sat. Emily and I had stopped all pretense at small talk, our
eyes riveted on Connie's tall figure coming toward us. Whatever I had expected, I was not prepared for the lightness of
his manner or the carefree way in which he greeted us.

"Hello, girls," he called as he approached, "any coffee left
for me?"

He came up the three broad steps to the terrace and sat
down beside his mother, one arm lightly around her shoulders. She reached up and caught his hand.

"To be sure, there is," she said. "I'll go get a cup for you."
Emily's voice was a match for Connie's. With no trace of the
anxiety we had shared all morning, she bounded up and went
into the house. Connie lit a cigarette and gestured beyond
the terrace toward the wide cleared meadow leading down to
a thick forest of trees. "I've got to get that grass mowed down
below," he said to me. "and remind me to get that scrub
brush taken out. It just blurs the view and stunts all the wild
dogwoods." Dumbly I nodded.It was not at all the kind of
talk I had expected.

Emily came back with a tray for Connie and poured his

coffee. "Where are Eldon and the kids?" he asked. I explained. My father had driven Vicki to her usual Saturday riding lesson and Geoff was in his room apparently asleep, for his grandmother and I had been mercifully spared the strident music which emanated with ear-shattering loudness from the expensive speakers Connie had bought him.

"I've got to have a talk with him," Connie said. "He spends too much time in that room. What that young lad needs is fresh air and a little exercise. He's hardly been outdoors since school ended except when a chum with a car comes over."

Geoff's behavior had indeed been erratic. Claiming an inability to sleep, he was keeping late hours in spite of our constant demands that he try to rest. In consequence, he seldom appeared before noon and his breakfasts were haphazard if he had them at all. He had become irritable and rude, sarcastically turning aside even the most innocuous question. More worrisome, he seemed perpetually to display symptoms of an oncoming cold: red eyes, runny nose, a low level of energy. Yet he resisted every attempt to get him to his doctor. He had refused Connie's offer to pay him—over and above his weekly allowance—to work on the lawns or help with the weeding, even though the allowance was usually gone within a day or two of his receiving it. Connie and I were puzzled and angry at the turn his behavior had taken since his arrival home from prep school for the summer holidays. Outwardly, he was observing the rules we had made regarding how late he could be out with friends, our requests to meet the friends, and to know what plans were afoot. But he appeared to seethe at such restrictions. I had tried to dismiss his attitude as a teenage characteristic—a drawing away from parental influence—even as I worried about whether such attitudes were indigenous to all sixteen-year-olds. I had, after all, been an absentee mother in many instances. Perhaps this sea change in his character and behavior were within the norm. But what if they were not? I had spoken to other parents whose concerns did not seem to match my own, and I had read some books and talked to a few professional people I knew. But nothing I had heard or read had helped to diagnose Geoff's actions satisfactorily to me.

Emily did not share our worry. "Didn't I raise five boys myself?" she said. "They go through these stages. Believe me I know. You think, now, you were an angel, Con, but you gave us some anxious moments all the same. Geoff will grow up to be a fine young man and a credit to both of you. You mark my words.

"It's Vicki you've got to watch," Emily told us. "She's going to be a little beauty and you'll have to beat the suitors away. It's amazing," she added softly, "how like Kathleen she is."

Connie's only sister, adored by him and all his brothers, had died tragically in 1958. A Pan Am purser, Kathleen had drowned swimming in the waters of Accra, Ghana. Connie was working on *The Longest Day* then and he had flown to Accra and with Pan Am officials had wrestled through the red tape formalities of that newly emerged nation to claim her body and fly it home to Dublin, where Connie delivered his sister to her mother and brothers. A memorial mass for Kathleen was held in New York shortly after Connie's return from Dublin. The church was filled with people. David Parsons of Pan American explained to me that many of the mourners were crews in New York at the time. "When one of us goes down, it affects us all," he said.

Connie was not present to thank and greet the strangers who had come to the memorial service. He had disappeared as soon as the mass was ended. I found him much later back in the small office we had rented in New York, working intensely on his book. He did not mention Kathleen or his experiences in Ghana for days, but he worked out his grief in dogged hours of labor on the book. His dedication for *The Longest Day* reads "For All the Men of D Day," and once it had carried a second line, "And especially for Kathleen." He deleted that part of the dedication. "She had her private D

Day," he said. "Each of us does. I loved her. Better to let it go at that." The ability to face hard facts squarely without an open show of emotion had always been one of his strongest characteristics. Now, in 1970, as in 1958 when Kathleen died, Connie appeared to be facing his own D Day—or "C Day" as I was to discover he had written in red ink in his diary for Friday, July 24, 1970—with the same decisiveness and tenacity as he had faced Kathleen's.

On that July Saturday after "C Day," sitting on the terrace drinking his coffee, he shared two of his decisions with his mother and me. First, Connie said matter-of-factly, he had reserved a seat for Emily to fly back to Dublin late that same afternoon. Emily and I both began to protest. She was not due to leave for another four days. But Connie was adamant. Second, he told us, he planned to be away himself and needed me close by the phones in the office.

For one frightening moment I thought he had decided to have the radical prostatectomy. "Remember that fishing trip I planned, Katie?" he asked. "Well, I want to get it in and then," he held up his hand with mock solemnity, "I promise I'll get down to work." Nothing Emily or I could say had the slightest effect on his decisions. Emily and I put together a hasty lunch and then went up to pack her suitcases, working around Connie who sat on the bed and regaled her with Irish stories, prompting her to a few of her own. But then, finally, she turned to him. "What about this illness, Con?" she asked. "You've not mentioned one word about it."

"I'm going to work that out."

"How?" Emily and I asked at once.

"Have I ever let either of you down?" We shook our heads. "Well, I won't now," Connie said. "It's going to be all right. I thought you knew, Mother, I'm on a ten percent commission with the Guy Upstairs."

"Don't be blasphemous," Emily scolded, but years seemed to have dropped from her face.

My father and Vicki had lunched out after her riding lesson

and Geoff was then up and about, silent but, thankfully, not at all grim. We spent a pleasant few hours until the car came to take Emily to the airport. The whole family trooped out to see her off, Connie and Geoff carrying her luggage. In her bedroom, checking for last-minute things, Emily suddenly came across and put her hands on my shoulders. "You promise, Kathy, you'll let me know about Con?"

"Of course." I was still puzzled by his attitude and the speed with which he had engineered his plans.

"You know, my dear, I think it's all going to be all right. You'll all be in my prayers continually. And please don't carry on so about the children. You want everything to be too perfect."

"I thought everything was nearly perfect up to now," I told her. Impulsively I threw my arms around my mother-in-law. "Thank you for giving me Connie. If I could raise a child to be a man half as generous and gentle and talented, I could never ask for anything else."

Emily's eyes misted over. "I love him, too," she said, "and I thank God the pair of you found each other."

We went down to the waiting car.

That same evening Connie and I had been invited to a dinner party. The mood he had sustained so long during his mother's presence had dimmed, and since neither of us had slept the previous night, I wanted to telephone our hostess, late as it was, and cancel. Connie wouldn't hear of it. "We carry on as usual," he said, "until we know more about where we're going and why."

"Will you tell me exactly why you sent your mother home today?"

"I don't think I could take it with her here. I don't want to have to pretend and God knows I shouldn't have to here in my own home. She'd be torn apart with worry. Now, at least,

94

I think I've relieved her mind a little. If she stayed on, I might not be able to carry it off. This way is better all around."

We went to the dinner party. I don't remember very much about it. I didn't want to let Connie out of my sight. He was moving among people, pausing occasionally to chat, seemingly enjoying himself as thoroughly as always. And yet, one thing about that Saturday evening, July 25, 1970, stands out clearly in my mind. In our early married days Connie and I had devised a secret signal between us. Whenever he wanted to talk with me privately, to get away from admirers or from critics of his books, to leave someplace early, he would touch his tie. Similarly, I would twist my wedding band. Those little gestures had more than once extracted us from some social or business relationship we chose not to continue at the moment. From across our hostess's room I saw Connie touch his tie and head for an open window away from the other guests. I joined him almost immediately. He was staring out into the night, his face unguarded, shrouded with sorrow. "It's so unreal, Katie," he said. "I can't believe this is happening to me. I really cannot accept it at all. But, yet, I must." He reached out and put his arm around my waist. He smiled, as though we were sharing a secret joke. "I'm going to beat this thing," he told me. "I promise you right here and now that in ten years' time we're going to laugh about the summer of 1970. I won't be beaten. You remember that."

$$\stackrel{=}{=} 10 \stackrel{=}{=}$$

CORNELIUS

Today is Sunday, July 26, 1970. Shortly before noon yesterday, a little more than seventeen hours since the conference with the urologist, I began work on the first tenuous outline of a plan to research this cancer. There are pitifully few guidelines for the victim to follow. You either place yourself in the hands of the first specialist who gives you the news or you strike out to find alternatives to his judgment.

On a yellow legal pad I've put down the decisions that have to be made rather quickly. Number 1 is, of course, the radical prostatectomy. Suppose other doctors support that opinion as the single, universal "cure"? At the moment, Pat Neligan is for a prostatectomy but only if two or three other urologists advise it. If that happens, will I submit to the operation then, believing as I do that it's not the answer? Or is it just one man who's made me so dislike the thought? I honestly don't know. I've got to get facts on similar case histories: men whose age and occupational pressures are not unlike my own; some idea of their productivity after the operation; longevity statistics—how many died of their disease and how soon? And where will I fit into the charts?

The New York urologist says I can live possibly fifteen years barring other illnesses or complications, although his definition of "cure" is five years, cancer-free. He's assuming that the malignancy is confined solely to the prostate. Suppose it isn't? He was wrong on his forecast of the biopsy results. He can very well be wrong about the containment of cancer cells to the prostate. That would considerably shorten my life span. I might have no more than three to three and a half years left. If that.

At this stage, even though I know very little about cancer, I think there is a strong possibility—given the stories I've heard of the hedgehopping nature of the disease—of its recurring someplace else in my body even if a radical prostatectomy was to be performed.

The second item on the list is who to tell and what to tell them. I've got colleagues and publishers in one column, friends in the other. One question applies equally to both: if I tell them, how will they take the news? Suddenly I've become protective of myself and my reputation. The word "cancer" triggers about the same kind of paralyzing fear as leprosy or plague. One might as well write off the victim. He probably can't be counted on in business or as a friend for any length of time.

Colleagues and publishers pose a mammoth problem. The colleagues can put you on the shelf and forget about you. The publishers might very well cancel contracts. Somebody's bound to say, "Well, we really can't ask Ryan to do this article or count on him to finish his book, because the poor bastard's got cancer."

Friends are probably going to react in just about the same way. Which ones do you really know well enough to predict their reactions, now that those reactions are crucial not just to you but to your wife and children? Can you really burden friends with a thing like this? Do you confide in hushed tones, leaving the underlying impression in their minds that you're begging for their continued support and companionship? Do you tell them straight off that you don't want their sympathy, only the continuance of the status quo you had before they knew? And how are they expected to maintain that after you divulge your little secret? People may keep their distance, as if they could catch cancer like a cold.

There are several friends I wanted to talk to, but each time I started to dial a number I stopped. Dr. Theodore Safford, who is a fine physician and one of the best friends I've got in Connecticut, is somebody I'll talk to soon. At the moment I just don't have enough to tell Ted, but it's some comfort to believe that your doctor friends are going to have a different outlook than those in other professions. Like Pat, Ted's friendship won't be changed by the fact that I have cancer. Maybe Mel Thompson, John Tower, and Red Gordon won't regard me as a pariah either. All three live here and Katie and I spend a lot of time with all these people and their wives. Mel, in the chemical business; John, in the pulp and paper industry; and Red, a Pan Am pilot, are all hardheaded realists. I'm gambling that when I can bring myself to tell them, they'll take the news in stride and their wives will be good outlets for Katie's emotions. They'll help her through the rough days I'm fairly sure are bound to come.

The friends I can't talk to just now are the ones I want most to call, but I know them too well. They'd react as I would if I heard such news from one of them. They'd start moving mountains if they thought it would help, and every day there would be a new scheme to bolster Ryan's morale. Pete Kriendler, Bill Hearst, Ben Wright, Ben Grauer, Walter Cronkite, and Joe Ryle in New York are among the oldest and closest friends I've got in this country, along with Herb Caen in San Francisco, Jack Thompson in Chicago, and Bob Considine, wherever he happens to be on a story.

With the exception of Kriendler, I've known the rest of them since the war and we've traveled a lot of country together. They're too close to me, too much a part of my life, and, by God, they'd start meddling with what's left of it if I told them now. I can just see the meetings at "21" to discuss my "complaint," and the suggestions put forth about the best way to defend me against the god-awful thing that has happened. I'll tell them in time, but not yet. If my research bears fruit, I won't have to tell them for a long time.

It's curious what tangents the mind takes in the wake of this kind of bewilderment and shock. Yesterday I called Annie Bardenhagen, my secretary, to tell her about the biopsy finding. Many of the extra burdens this cancer imposes will fall on her because she'll have to carry the office work almost single-handedly until I finish getting the medical opinions I must have in order to decide what to do. Additionally, I needed Anne's good counsel and sensible views. Her phone rang and rang. Then it dawned on me. She and her family are away on vacation. Anne won't be back until August 5. She doesn't even know I've been in hospital.

Throughout yesterday and continuing into this morning there have been numerous telephone calls with Neligan and with Paul Gitlin, my lawyer, the one friend I had to tell. Of the four of us, I would say that Paul and Pat are more shaken at this point than Katie and I. But we have reached some vital decisions. They both agree we should get more opinions, find out all we can about other courses of treatment and where they're located.

Incredible as it may seem, I'm going to start my end of the research by going fishing. The third item on my legal pad, "fishing trip," is the only one that has no question mark. Yet on Friday night, after the urologist's disclosure of his findings, I had absolutely ruled it out of my thoughts. Yesterday morning, Saturday, as I was making the first of these tapes, I made up my mind to go, and today I'm more than ever convinced that I'm right. So tomorrow, Monday, July 27, I won't be shut away in hospital awaiting the surgeon's knife and the end of an active, normal life, the sure end of my sexual potency, and the frightening chance that my mental faculties will never again be acute. I may have to face that in just a few weeks, but for now I want and need the pretense that all is right with my world.

It has been three years since I fished the Alta River, 250 miles north of the Arctic Circle and, to my mind, the greatest salmon stream in the world. It's the most magnificent place I've ever fished. Great stands of pine and birch line the banks and in some places sheer granite cliffs rise into the sky. The water is white and noisy at the rapids, black and quiet in the deep, still pools where the great salmon live. If I should be so unlucky as never to see the Alta again, that is all the more reason why I have to go tomorrow.

When I get to Oslo, the first leg of the journey up to the Alta, I'm going to start checking by phone to find out where the outstanding urologists in Europe are located. If I can get a list or even two or three top names, I can arrange appointments after I get back from the river. Pat is picking up the pathological slides today so that I can take them with me if I decide to see any doctors in Europe. Neligan points out that although he does not question the laboratory report, the difference between inflammation and cancer can be as little as 1 percent on a pathological slide. After all our mental anguish, it would be funny as hell if the hardening in the right lobe is just an infection after all.

But Neligan is not encouraging me to that point of view, and he's already started to track down doctors here in this country. One of the names he's come up with is Dr. Joseph Ward, a friend of Pat's from medical school in Dublin but now in New York. Dr. Ward wants to see me on my return from Norway and he, in turn, has given Neligan another source. Ward suggests I should also see Dr. Willet Whitmore, Chief of Urology at Memorial Sloan-Kettering in New York. So while I'm away Pat will start to set up appointments with these two doctors and I'll try to get information on the European side. We are on the move.

I feel guilty about how this news of cancer appears to affect Gitlin and Neligan. Each telephone call between us reveals an increasing involvement in my situation on the part of them both. There is simply none of the usual banter in our conversations. I'm getting very strong emotional vibrations from Paul, along with protective and practical advice. Pat's attitude is about the same. He said at one point he wished to God he'd never found the small hardening in the prostate. Well, so do I, but I can't have him feeling remorseful about it. We played out a piece of black comedy in which I found myself telling Neligan that, after all, if you've got to get cancer, the prostate is probably one of the best places to have it; and some men live long productive lives without even the knowledge that a small malignant tumor is there. His reaction to my medical "knowledge" was ungracious to say the least, but for the time it took his mind off the fact that he had discovered the lesion.

At this point the only positive action I've taken has been to send Mother home to Dublin. She left for the airport about 4:30 P.M. yesterday. She was confident and relaxed; all traces of the agitation she felt when she first heard the news appeared to have gone. I believe she is now convinced that the specialist was wrong in his diagnosis and even if it should turn out that I have "a spot of difficulty," I'll overcome it. Mother's saints, I expect, will see to that. On the front steps we held each other tightly. She is a woman of great elegance and considerable charm. Katie and I saw her into the car. She smiled out at us, her eyes clear and free of worry. "God will protect you, Con," she said. "You're a young man. Mark my words, all will be well." Then she asked if there was anything she could do for me in Dublin. I told her no. I didn't see what anyone could do. We were talking about two entirely different things because she said, "Well, I may just drop in and ask Mr. Grogan to send you along some samples." Mr. Grogan is a Dublin shirtmaker. We waved until the car had rounded the driveway and was out of sight. I wonder if I'll ever see her again.

There are at least three depressing aspects in a search for opinions about how best to treat this cancer: time, money, and getting to the top men in the field. I know the clock is running but I don't know if time is on my side. The most pressing problem, I think, is whether one has the money for research and consultations. Travel, appointments, tests, are only the beginning. The astronomical figures can surely be expected once you've decided which kind of treatment to undergo. And if I'm overconfident about the time I've got, I could leave Katie and the children penniless—the new book unfinished, the royalties of *The Longest Day* and *The Last Battle* eroded by doctors' fees, hospital costs, and medicines. Have I the right to gamble with their future? It may be totally illogical but I think the answer is yes. If I find the most feasible procedure for my case, I'll hold back time with one hand and finish the book with the other. Somehow.

The most urgent aspect of my decision is to locate the top urologists wherever they're to be found. I have to do this without prolonged expenditures of either time or money and in this, I believe, my career becomes of utmost importance. I've traveled around the world for twenty years researching, interviewing, reporting. I do these jobs as well as anyone around. But I never thought I'd put these skills to use for myself alone. Ryan researching Ryan's cancer is a project so strange that I am immediately aware of the danger of one pitfall: I am going to have to maintain maximum objectivity and a detachment I have never felt about my books.

This battle I'm about to research didn't take place twenty-five years ago. There's no time to read background and assemble statistics over a period of years. This battle is immediate. I'm squarely in the middle of it and my knowledge of the enemy's strength and probable movements is, as of this moment, pathetically slim.

Part Two
THE PLAN
August–October 1970

÷ 1 ÷

Dear Doctor:

The bearer of this letter, Mr. Cornelius Ryan, was diagnosed as having Adenocarcinoma of the Prostate, following the performance of a Silverman Needle Biopsy . . . of the base of the right lobe of the prostate on July 23rd, 1970.

On digital examination there is no nodularity of the prostate . . . I referred Mr. Ryan [to a urologist originally] because I noted a small firm hard area in the base of the right lobe. Intravenous pyelography and cystoscopy performed concomitantly with the needle biopsy were normal . . . Reports of blood studies performed are enclosed. Mr. Ryan did not have a metastatic series performed. The report of the pathological specimen is enclosed herewith and Mr. Ryan has the actual slide specimens with him.

Mr. Ryan is referred to you for consultation and opinion as to the best method of treatment of this prostatic malignancy in this fifty-year-old otherwise healthy male.

Both Mr. and Mrs. Ryan are aware of the diagnosis and have discussed openly with me . . . the various modalities of therapy . . . your considered opinion expressed freely to Mr. and Mrs. Ryan as to the best form of treatment, the anticipated complications, prognosis, etc. is requested. Mr. Ryan must then decide his course of action.

With my grateful thanks for your help in this unfortunate situation.

Very truly yours,

Patrick Neligan, M.D.

KATHRYN

On August 3, Connie returned from Europe. He had been gone exactly a week. Bad weather at the Alta River forced him to cut short his salmon fishing and, as a result, he was able to spend several days telephoning cancer research centers whose names he and Pat had hurriedly collected before his departure. Pat, who had begun his medical practice in Great Britain, came up with some European sources, and Connie found still more by employing a method he often used to save himself footwork on a story. He telephoned several European cities and simply asked the operator in each place to check the directory—in this instance for a listing of cancer research institutes and libraries.

Back from the salmon stream, he shut himself into a hotel room in Oslo and, working from the list he and Pat had compiled, he telephoned one center after another. He was fortunate in finding English-speaking directors, technicians, or doctors at almost every place. Identifying himself as a freelance writer who planned to submit an article on cancer to British journals, he asked a variety of questions about the work being done at each institute. A few of them, he learned, were engaged solely in research. Some were renowned cancer libraries. And still others were prestigious centers for both research and treatment. In spite of the work being done at each institution, at all of them Connie asked one question that was always the same. It was his key query: "Where (or where else) in your opinion is the most advanced work on prostatic cancer being done and by whom?" As he had done in previous research, Connie was looking for a kind of endorsement: a name backed up by two or three other sources. He got far more than he expected.

To his astonishment, the names of two institutes and two specialists were mentioned by six of the eleven people he talked with. Nearly 55 percent of the group—far more than he had hoped for—had, in part, given the same answers to that question. It seemed almost too good to be true, he told me later, for the names the majority of the European experts ranked high on their recommendations were those of two U.S. hospitals and doctors. They were: Memorial Sloan-Kettering Cancer Center, New York City, Dr. Willet F. Whitmore, Jr., Chief, Urologic Service; and Brady Urological Institute, Johns Hopkins Hospital, Baltimore, Dr. Hugh J. Jewett. Connie could not have been more impressed by his findings. As he put it, "I had to go to Europe to find that two of the top experts are in my own backyard."

Awaiting him at home was a telephoned message to Pat's letter. Dr. Ward, the urologist who had gone to medical school with Pat in Dublin, called Dr. Neligan on the afternoon of the third, a few hours before Connie got back. Pat arranged an appointment for Connie and me to see Dr. Ward in New York, Wednesday, August 5, at 2:00 P.M. Our mutual journey to find out all we could about cancer was about to begin, even as the first of Connie's trips was ending.

He arrived home in the late evening of the third. The driver of the long black limousine Connie used in those days for airport trips sounded two beeps on the horn, our family's signal that Connie was either departing or coming back. Immediately I threw on all the outdoor light switches and Geoff and Vicki raced out the front door and down the steps to the car.

I watched through the screen door as our children swirled around their father, interrupting each other to ask him how big the salmon were and how many did he kill and how was the trip. I would have liked to have raced down to him myself but I stayed put. Sometimes one memorizes a scene without knowing why, but I knew too well the reason I wanted to fix that homecoming in my mind. Even then I was beginning to store up memories against the time when there might be no others.

The spacious interior of the car was softly lit, the children having opened every door, and silhouetted against the light was Connie, one arm draped languidly on the car roof. He was directing the removal of his luggage, playing his customary game with Geoff and Vicki, who had to guess which of his suitcases held our gifts (there was never a time he came home without some), and listening while the children tried to decide which bag should be carried up to the house with care.

They knew the game as well as he did. Every suitcase held at least one gift for someone, but Connie, pretending they were all in a single bag, used the ruse as a good way of getting his luggage quickly up to the house. Only the fishing gear was Connie's alone to carry. I watched as he reached into the car and picked up the big aluminum tube that held his rods. He placed it carefully against the car while he went back to the trunk to help the driver take out the leather bag that stored his tackle, reels and hand-tied salmon flies. His voice, floating up to me as he chatted with the driver, was light and cheerful, and I could hear snatches of a conversation that told me two kindred souls were ending a mutually agreeable talk about fishing. The driver seemed to be as enthusiastic about the sport as Connie was.

Geoff came up the steps with a suitcase and I held open the door for him. Passing me, he said quietly, "Mom, he seems fine." It was the first time Geoff had referred to Connie's illness since that night, ten days before, when we had gotten the news of it ourselves and I had told that news to Geoff. I was surprised and touched by his remark.

Upstairs in our bedroom the children had already begun to open suitcases and hunt out presents. I stayed in the foyer while Connie said good night to the driver. Then he bounded up the outside steps and I rushed down to meet him. He threw his arms around me.

"Gosh, I've missed you, Katie," he said.

"And I've missed you," I told him. "You'll never know how much."

We'd been apart for longer times but none of those had ever seemed to drag interminably.

Inside our house Connie put his hands on my shoulders and held me away from him.

"Let me look at you," he said.

That, too, was a part of his "coming home" procedure, but the familiar words had taken on new meaning for us both. We studied each other. Our eyes met and held steadily, and I remember Connie smiled.

In the next instant he hugged me tight. With his mouth to my ear, he whispered, "Jackpot!"

"What?"

"I hit the jackpot. Where would you guess the top men are?"

And then he told me everything.

$$= 2 =$$

CORNELIUS

I came back from Norway on August 3 to learn that Neligan had set up the first of our consultations—with Dr. Joseph Ward in New York. On Wednesday, the fifth, Kathryn and I drove in to see him. I found Dr. Ward charming, elegant, very Irish, and very efficient. He sent me for laboratory work and he gave me a thorough examination.

At the end of it, I joined Katie in his consulting room. Here was no austere, forbidding setting. The office was as pleasant and as comfortable as the man who occupied it. Dr. Ward postponed getting to the reason for my visit until I was seated and we had exchanged some small talk. Then, as gently as is probably possible under such circumstances, he gave us unsettling news. Not only did he confirm the first urologist's diagnosis of cancer, as did Dr. Gaetz, a pathologist at St. Luke's Hospital with which Dr. Ward is associated, but Ward's assessment of my problem carries far more serious overtones. He believes the cancer is not just confined to the prostate. it may well have spread outside the gland. In a letter to Neligan* which he dictated, he wrote:

On examination, I think that the hard area on the right lobe of the prostate is very close to the prostatic capsule and, in fact, I have a suspicion it may have gone outside the capsule on the right side.

The hardening, he told Kathryn and me, appears to be extending rather high up from the right base and may also be either close to, or involving, the seminal vesicle on that side.

I experienced another one of those moments of sheer terror. This news not only sounded more serious than I had been prepared to hear but the medical terms made it impossible to understand just how serious it was.

Prostatic capsule. Seminal vesicle. These were words that I had never heard before or, if I ever had, they had meant nothing. They seemed to have importance now and I wanted to find out just how great that importance was.

This urologist, sympathetic and forthright, did not object to my questions. Dr. Ward sketched the prostate for Kathryn

---

* Both doctors have kindly given their permission to use their correspondence, as have the other specialists named throughout the book.

and me, talking as he drew. In size and shape, the gland is a lot like a chestnut, and weighs about twenty grams. It rests on part of the rectum, which is why its contours can be examined by gloved finger. Its base, strange as it seems, is up, not down—just below the neck of the bladder. The front surface is slightly convex. The entire gland is enclosed by a thin, firm, fibrous covering—the prostatic capsule. And it is through that microscopically narrow coating that Ward believes the cancer may have penetrated.

I interrupted the doctor's explanation. It was a very hard question for me to ask but if the thing was growing fast, I wanted to know if I had wasted precious time during the past eight days in Europe.

"Could this lesion have gone outside the capsule since the diagnosis thirteen days ago?" I asked.

Ward's eyes were sympathetic. "I didn't do the original examination or the biopsy, Mr. Ryan," he said, "so I don't know what I might have added at that time. All I can really tell you is what I suspect as of this moment."

"But do you think it could have spread that much since the biopsy was done?"

Very quietly he said, "I think it was already in the area we're talking about. As I said, I can't be certain it has invaded the capsule or gone beyond it. I just have very strong feelings that this is so."

We looked at each other for a minute and then he proceeded with his drawing, holding it up and marking in lines so that Kathryn and I could see the picture taking place as he worked.

He was drawing the seminal vesicles. They are two rather rounded or bumpy membranous pouches holding a fluid that forms part of the semen. They snake, right and left, from the base of the bladder to the rectum. Each vesicle has an elongated, slightly pyramidal shape. The broad end is backward, behind the bladder, and the pointed end juts forward into the prostate, where each of these pouches joins with a corresponding excretory duct of the testes to form the ejaculatory duct.

In the completed sketch the prostate resembled a tiny, cuplike vase set under the base of the bladder. The excretory ducts of the testes look like two fern fronds rising right and left from the prostate into the bladder base, while the seminal vesicles, to either side of the fronds, are somewhat twisty and branchlike. The ureters (the tubes that carry urine from the kidneys to the bladder) are to the outside of the seminal vesicles. They all come together in the prostate—right ureter and right seminal vesicle run into the right of the prostate base, the corresponding left ureter and seminal vesicle disappear into the prostate on the left.

Pointing to the right seminal vesicle, I asked Dr. Ward the significance of his feeling that the lesion might be close to or involved with that little pouch or sac. He was silent for a moment. Then he said:

"Dr. Neligan has asked me to speak frankly with you both. I want to do that so I have to say that our indication for a radical prostatectomy is one where there is a solitary nodule which a surgeon has an excellent chance of removing in toto. In your case, Mr. Ryan, I suspect that the hardening has probably extended beyond the confines of the prostatic capsule and may be involving the right vesicle." He paused and looked directly at me. "If that is so and the functions of the vesicle are being invaded, in my opinion a radical prostatectomy would not be justified."

My feelings were mixed then, and now, twenty-four hours later, still are. The first urologist never suggested that the firm area or hardening might be extensive. But Dr. Ward believes that not only its position but its probable involvement outside the prostate would make a prostatectomy useless. I keep thinking about what I was told of the aftermath of a prostatectomy—the bladder spasms, the postoperative weakness, the chance of a lessening of my mental faculties, sexual impotence, the incontinence that would undoubtedly occur. My God! I would have had to suffer all that—for nothing!

I simply cannot believe that this invasion of the seminal vesicle, this new growth, has come about in just fourteen days, between July 23 and yesterday, August 5.

Suppose that should be the case. Dr. Ward's suggestion for the measures I could take now is interesting. He believes that I am a good candidate for hormone therapy. That opinion, too, is directly contrary to that of the first doctor who put the notion aside like so much fog—a smoke screen employed by his "opponents" to mask the real "cure." Yet Dr. Ward tells me that great advances have been made in treatment by hormones. Since testosterone, the male hormone, stimulates the prostate, estrogen, the female hormone, can shrink the gland and inhibit its activity. Spread might be checked for quite a long time. Additionally, Ward says that work is being done to match the correct dosage of female hormones to the individual involved, so that not only are the manufacture of male hormones stopped but the feminine-like changes to the body that could occur due to injections of female hormones are minimized.

Well, that all sounds iffy and not a very pleasing prospect— I'm damned if I want to develop a bosom—but it would be far easier to bear than living with the knowledge that one had submitted to a prostatectomy that should never have been done.

At one point in our conversation, Dr. Ward leaned across the desk to me and said, "If you were my own brother, given these circumstances, hormone therapy is what I'd advise for the present time. If needed, you could go on to other treatment later. But whatever you decide, I honestly believe a radical prostatectomy is useless in your case."

I now have two opinions and two totally opposite points of view. Dr. Ward's suggestion is a little more intricate, or sophisticated if you will, involving perhaps other modes of treatment as time goes on. But, of course, one wants to get this thing over and done with. One wants, most of all, to forget about it, to have it all in the past. But obviously, if Ward is right, a prostatectomy, with all the drastic effects to one's psyche that it conjures up, cannot be just relegated to the back of the mind once it is performed. Too many physical and emotional problems could surface as a result of the operation, and if it proved not to be the "cure," one would be approaching stopgap treatments, as maimed in mind as in body.

I was aware of all these thoughts even as I said to Dr. Ward, "I think I've got to push further. Is there anyone else you think I should see?" I did not mention the names I had heard about in Europe.

Ward did not even hesitate. "Absolutely," he said with conviction. "I definitely think you should get other opinions. I have two men in mind whom I believe it important for you to contact." He began to scribble rapidly on a prescription pad.

"The first," he said, "is Dr. Hugh Jewett at Johns Hopkins in Baltimore. He is probably the world's greatest authority on the radical perineal prostatectomy. I worked with him for one year and I can in all honesty advise that you consult him. I have told you that I would not operate, but I value Dr. Jewett's opinion.

"The other man is here in the city and you should see him as well. Dr. Willet Whitmore at Memorial. Don't make up your mind about anything until you consult these men and please let me know whatever I can do to help."

I felt Katie's touch on my arm and turned to her.

"Jackpot!" she whispered.

She was right. Out of all the specialists he might have named, Dr. Ward had picked the two men whose names I had heard over and over again in Europe. The number of cancer experts who had given me those names had risen now to seven out of twelve. The percentage rate had jumped a good four points.

Kathryn and I left Dr. Ward's office enlightened and perhaps even a little optimistic. With hormones and whatever other treatment might become necessary to supplement them, maybe I had a fighting chance. I would be impotent, of course, and the side effects of female hormones did not exactly appeal to me. Still, I thought we had been given a brighter picture.

I did not tell Kathy the agonies of doubt I had suffered during my week in Europe. I had had almost no sleep, other than a couple of restless hours each night. I'd get into bed and stare sightlessly into the dark until the fears became too great to bear, and then I'd turn on the light, smoke a cigarette, and pace the floor. I am finding that by day I can control the fear but, try as I will, I dread the coming of dusk. It brings terrors that are hard to submerge or contemplate rationally. Keeping a light on helps a little—it seems to hold the demons at bay and makes them less menacing—but none of the books or research I have at hand are any use of all. I simply cannot remember what I read. My mind is far from statistics and history. It is on pain and death.

After our visit to Ward we talked a little about it on our way to see Michael Korda, editor in chief of Simon & Schuster, the company that publishes my books in the United States. I had put Michael off too long. He was anxious to know how the book was coming along, eager to have the first pages in hand. How could I tell him there was nothing to show? I know I must do the book but, as time goes by without some copy, Michael is bound to wonder why. Yesterday, as Katie carefully avoided looking at me, I told Michael the book was coming along beautifully; I just wasn't ready to show it to anyone yet.

I don't know how I managed it, but I drew on my original outline for the book, embellishing it with dramatic vignettes of interviews I'd done in England and Holland, and Kathryn matched my stories with some of her own, drawn from her memory of the long-finished American files. I think Michael was impressed. I hope he was. We were practically writing the book right there in his office.

I felt charged up as I talked. Excited. It was the first time in months I hadn't thought solely about myself and my physical problems. Like a cathartic, talk of *A Bridge Too Far* was erasing the gloom and despair. I suddenly began to get the feeling that it can continue to do so.

After our session with Michael, we had a drink with my lawyer, Paul Gitlin, and brought him up-to-date. Then we drove home to discover that Pat, as a result of my briefing to him about the Norway trip, had obtained an appointment for us with Dr. Willet Whitmore at 1:00 P.M. on Wednesday, August 12. I told Pat everything about my conversation with Dr. Ward, including the fact that Ward would be sending Pat a letter on his findings, the contents of which I knew in part.

Today, Thursday, August 6, Pat and I had a longer talk about Ward's opinion. Pat, at this point, is still holding to the view that a prostatectomy may still be the right course of action. He, Katie, and I are all a little confused because we now have gone from one urologist to a second. The first has said, "Get the prostate out," while the second says, "There is no justifiable reason to take it out. Think about having hormone treatments."

What I am thinking about is that Pat has now set up an appointment with one of the two men I am most anxious to see, and now I want to get in touch with the other one.

Just a few minutes ago I telephoned the Brady Institute at Johns Hopkins and asked to speak with Dr. Hugh Jewett. I was put onto a man named Lanahan who asked me a few pertinent questions. I answered as best I could and Lanahan has given me an appointment with Dr. Jewett for September

1 at 11:00 A.M. Even if the thing is growing, I don't know
what else I can do for now. Except wait.

Pat just called back and I gave him the news about the
Jewett appointment. He has just told Dr. Theodore Safford
about the cancer. I had wanted to tell Ted myself before I
left for Norway, but all the news was so depressing that I
hesitated to make the call, even though Ted is a good friend.
I'm glad Pat made it for me. Ted is close to me and, like Pat,
such an involved and dedicated doctor that I want him apprised of our findings as they happen. He is also Katie's
doctor and looks after the children as well, so it is a great
comfort to me that he will perhaps be able to help them in
times when I cannot.

Just a minute ago the phone rang again and it was Jean
Safford, Ted's wife, on the other end. Jean is one of my favorite people, too, a sturdy-minded, practical woman. She can
sound brusque but she didn't just now. In the most common-
sense call I've had, she asked, "Connie, how are you?" and I
replied inanely, as one always does, "Fine." There was a
pause and then Jeannie said, "Good for you, lovie. May I
speak to Kathy?" I switched on the intercom and got Katie up
at the house. The girls are talking now. That takes a load off
my mind. Is there anything better than good friends?

⹀ 3 ⹀

IT IS LATE SATURDAY afternoon, August 8. We have just gone
through such an incredible experience that I want to get it on
tape as quickly as I can. Katie has gone up to the house to do

some typing (she is working on a book, entirely on her own, and independent of *Bridge*. Thank God one of us is working). I think she is under the impression that I am in the office beginning, at last, to plot out the salient parts we will need as guidelines for *Bridge*. I will begin to do that soon because I must, but today I want to record the events of this afternoon while they are still fresh in my mind. Because I have learned a very important lesson.

Up to today the list of friends and family who know about my illness totaled eight: Pat and Vera Neligan, Kathy's father and my mother, Paul and Zelda Gitlin, and Ted and Jean Safford.*

The Neligans, the Saffords, and the Gitlins are so close to being family that I know my secret is safe with them. We have two other friends almost, I thought, like family, too, whom we have known for many years. We have been the recipients of their hospitality in their handsome Westchester County, New York, house far more than they have come to us, and we often have felt guilty about that except that we entertain rather informally when we are working—while their dinners and lunches are invariably two-to four-course repasts with all the stops pulled out. Often they have a mix of people of varying interests and occupations in their home.

Today only Kathy and I were asked for lunch. I don't know what possessed me to tell them what has been happening in our lives. Perhaps I felt I owed some explanation for the fact that we have been out of touch for several weeks. Katie has been avoiding social contacts. Her voice and her face are nearly always dead giveaways to whatever emotion she is feeling, and she has not trusted herself to see or to speak to many people outside those who know about my problem.

So we had not seen these friends in days, and when the invitation to lunch was tendered while I was in Europe, Katie accepted. She couldn't think of a reason not to and she did

---

* I had not yet told Connie that Geoff knew as well.

not want to be caught up in a lame excuse. Just shortly after lunch I caught Katie's eye and indicated I was going to tell our friends of the turmoil we are passing through. Kathryn half shook her head and then nodded her agreement as though to say, "If that is what you want."

We left the table and went outside to a screened porch which overlooks a beautiful swimming pool and animal statuary set like live things in high meadowlands beyond. It's been warm all day but crisp, too, with no humidity, and the four of us sat in companionable silence for a few minutes.

Then I said, "We've had a rough time these past two and a half weeks and a lot of problems going back to April."

Our friends looked uneasy and worried, as if I might be going to announce that the problems were between Kathryn and me.

"It's not a domestic matter," I told them, "although in time it's bound to occupy more and more of our attention at home." I hesitated and then plunged in. "The fact is," I said, "I've got cancer."

I know I didn't imagine the sudden change in atmosphere. I sensed that Katie noticed it as well. It was as though I had, in an instant, become a totally different person in our friends' view. I felt as though I had committed some unpardonable gaffe, some serious breach of social etiquette. They averted their eyes. There was silence and then they embarrassedly expressed regrets. I had become—apparently all in an instant —what from the first I had feared I might become in the eyes of some people when the word "cancer" was mentioned: a pariah, set outside the mainstream of life. Both husband and wife seemed appalled. I felt a gulf between us which might never be forded. It grew wider with each second.

Finally, our host spoke. "Jessica, tell Connie about your sister."

She was silent so long that Kathy asked, "What about your sister, Jessica?"

"Charlene's the odd one in my family," Jessica told us

curtly, her eyes, I thought, sliding away from mine. In all our years of friendship, I had never heard Jessica mention a sister named Charlene. "Rupert and I haven't seen her in years. She can be terribly difficult." Her hands sketched a square in the air. "She has cancer, too."

I was beginning to feel angry. Her manner of looking (or not looking) at me, her tone of voice, the square drawn in the air, were unsettling. "Well, if she's got cancer, that's probably why she's odd," I said smarting from the hurt that I was feeling.

"Oh, no. She's always been that, even before our family left England to come here," Jessica said. "She's had cancer for about fifteen years. She was odd long before that. Of course we haven't seen her in all that time and rarely before. No more than necessary. But we do hear from her rather often. I'm wondering if I can lay my hands on one of her letters." Why, I wondered, given her assessment of her own sister, did she bother? However, she got up immediately and went into the house.

I turned to Rupert. "Where is Charlene's cancer?"

"I'm not really sure I know, old boy. But I think you'll be interested in what she's done about it. Her letters to Jessica are sure to have some mention of it. That's really all she ever writes about." Rupert paused. "I will give her credit for one thing," he said. "She didn't waste time on these cancer doctors. She found a way to control her disease and keep it at bay. I'm sure that's why Jessica wants to get one of her letters."

One can know a couple for years and suddenly find them strangers. Every instinct told me to get out of there and go home. My news had made a rupture in our relationship that, I felt certain, would never be repaired. I felt vulnerable, exposed, and very surprised at the turn our conversation was taking. Our friendship has stood the test of time for over fifteen years, although politically and in other matters we have been often at opposite ends of the pole. Still, always before, we have, all four, respected one another's opinions, and our different points of view have made for good conversation. Now, I think that has ended for all time.

Jessica returned to the porch bearing a bulky envelope laden with stamps. She took her chair again. "Charlene has been living in the Southwest for many years now," she began. "About 1955, around the time we first met you when we all lived in New York, a doctor in Austin told her she had cancer. Almost the only thing Charlene has in common with the rest of the family is a distrust of doctors. Only proper foods, vitamins, sleep, and exercise, plus weaning oneself from poisons or chemicals that harm the body's system"—she stared at my lighted cigarette—"can eliminate the need of doctors."

"Even if one breaks a hip?" Katie inquired with false innocence.

Jessica stared her down. "I didn't say they weren't useful for some things, dear," she said. "Anyway, I gather the outlook for my sister was rather appalling. But about fourteen years ago Charlene began to pull herself together and she went onto a diet of natural foods and vitamins. They helped her tremendously. Certainly her strength came back. And then, a few years later, she heard of a place in Tijuana where a *real* cancer cure existed. The cure is called Laetrile and, taken by injection and supplemented by a nourishing diet and vitamins, it can work miracles. Charlene goes regularly to Mexico and she is cancer-free as a result of this incredible discovery."

"But what is it, this Laetrile?" my wife asked.

"Crushed almond pits and cherry laurel leaves. Apricot pits, too, I believe."

I was beginning to feel not only angry but ill.

Jessica took no notice. "You can see that the medical profession is not only far behind the times but jealous of any cures they do not discover by themselves."

"Can't Charlene get this medication in the States?" Kathy asked.

"No, dear. Obviously the cancer societies and Drug Administration are against anything they haven't discovered or promoted."

"Perhaps they have, and found this substance useless," I ventured.

"Nonsense. These agencies are all aligned together and, of course, it's the poor public who suffer from their sins of omission," Rupert said.

This was definitely one argument I didn't want to pursue. From the outset, ever since I made the mistake of telling them what I had, I knew cancer was one topic that I would never again bring up in front of them.

Kathryn obviously wasn't letting up. "Where was Charlene's cancer?" she asked.

"Does it matter?" Jessica said. "She's been cancer-free now for years and she believes she'll stay that way as long as she takes the Laetrile injections in Mexico and sticks to her diet.

"Kathy," Jessica went on, "I want you to copy her diet down. I'll read off the important things." She gave Katie Charlene's large envelope to write on.

"Now," she said, settling her eyeglasses, "no salt and no products containing salt. No smoked meats, pork products— that includes bacon. Also only a quarter pound of meat per day. Even less would be preferable."

Jessica looked up from the list. "Did you know, Connie, that the reason the mortality rate worldwide is greater for men than for women is because men eat more meat?"

"Tell him about Eskimos too, dear," Rupert said.

Before Jessica could continue, he went on to tell me about them himself. "They drink a cleansing soup made from the bloods of animals and mixed with the stomach and intestinal contents as well. They're hardly ever ill, you know. Very hardy people, Eskimos."

"Rupert's right," Jessica told us. "Now, dear," to Kathy, "no food in cans, concentrated milk, and absolutely no com-

mercial breakfast cereals. But you can have homemade oat-
meal, brown rice, pea pods, rare beef, or lamb only if you
must have meat daily. And, of course, fresh fruits and vegetables—but no sauces on anything, ever. And no foods like
corn, mushrooms, tomatoes, cranberries, or bananas."

Jessica has always set a good table but I have always found
the lamb and beef too rare, the food overly bland. I glanced
at Katie dutifully writing away. I wondered if she planned to
retire her Cordon Bleu apron.

Jessica had one more piece of news for me. If I can't get to
Mexico right away, although she strongly urges it, I might
write immediately to a Dr. Josef Issels, head of the Ringberg
Clinic in the Bavarian town of Rottach-Egern. He, she tells
me, also believes that proper diet and "whole body therapy"
can help people "like me." It seems the doctor applied a
poultice of cabbage leaves to a terminal cancer patient on the
theory, as nearly as I could judge, that it couldn't hurt and
might help psychologically. "He is said to instill people with
the will to live," Jessica said.

"I've got the will to live, Jessica," I told her. "More so than
you can guess."

"Do you still have your tonsils?" she asked me.

Startled, I said that I did.

Jessica shook her head. "Get them out. Dr. Issels believes
teeth and tonsils are a constant source of infection."

Today is the first time in weeks that I have seen my wife
want to laugh and, had we been alone at that moment, the
release for us both would have been instantaneous.

"Get your teeth out, too, CJ," Katie said. "You can drink
the Eskimo soup without them and when your gums get
harder you can crush pea pods by yourself."

I did laugh and Katie started to giggle. Our well-meaning
friends permitted themselves the semblance of ghostly
smiles.

To stop what could have been a dangerous outlet for our
pent-up emotions and to get back to the point, I asked Jessica,

since Rupert didn't know and Kathy hadn't discovered, just how and where Charlene's cancer had been detected those fifteen years ago.

"She had a lump in her breast and this doctor she saw in Austin wanted to do a biopsy. Charlene wouldn't hear of it; quite right as it turned out. Laetrile and her sensible diet dissolved the lump. She's had a few more tumors since that time but she knows now how they must be treated."

"Did it ever occur to you, Jessica, that maybe she never had cancer that first time? And couldn't she have benign cysts now?"

"But of course not, dear. She knew what she had and has. And so do her nutritional experts and the Laetrile people."

It was time for us to go. It is a good hour's drive from their house to Ridgefield. Jessica and Rupert walked us to the car. "Well, you've got a lot to think about, old boy," Rupert said. "Let us know how we can help."

Jessica spoke up quickly. "Darling, that's up to Connie. Only he can help himself. He's just got to keep away from all these doctors. The fees alone must be appalling."

We thanked them for the lunch.

"Glad you could come, dears," Jessica said. "We must do it again sometime."

I don't know if we ever will. What have we possibly got to talk about?

= 4 =

TUESDAY, AUGUST 11, 1970.

Ever since our luncheon with Jessica and Rupert I have been overwhelmed with regret for having brought up the subject of cancer with them. Yet there comes a time when the burden of worry is so great that one feels the greatest compulsion to pass it along to others in the hope that, by doing so, it will somehow lessen one's own load. This attitude is most unkind to others.

Outside of Mother, who I wish with all my heart had not been here during those first crucial hours after I got the news, I do not intend to tell anyone in Ireland. I hope I have convinced Mother that all will be well and that she can have so free a mind about me that she will not discuss the little she knows with her other sons. My brothers are the last people whom I want to know about my condition. With the Irish mysticism which so often goes hand in hand with despair, they would surely descend into depression, start burning candles, and holding vigils for me. I prefer to save all that until later.

My brothers are often overly dependent on me. They see me as the problem solver, the moneyman to underwrite their ambitions, just as they did when they were children. Now, they want my judgment and seek my advice though they have families of their own and I am an ocean away from them. They have never been able to understand—with the lone exception of my brother Joe, the second eldest, who does try to understand me—that my heart, my allegiance, and my love are now with a different family, my own Katie, Geoff, and Vicki. Because of worry for them I have not been sleeping; I cannot concentrate. Yet, somehow, I must. *Bridge* has to be written. My children and Kathy have got to be cared for. To think of them alone without me is the fear that grips me through the nights.

The thought of never seeing my children grow up haunts me more than anything. Not to watch them stretch, mature, expand, strike out on their own, is difficult to face.

I think of Vicki, and the men who will someday cluster about her. I don't think I am jealous, but I am certainly protective. I think of the wedding I will undoubtedly miss—that time, perhaps not too far distant, when *I* should be walking with her up an aisle of a church, her hair spun silver, her decorum gentle, her beauty incredible. I dislike the bridegroom, unfairly, because right now she belongs to me and he will undoubtedly wed her in a time and place I can't inhabit. This stranger who is bound to come along—will he ever really know Victoria? Can he match a father's love, provide a father's protection, encourage her ambitions? There is a quality in Victoria, as positive as her name, and so far I think I have been able to preserve that specialness, to encourage disagreement (unless it is with me), and to make her think and feel and work for breakthroughs as I worked so many years ago.

And there is Geoff, my only son. He is too introverted and he has reached the age where family count for less than friends. We should still count for something, but at least I know some reasons for his resentment toward his mother and me. I've been out of touch with him. So has Katie. He's been away in school and when we get together that time is always a private donnybrook. I've seen him unable to eat a dinner because of scoldings. Katie and I have always been so busy in the office that we expect each child to exhibit an adult approach to work and play. Sometimes I think we've blotted up the kindness and the love he had to give with command after command and rule after rule. But he has paid us back for that and does it even now. I cannot find it in my heart to blame him. The blame is mine and Kathryn's.

Geoff wasn't always sullen and withdrawn. When he was four or five there was a constant happiness caught often by my camera, a joy of life and love of people. Did we stamp it out? Did I try too hard to make him a fisherman, a hunter, an athlete? Did Kathryn try too hard to make him a scholar? We wanted only the best for him but on *our* terms; it was always *our* view of what was best. When he tried and failed to manage a task we'd set, we'd put him over the jumps again. Is it any wonder we find him, now just past seventeen, sullen and antagonistic?

I love the boy. I loved him on the day he was born and I came into hospital to find him already a little person, squawking his way into life. I loved him this August 2 when he turned seventeen and I, as usual, was away. If it hadn't been for the calls I wanted to make, I would have taken him with me to the Alta where we might have found some common ground for talk.

Today, we've had a talk, for all the good it's done either of us. He is as unyielding as a boulder. His eyes blaze with an emotion very close to contempt. He worries me. I am concerned about his future. I don't know if I can protect him from himself and I don't think he gives a damn one way or the other.

I decided to tell Geoff this afternoon what is wrong with me and what I am trying to do about it. As it turns out, Kathryn had already told him. I wish she had left that to me. He must have wondered why I've kept him in the dark about it, shutting myself away, taking off on trips, barely taking notice of him and his sister.

An hour ago I called him on the intercom to his room and got a blast of rock music. It took full volume on the intercom and several shouts before he heard me.

He came down to the office, looking sleepy, unkempt, dressed in today's 80-degree heat in a long woolen shirt and a pair of jeans so frayed that he steps on the long strings of fiber that hang down from his pants.

Seeing him this way, my own tensions and worries accelerate.

He slouched down in a big chair across the room. "Come on over here where we can talk." I pointed to the leather chair beside my desk. Reluctantly, he came.

"Geoffie, I want to tell you about something. I've not been feeling too good lately, still don't, but we haven't had a good man-to-man chat in a while and this seems as good a time as any."

He fiddled with the welting on the chair.

"Please give me your attention," I told him. "This is important to all of us."

He stopped plucking at the chair and stared at me. The boy does not look well. His color is off, much too pale for summer. His eyes are red-rimmed and he sniffles. I gave him my handkerchief.

"Blow your nose," I said. "Have you got a cold or something?"

"I haven't got a cold," Geoff said. "Or something."

"Look, Geoff, can we have a talk or can't we?"

"Sure," Geoff said. "Our 'talks' are when you lecture and I listen." He leaned forward. "Go on," he said. "Lecture! That's the only kind of talk you know."

"Stop baiting me, Geoff." I put my head in my hands, breathed deeply. "Look," I said, "I'm going through a rather rough time just now. I don't mean to lecture all the time. I'd much rather talk *with* you, not *at* you." I put out my hand. "Let's get along. O.K., Big G?" That was a name my friend, the British actor Kenny More, had given Geoff some ten years earlier.

He shook my hand. "O.K." But he was wary.

I lit a cigarette and settled back in my chair. "I've been under the weather physically for several months now and I didn't know why. It's caused me a lot of anxiety and that, in turn, has made me sometimes irritable with you and Vicki. Your mother has had to bear the worst of my worries. She still does, and she'll have to keep on bearing them. I want you to help her all you can by not worrying her, by knuckling down to school—your grades are nothing to write home about. I'm tired of spending money every summer to tutor you in math when you could do the work by paying attention in your classes. You don't go to the cheapest prep school in the world. You add the cost of tuition, room and board and then tack on this tutoring every summer and you begin to get some idea of what it's costing for you to get an education."

Geoff stared at me. "What else did you want to tell me?"

"That the docs say I've got cancer."

He began to pluck at the frayed legs of his jeans. "Mother told me."

That was news to me. "She did? When?"

"The night you found out. She told me then."

I was surprised and a little angry. "I didn't know. You must have thought I was a real jerk not to mention it."

"No," Geoff said, "I never thought you were a jerk."

"Well, all I can tell you is that I'm trying my best to find out everything I can about this disease. I'm not going to be beaten by it. This family isn't going to be beaten by anything."

"I know," Geoff said wearily, "I've heard that all my life."

"Don't you agree?" I asked.

"It's O.K. for you, I guess," he said. "The old unbeatable attitude."

"What about you?"

He shrugged. "I don't know."

I changed the subject. "Your mother says you had some chaps in the night before your birthday and you camped down in the woods."

"Yeah."

"She was a little worried. Not about the camping out. But she didn't know these guys and didn't much like their looks. She thought you all acted a little peculiar."

"Peculiar?" His voice was scathing. "She's a snob. What do you wear for camping out? Gray flannels and a shirt and tie?"

"Geoff, don't be sarcastic."

Again, he shrugged. "O.K. Believe what you want to. You will anyway."

"Who were these fellows?"

"Friends."

"Friends from where?"

"From around."

"You're not making this very easy."

"I didn't know I was on the witness stand." He sniffled again and wiped his nose on his sleeve.

"What the hell *is* wrong with you? I gave you my handkerchief. Use it. And would you mind telling me why you're wearing a wool shirt in the middle of a heat wave? You've got lots of summer shirts and decent pants upstairs. Why don't you ever wear them?"

"I like these."

Suddenly I was frightened for him. I grabbed his arm and pushed his sleeve back. He sat impassively, glaring at me.

"Like, look, man, no needle marks," he said.

I didn't answer. I felt ashamed.

"That's what you were looking for, wasn't it?"

"I want to know why you seem to have a cold, why you dress the way you do in temperatures like this, why you're so lethargic all the time, why you never get outdoors."

"And why I'm not like you," Geoff said. "That's really what bugs you, isn't it?"

"No, it isn't." I didn't want him to be like me. Like me was to have cancer. I wanted him to see his dreams—whatever they were—come true. I wanted him to be a good man. I also wanted the answer to a question which, if affirmative, might stop his future as surely as cancer might be stopping mine.

"Geoff, are you on drugs?"

He laughed. "Boy, you'll think of anything, won't you?"

"Are you?"

He got out of the chair and started to walk out of the room.

"Geoff, come back here."

Over his shoulder he said, "Think what you want."

"I want the truth." But he had already slammed the office door.

I've been sitting here ever since forcing myself to put this down on tape. I think he is on something and I've got to get him off it before it ruins his life. Maybe all that's wrong is pent-up resentment but that's bad enough. I've caused plenty of it in him and so has Kathryn. Somehow, before it's too late, I've got to find a way to help him.

Last summer I know he was all right. This school year it seems to me that every time he's come home he's changed a bit more, become more secretive and withdrawn, and God knows, more bad-tempered. He hasn't had much of a mentor in me in that department lately.

Maybe the best part of my life is over, but his is really only just beginning. If I could make a choice between protecting him and being rid of cancer, I'd take the first. I can't stand by and see him be destroyed.

= 5 =

KATHRYN

In the ten days after Connie returned from Europe with the names of Drs. Whitmore and Jewett, we lived in a state of suspended animation awaiting appointments with them. Their opinions might make the difference between hope and despair.

Dr. Ward, too, had recommended that we see these men. He was a source close to home via Pat and, although we had seen him but once, we trusted him. We were counting the hours and the days until both conferences with these illustrous doctors were completed. We had an appointment to see Dr. Whitmore on August 12; Dr. Jewett had no opening until the first of September. The interval between those times would be an anxious one. We could not begin to assess the approach to treatment until all the crucial returns were in. But the time weighed heavy. For all we knew, the cancer might be growing in the interval between its discovery on July 23 and each succeeding appointment. It was this that worried me most of all.

Dr. Ward had not voiced that view, but his suspicion that by August 5 the malignancy was already too extensive for a radical prostatectomy made us wonder if it had been all along.

In those early August days we played a macabre guessing game. If Pat had sent Connie to Dr. Ward at first, would he have told us on July 24 what he did on August 8? Would we then have tried to fix appointments with those men who figured so prominently on Connie's list? Would Connie have bothered compiling a list in Europe at all? We both thought he would have. But it was really Dr. Ward's suggestions that played a crucial role in our decisions. He is a man who values opinions other than his own. The patient's welfare, not his personal vindication, is his prime concern.

Whitmore and Jewett, stars in the field of urology, might not feel the same. In the medical world their fame preceded them like a flourish of trumpets so that the alacrity with which each of them agreed to see us surprised us. That led us to hope that they, like Dr. Ward, were men of compassion. We had been so bruised by our first encounter that, even after seeing Dr. Ward, we were fearful of the reception we would have at the hands of these renowned specialists. We would know more about that soon. At last, we were to meet them face to face.

On Wednesday, August 12, Connie and I drove into New York for our appointment with Dr. Willet Whitmore. It was a scorching summer day. We spent most of the drive into town discussing Geoff. Connie was upset that I had told our son so quickly about his father's cancer which, quite properly, Connie felt was his prerogative. He described the conversation, or lack of it, with Geoff the day before, and we decided, no matter what the future held regarding Connie's health, that we must spend more time with both our children, especially to discover the reasons for Geoff's lethargy and the secretiveness of his nature which seemed to be growing day by day.

We agreed that we would offer once again to pay him for outdoor work, more as a ruse to get him away from his room and outside into the sun, than for any help we expected him to do around the lawns and gardens.

I did not tell Connie, for he would never have agreed, that regardless of the many books on teenage behavior that urge parents to respect their children's privacy, I hoped to have an opportunity to get into Geoff's room long enough to examine its contents thoroughly. Something about him, we both knew, was very wrong. I didn't think we would find out what it was from Geoff himself. If I could get him out of the house I intended to conduct a search of his room. If any evidence existed that could account for his seeming poor health and antagonistic attitude, I felt I could expect to find it there.

Connie was hurt and confused by Geoff's attitude. I was having doubts about both our children. There were many arguments between them and more than once I had overheard one or the other threaten "to tell them about you if you say a word about me."

The problems of adolescence weren't all Geoff's. Vicki was maturing, too. At thirteen she could have passed quite easily for sixteen, and her days and nights seemed to be filled with seemingly endless telephone calls to and from the house. Many of the callers were young boys. I always asked their names and was often surprised and not a little concerned when, on hearing that question, the caller hung up.

I was very close to the end of my book, *The Betty Tree*, and the patterns of behavior I was writing about from memory were proving different in ways I had not thought about from the actions of Geoff and Vicki and their friends.

While worried about Geoff, Connie seldom found fault with Vicki. I found possibly too much fault with them both. It was a time in our lives when we could have used some peace at home but, as events would show, that was not to be our lot.

Family worries were perhaps a blessing in disguise that August 12. Otherwise we might have made the trip to the city in silence, each of us deep in thought about the man we were to meet, speculating about him and the great esteem he commanded in his profession, and, worst of all, theorizing about what he would say to Connie.

In 1970 the vast complex of Memorial Hospital for Cancer and Allied Diseases at 444 East Sixty-eighth Street and the Sloan-Kettering Cancer Center on East Sixty-seventh Street between York and First Avenues together occupied a full city block. There was the hospital itself, research centers, laboratories, radiation treatment areas, and outpatients' departments. Across the street was the still larger two-block sprawl of buildings, including New York Hospital, the Cornell University Medical College, the Lying-in Hospital, the Payne Whitney Clinic and other departments.

The entrance to the outpatient department on Sixty-seventh Street is through automatic sliding doors which lead onto a ramp designed for wheelchairs. Solicitous doormen wheel many patients up the ramp, past wide windows overlooking the street, to the spacious counters on the information floor. The doormen treat everyone with a courteous, warm attention. Their attitude takes some of the fear away, though never all of it.

At the information desk we were directed back along a hallway opening into a huge bullpen where white-clad secretaries worked at files and notes. Examining cubicles ran through corridors which intersected the long passageways on either side of the building, and rows of chairs were placed along the passageways, nearly all of them occupied.

It seemed an endless time before we reached the section given over to Dr. Whitmore's department. A pretty dark-haired girl, seated behind one of identical desks which filled the giant bull pen, told us that the doctor was running late. It might be some time before he could see us. She suggested we wait in the large lounge near the front entrance. We elected to stay close at hand, although there was no place to sit. The chairs were taken, mostly by men, but I noticed a few worried-looking women, too. They sat beside their husbands, the couples occasionally holding hands and whispering softly to each other. The men, I noticed, were of all ages, some quite young, some perhaps Connie's age, others obviously elderly. There is a kind of silence in these cancer centers that is not really silence at all. The air is full of tension and soft, sibilant whispers. One notes immediately that eyes are hastily averted to shut away the sight of tears. Everywhere there is the shocked look of people who have been hit by sudden disaster.

We stood beside the girl's desk and, in time, struck up a conversation with her. She was Dr. Whitmore's daughter, substituting for his regular secretary, away on vacation. She asked Connie to fill out a medical form which included a listing of his occupation. As soon as she read the name, the girl said, "You wrote *The Longest Day.*" Connie was pleased. He nodded. She had loved the book, although she was far too young to regard it as anything but ancient history. Yet she remembered it well and asked Connie a number of questions about the book.

Finally, a couple of chairs became available. Patients had come out from the areas of the examining rooms, but of the doctor there had been no sign. Each time we saw a man dressed in a business suit under a white coat, we guessed he might be Dr. Whitmore. But none of them spared glances for any of us.

At one point I had the briefest glimpse of a tall, slender

man in operating greens streaking by. He flashed a brilliant smile but was gone so quickly I did not really see his face. But I remembered the smile.

We sat on. I was next to a well-dressed, handsome woman who was holding hands with her equally attractive husband. She whispered to me, "What has your husband got?"

Startled, I mumbled a lie. "We don't know yet."

Her smile was sad. "Then I hope your news will be good," she said. She sighed and tightened her clasp on her husband's fingers. He, I noticed, was staring into space, oblivious to our hushed talk.

I leaned toward the woman. "I hope your news will be good, too."

Tears shone in her eyes. "We've already got our news," she said. Bending closer to me, she whispered, "My husband has cancer of the bladder. We've come from Virginia. Dr. Whitmore plans to admit Charles today after the last test he had run comes down from the lab."

I was too shocked to even offer her my sympathy for whatever use it would have been. This was the first time Connie and I had been in a room together with other cancer victims. Instead of kindness, I asked the first thing that came into my head. "Has everybody here and in the lounge come in because of cancer?"

"Of course," my new friend told me. "This is a cancer center, probably one of the best in the world."

I looked along our rows of chairs and then across the bull pen to the opposite wall where still other lines of people waited, some in wheelchairs. A new life was beginning for us, and new friendships we would make in an instant, sometimes never to see the people again but to remember them always. In time they would become more memorable and closer to us than many of the people we saw daily.

There are no strangers among those whose lives have been shattered by cancer. In a cancer hospital, outside lives are left behind, checked at the door. Once inside, one quickly encounters the decency and understanding of people with a shared problem. I know of no other place where these qualities seem more noticeable. Frequently people never come to know each other's names and names are not important. The interest and concern that people show for one another wipe out a need for introductions.

By 3:00 P.M. we had been waiting a little more than two hours. My neighbor and her husband had left, accompanied by one of the men in white. As they headed up on the passageway which I was later to find connects the Sloan-Kettering offices with the main floor of Memorial Hospital, the woman turned back to wave to me. I blew her a kiss. She smiled faintly and turned back to link her husband's arm in hers.

Connie and I sat on, not talking. He was as silent now as he had been on the Friday night we waited in the first urologist's outer office for the conference that had started us on this fearful journey of discovery. I put my hand over one of his and he patted my hand absentmindedly, staring across the bull pen but, I think, not seeing the rows of people seated against the far wall. He was seeing deeper and darker figures. He was perhaps imagining the future.

We were both startled when Dr. Whitmore's daughter came over to us. "Please go into the second room on your right," she said, pointing to the intersecting corridor near where we were seated. "Father will be right along. I'm so sorry you've been kept waiting."

The room, I thought on first glance, was barely large enough for the green metal desk and the three chairs which occupied it. Then I noticed that its looks were deceptive. A long white curtain, like those used to separate beds in a ward, was half drawn, revealing an examining couch, a basin, a cabinet arrangement, and some wall-hung clothes hooks.

Tentatively we took seats before the desk, Connie directly facing it, me at an angle to the chair behind it. A white phone with a battery of buttons, several lit, was the desk's sole appointment.

Connie turned to me. "Did you bring your notebook?"

I nodded and started to open my handbag.

"Never mind," he said. "I've got mine," pulling it out from his breast pocket and rolling out the point of lead on the gold pencil he was seldom without. "You just listen. We can compare notes afterward."

Again I nodded. We sat on.

The voice and the rush of air came together. "I'm sorry we're running so far behind. How are you both? My daughter tells me she's had a marvelous conversation with you. Mr. Ryan, I think you've made her day. I'm Dr. Whitmore."

He was already seated by that time, extending his hand across the desk first to Connie, then to me. He was the man in operating greens whom I had noticed earlier. The same flashing smile, the swift, quiet speed and now—close up—a finely chiseled face, high cheekbones, straight handsome nose, sandy hair. His face, even in repose, seemed to be smiling. I noticed those lines were permanently etched into his features, lifting the corners of his mouth. An intensity of spirit, health, charm, vitality radiated from the man. He seemed like a thoroughbred eager to race. In his wrinkled, green operating room garb—I have seldom seen him dressed in any other way—there was a quiet authority about him as though he needed no trappings to set off his distinction. No wonder, I thought, his fame had spread so far. His looks and charm would make people remember him. I saw Connie write a note on the top page of his small, spiral-bound book. He turned it toward me. On it he had written, "The Cary Grant of medicine."

From the desk Dr. Whitmore picked up a folder he had brought to the room and took from it a letter we recognized:

Pat's. "Did you bring the slides, Mr. Ryan?" The voice was low, pleasant, devoid of any regional accent.

Connie handed them over. Whitmore sprang to his feet. He seemed almost to bounce in the white tennis-type shoes he wore. "I'll just be a minute," he said and disappeared through the door. In seconds he was back.

"Now," he said, "I'm going to ask you to go over there by the table and get undressed." Connie groaned. Dr. Whitmore's smile was sympathetic. "I expect you're a little tired of examinations."

"Yes," Connie said. "Every time it feels a little more like somebody's drilling a well."

Again the quick flash of Whitmore's smile and the sudden light jump up from his seat. "I'll show you where you can hang your clothes and you'll find a fresh gown on the table. You know exactly how to put it on by now, I expect?"

"I'm an expert," Connie told him. "If you ever need me to demonstrate to a class, I can do the whole process from untying my shoes to getting into the examining robe blindfolded."

Whitmore grinned. "I don't think I'll ask you to do that. I'd much rather hear you lecture about your books and how you do *them*." He closed the curtains around Connie and came back to the desk.

"Now," he said, his attention, it seemed, completely focused on me. "You tell me how this all began, what you felt, what you are feeling, and a little bit of family history. Children, any illnesses you've had, all that. All right?"

I smiled. One cannot help smiling at Dr. Whitmore. "Connie's the patient," I said.

"Just a few details," he urged. So I talked for a few minutes as Whitmore listened carefully, giving me his full attention.

Connie called, "I'm as ready as I'll ever be, Doctor," and Whitmore excused himself. At the curtain he turned back to me.

"If you'd prefer to wait outside, please do. I expect my daughter or one of the girls could get you some coffee, although I won't keep him very long. I quite agree with him. He must be very tired of these examinations."

"May I stay?"

He looked quizzically at me again. "Do you want to? I'll be asking him some questions that he might prefer to answer in privacy."

"Connie, do you want me to leave?" I called, remembering that I was to be the ears whenever he would not be able to take notes.

His voice was more reassured than I had heard it in weeks. "Stay, Katie love," he said. "As Dr. Whitmore will learn, we don't have many secrets from each other. Also, we work together."

"We're a team," I said to Dr. Whitmore and felt tears sting my eyes. He smiled and nodded and disappeared inside the curtain where Connie was hidden from view.

Whitmore's questions and Connie's responses were repetitions of what had gone on before. As the previous doctors had done, Whitmore said that Dr. Neligan must be a fine, thorough internist. "It's amazing," I remember him saying, "that since the hardening is so small, anyone discovered it at all. One has to work to find it."

Connie groaned. "I know."

"Only another few minutes, Mr. Ryan." Whitmore's voice was soothing. "Your research must take you to a great many countries."

Connie said it did. I thought of the last piece of research he had done which had led him to this place and this man. We did not detail to Dr. Whitmore how we came to contact him. Dr. Ward's recommendation and Pat's call to him would probably have been reason enough. He did not know that he was a brilliant star in our rather shaky firmament, that Connie's statistics had turned out his name often among a list of many experts in the field of genito-urology.

140

As quickly as he had gone in, Dr. Whitmore darted out from behind the curtains. Passing me he put his hand briefly on my shoulder. "I'm going to pick up the slides. Be right back," and with that silent sprint of speed which continued to amaze me, he was gone.

Connie was dressed and back in his chair when Whitmore returned. His absence had given me only time to say, "Nothing new on the questions, except that he wanted a bit of our family history and my health."

Connie nodded. "I know. What's your impression of him?"

"You mean besides what you wrote?"

He grinned. "Don't you agree? About the Cary Grant thing?"

"Yes, but we can't make judgments on that. We have to get through the next part."

"I know, Katie, but I like him. I can identify with him. It's not just the coincidence of his name turning up so often. He's good. One can sense that."

I agreed with Connie. There was a charismatic aspect to Whitmore's character. There was an electrifying aspect, too. The little room where we sat seemed charged with the power of his personality. Suddenly, as he had done before, he bounded silently into the room and came around to his chair.

Carefully he lifted up the slides. "Well, there's no doubt about it. I looked at them while I was on my way to pathology. Our boys here agree. It is definitely adenocarcinoma of the prostate with perineural infiltrate."

"Cancer," Connie said flatly. "What's the last part mean?"

"It means involvement of nerve fibers in the area between the scrotum and the anus."

Taking paper from his desk, Whitmore began to draw lines such as a chartist might make. "Let us assume now that the average life expectancy, given your age, with this kind of ca. is fifteen years." The top line he labeled "15." He continued: "You've got a tumor in an area where cancer is traditionally slow-growing. In my opinion you could do nothing at all and probably live out the fifteen years. Certainly I would expect you could live five years before any treatment might be indicated." He drew another line. It was shorter. Too short.

Connie broke in: "Dr. Ward, who you know we've seen, talked with me about hormone therapy."

"Let me tell you about hormones," Dr. Whitmore said. "Hormones can be beneficial. You can take them at the beginning, you can take them in the middle, or you can take them at the end. What they can often do is extend longevity to the hypothetical statistical fifteen years we are projecting here."

"What do you think I should do?"

Again Whitmore smiled. "I hope I won't shock you. I advise you to do absolutely nothing."

Our silence was total. Finally Connie said in a voice I did not even recognize, "Doctor, one can't imagine doing absolutely nothing."

"I know," Whitmore said. He leaned back in his chair. "Let me explain. I have probably performed more prostatectomies than anybody in the country, with the exception of Dr. Hugh Jewett in Baltimore." We glanced at each other. "But my approach over the last few years has been to veer away from prostatectomies. They often produce greater surgical complications and mortality than the cancer itself.

"Now I'm leaning toward a concept of studying the development of the carcinoma cells, learning all I can about their growth in the individual. In some cases a malignant cell in the prostate might multiply or spread every two years or, for that matter, every two days, or every few months. But until we find a growth factor in each individual, I am not of the opinion that anything should be done except constant check-ups to see how the cancer is behaving."

I think Connie and I were equally attuned and in equal confusion. The first urologist had said prostatectomy and prostatectomy *now*. Dr. Ward had said that if Connie were his brother, hormones would be the route he would advise him to take. Our friends, certainly not medical experts, had advanced the idea of using a Mexican-manufactured drug called Laetrile, cabbage poultices, and—the thought made me ill—Eskimo blood soup. Here was one of the men Connie had tracked across an ocean telling us calmly that it might be wise at this point to do absolutely nothing at all.

I was obsessed by one thought: would any two experts ever agree about a single course of treatment? The only points of reference each specialist had in common was that yes, Pat had discovered a slight hardening along the right lateral lobe of the prostate, so slight that every doctor had been impressed that he had even found it. And yes, each of them agreed that the biopsy report was accurate: adenocarcinoma of the prostate. Beyond that lay a forest of opinions that shook our confidence—the confidence that, in historical research, we had always found in discovery of back-to-back agreement. There was only one consolation and it was small: only the first urologist advocated the radical prostatectomy. The views of the other two doctors—Ward and Whitmore—were opposed to haste and drastic measures. Could we live with this diversity of opinion? Could the children? Connie and I had always had a master game plan. How could we now start to play blindly? The divergence of medical views ran contrary both to our natures and our work methods.

Our consternation did not escape Dr. Whitmore's notice. "Mr. Ryan," he turned to Connie, "while you were waiting to see me did you notice the men around you?"

"Not really. There appeared to be one about my age. Katie spoke with his wife. I also saw a youngster. I don't remember the others."

"There were three men out there I wish you had looked at. The youngest is fifty-seven, the next is sixty-three, and the oldest is seventy-nine," Whitmore said. "Each of those three has prostatic tumors. They have been under observation by me for some years now. I have done absolutely nothing in the form of treatment at all for any of the three. They come in very regularly for evaluation. So far, there has been no need to do anything other than examine and observe."

"It's both liberating and exhilarating, that kind of news," Connie said, "but I wonder if that method would work with me? My next book is very important. I have to have a worry-free mind. I know myself rather well. All the time there would be a nagging feeling that while you might be watching the growth factor of the cancer, a day or a week before my next appointment, the thing might get larger. It might be spreading to other parts of my body before you saw me again. I don't know if I can live with that uncertainty. Let's assume that I could. Somehow. What would you do if you found that a time had come when something should be done?"

The smile lines were still on the doctor's face. "Well," he said gently, "at that particular point, you might be put on hormones which would arrest to a degree. Contain. Allow us more time. But I think if your condition came to that, the cancer would override the beneficial effects of the hormones in the end."

He paused. "There is a third therapy, one we have developed here—the implantation of radiation seeds into the prostate. These seeds both shrink the gland and kill a very high percentage of cancer cells."

"I've never ever heard of such a procedure," Connie said.

"No, Mr. Ryan, undoubtedly not," Whitmore said. "There's a reason. I would like to be able to tell you that I have statistics proving that this is a definitive therapy and that it actually does kill the cancer, but I do not have such statistics. We have only been doing this particular kind of treatment for about three years here. We have performed it on about ten to twelve patients. Every one of them is still alive. We have had no mortalities and everybody is going great guns. But three years is much too short a time for me to be even faintly positive that this is a workable idea in a majority of cases. Still, if the time comes, if you elect to stay with me for treatment, I would like you to consider all these modalities."

Connie finished taking notes. He put his pencil inside his breast pocket and shut the notebook. "I haven't mentioned it before," he told Dr. Whitmore, "but I have an appointment with Dr. Jewett, whom you mentioned, in Johns Hopkins on September first."

"I think you will find that Dr. Jewett will be against my advice to watch and do nothing before doing anything. But I respect him greatly and I think you would indeed be making a mistake if you did not take the opportunity to see him and be examined by him. It is quite clear that you, in your work and by reason of your personality, are quite capable of making up your own mind in a way that will be beneficial and interfere as little as possible with your writing. I shall be most interested, as my daughter has been impressed, in seeing you again if that is what you would like, but I respect your judgment too much to do more than tell you what I think we can do here and what I suggest. Just remember," he said, "the door is never closed."

We thanked him and he walked out to the bull pen with us, watching with a smile as we said good-bye to his daughter. I think I remember Connie autographing a piece of paper for her. At any event it was obvious that he was delighted by his meeting with her and that Dr. Whitmore was delighted by our appreciation of her youth and charm. In some ways they were very alike.

Out on the street we hunted for a coffee shop. We were not ready just then to sit in Memorial's restaurant. Connie still held the same dislike for hospitals that he had always had. We found a small, rather dingy place not too far away. At a luncheonette table Connie took out his notebook and we went carefully over his notes, comparing them with my memory of the appointment. Neither of us had thought to ask much about the radiation implant theory and it left a large gap in our research. In normal interviews we would not have overlooked the thread that could lead to a larger, fuller design. But, as Connie said, we were not really interviewing. We were being interviewed and that was unfamiliar ground, particularly in these circumstances.

"He did say he would do nothing?" Connie asked, flipping back through his notebook.

"He said for now. He said if regular examinations gave cause for alarm, then he would go to treatment."

"He didn't say 'cause for alarm.'" Connie corrected me. "He said that until we find a growth factor he was not of the opinion that anything should be done except for me to have constant checkups."

"Doesn't that make you feel better?"

"Yes. Yes. Yes. And no," Connie said.

"That's three out of four," I told him. "Back up! You feel better. I can see it."

He actually smiled, a relieved, bright smile. Almost a Connie-on-top-of-the-world smile. "It's the best statistic we've got so far," he said.

That moment was almost like the good old days—the ones I thought would never come back.

Doctors' handwritings are alleged to be notoriously difficult to read. "Alleged" is the wrong word. They are notoriously difficult to read, including their own medical shorthand. In his own notes of August 12, 1970, Dr. Whitmore wrote the following.* I quote in part:

8–12–70. GU note [genito-urinary notation]. 50 yr. old author (white ♂). Denies F.H. [family history] of GU disease, ca, diabetes. PH [past history] essentially negative. At age 7—appendectomy . . . No major illnesses. In April 1970 slight urethral discharge and sticky meatus, diagnosed as prostatitis and treated by massages c̄ [with]

---

* I have added explanations in brackets following medical terms and abbreviations in the hope they will make the notes easier for the reader to follow.

improvement but residual induration persisted and aspiration biopsy . . . → [indicates] adeno-ca. Comes for further opinion . . . No wt. loss, bone pain, sciatica

PX [physical exam] BP [blood pressure] 125/75 WD, WN [well developed, well nourished] athletic white ♂ . Not ill.
Neck: No adenopathy [enlargement involving glandular tissue]
Breast: No gynecomastia [abnormal enlargement]
Abdomen: LSK [liver, spleen, kidneys] not felt, no masses
Groins: Negative. Femoral pulses good = [equal]
Genitalia: Uncircumcised. Penis normal
Testes: Epididymis and cords normal [structure and condition of small oblong tube lying on and beside back of the testes]
Extremities: No edema
Rectal: Small < [less than] 15 gm. symmetric prostate. Rt. lobe scaphoid [boat-shaped] c̄ [with] mildly indurated border laterally. Lt. lobe rounder and more elastic. Doubt that I would have suspected it.

Rt   Lt

I.V.P. [intravenous pyelogram]
CBC [complete blood count]
Urinalysis
BUN [blood urea nitrogen], Blood sugar,
Acid, Alkaline, p'tase

} All normal at time of biopsy . . .

Rt   Lt

Impression: Stage C carcinoma of prostate. RX [treatment] Pros and cons of no RX, endocrine RX, irradiation, radical excision, discussed with patient. Recommend observation

Dr. Neligan referred pt.

Dr. Whitmore's follow-up letter to Dr. Neligan which both doctors have given me permission to use explains in more detail the substance of the conversation Whitmore, Connie, and I had on August 12 at Sloan-Kettering. Again, it is reproduced in its pertinent parts.

Mr. Cornelius Ryan . . . is a 50 year old white male who has enjoyed good general health and in whom the development of a urethral discharge in April 1970 led to a urologic investigation which uncovered a prostatic induration proved by biopsy to represent adenocarcinoma of the prostate. At the time of my examination . . . he was essentially free of urinary symptoms except for a persistent mild urethral discharge and specifically had no obstructive urinary symptoms. He had had no weight loss, bone pain, sciatica, peripheral edema, or other symptomatic manifestations to suggest dissemination. On examination he appeared to be . . . well developed, well nourished. There was no gynecomastia, no significant abdominal findings and no genital abnormalities except for the findings on digital rectal examination. The prostate was not significantly enlarged but there was slight asymmetry, the right lobe being slightly more prominent than the left with a mild but distinct degree of induration extending along the entire right lateral border of the gland from apex to base and with the suggestion of induration in the lateral aspect of the base of the right seminal vesicle. Review of the pathologic slides confirmed the diagnosis of adenocarcinoma of the prostate with evidence of perineural infiltration.

The pros and cons of various forms of treatment were discussed with the patient quite frankly, admitting the uncertainties regarding the natural history of this disease and regarding the influence of various forms of treatment upon it. My personal recommendation was that he have no immediate treatment until such time as serial digital rectal examinations provided some evidence of a local growth of his tumor and that, at that time, irradiation be given as the first form of treatment. This could be either in the form of external supervoltage irradiation or in the form of a retropubic I-125 implant. We are currently exploring the latter technique although it would be premature to make any claims for the method.

. . . Many thanks for the opportunity of seeing this patient.

Sincerely yours,

Willet F. Whitmore, Jr., M.D.
Chief, Urologic Service

What is so amazing about both Dr. Whitmore's handwritten report, on the day of Connie's visit to him, and his subsequent letter to Pat is that neither Connie nor I had picked up his words about "supervoltage irradiation." We recalled only his mention of the radiation seed implant I-125. Next to (a) observing Connie before doing *anything,* and (b) the possibility of hormone therapy if the cancer showed signs of progressive change, we remembered only that Dr. Whitmore had called the implant treatment *"a third therapy."* Yet, in his own notes, he mentions "irradiation" as a form of treatment (presumably using the term between the two forms of radiation treatment interchangeably). While in his letter to Pat he mentions "irradiation . . . as the first form of treatment" if the tumor was found to be growing *locally* and breaks down that description of this treatment into two parts: supervoltage irradiation *or* a retropubic I-125 implant.

In light of what we were later to learn about Connie's true condition, our failure to pick up the words "supervoltage irradiation" and the words "local growth" were to have serious consequences, especially in light of the differing views of doctors as to the workability of the techniques and forms of treatment then available. Mortals cannot be omniscient. That is a tragedy for doctors and patients alike.

$$\doteq 6 \doteq$$

CORNELIUS

Saturday, August 29, 1970.

Seventeen days have passed since we saw Whitmore and

two days to go until we see Jewett. The interval is agonizing. I can't work. The words refuse to fall in order. I have this disease and, for all I know, it is growing. I could be using up my days collecting opinions—each one, it is turning out, more diverse than the last. I still can't believe in Whitmore's "wait and see" attitude. I'm damned if I want to be a human guinea pig for him or anybody else in the medical profession. It's bad enough being a statistic, one of the 600,000 in whom cancer will be found this year.

I don't think I'm imagining how often I've heard the word "cancer" of late. In the past I know I must have used it myself without giving it a second's thought. Now that the connotation has taken on such a personal meaning I feel a raw ache, as if a wild animal had clawed and mangled my body, whenever the word is mentioned. I've had occasion recently to hear it rather frequently. Kathryn and I have seen a number of people socially since our visit to Whitmore, more than is customary for us when I'm working. Except that I'm not working. Not well. I thought outside activities—lunches, golf games, dinner parties—might lessen the shock of the findings of this malignancy. No one diversion has succeeded. "Cancer" follows me everywhere like a stray dog one hopes will just go away.

A few nights ago at a dinner party a woman was talking about her son who lives in Canada. He has gone there to escape the Vietnam war. But he is unhappy and work is hard to find. "Still," the boy's mother remarked, "he's safe. I'd rather he had cancer than be in Vietnam." A man down the table spoke up. "Either way, he'd be just as dead," he said. A few people laughed. Such talk continued. Kathryn and I went home early.

I don't like to discuss Vietnam even when it is not equated with cancer. I like still less the intensity of this war's supporters and the sick jokes proffered by some detractors. A lot of editors urged me to go have a look at the war and I was tempted, but I remembered the area when it was Indochina and one of my best friends, the photographer Bob Capa, was killed there in 1954—four years after Katie and I were married. Bob had gone with us on our honeymoon to Europe. I'd known him all through World War II and he had told me, after a look at Katie, "This innocent is not going on a honeymoon with you alone. I tell you that." And so he went along, a not very vigilant chaperon, and then four years later on a tour of the battlefront, which is where Capa could always be found in war, Bob was killed. Cancer or war. Either way, the man at the dinner party had said, one would be just as dead.

Two days ago I played golf with a famous actor who is an on-again, off-again friend of mine. He was nursing a hangover and grousing about a producer. "He's so goddamn mean," my irritable companion said, "that the sonofabitch wouldn't even give away cancer."

It's ridiculous to dwell on such remarks, but I think they tend to show how sensitive a cancer patient can become to trivia. I am becoming more and more aware that I must know and trust someone extremely well before I will ever feel free to discuss my illness.

To pass the time, and because I must, I have been trying to start the book. I wrote a dedication for *Bridge* that I showed to Katie. It goes: "For the soldiers and civilians caught up in the conflict whose courage, compassion, and despair are so integral a part of the human condition." Katie x-ed through it. "CJ, it's true, but I can't bear to have you use it," she said. "It's too much a part of what you're going through right now." She wrote three words: "For them all." I looked at her offering. "Does it say enough?" She put her hands over her face. "I don't know," she said. "It's better than 'for *us* all.' "

"I should hope so," I said. "If you didn't like my version, think how self-pitying that one would be."

"The men and women we've interviewed will know what we mean if we used the term 'them.' "

"And the reader's got to guess?"

"If this is the book it can be and will be, the reader will

know a great deal about 'them' and their courage, compassion, and despair. I just wish those words were integral to all people."

I didn't tell her that I wished the first word, "courage," was integral to me. I'm trying very hard not to let Katie see how very frightened I really am.

I've left the dedication for the moment and gone on to the lead. I've got about thirty-odd pages and maybe two hundred false starts. I know how I want to open but I can't seem to get it down on paper. The lead has got to be slow and build up suspense and then, very gradually, I've got to let the reader in on what the suspense is all about. It seems so very simple, but is so terribly difficult. I've got "soft September darkness and early morning mist." I've got a flat-footed "something was different" and a tortuous "something was curiously different." Then there are all kinds of variations on that. I need a cracklingly crisp first sentence that makes the reader want to go on to the next one, and it, too, has got to broaden the picture a little, but just a little. And by the end of the first paragraph I've got to hook my reader or I am lost, and worse, I will have lost him.

The little Dutch village is the best place to start. Put the reader where I want him to share the experience of the people there immediately. I know I've got to start in Driel, but I can't seem to put the words together. Why Driel? Driel is the village of innocents, the Dutch who live there have been bypassed by the war. They are bobbing in the backwater. They don't know that the wave of battle will come back and smash them. On the day on which I want the book to begin, the people of Driel are safe, unharmed—and then a few weeks later they're in the middle of a holocaust, suffering as much as the soldiers and, like the soldiers, having to take the punishment, the brutality, the stark, awful fact of war.

I love the soldiers and civilians who have made my books possible. I love their trust and their cynicism, their terror, their faith, their incredible ability to laugh when there's nothing to laugh about, and so they summon up a wild, desperate humor because with death and destruction all around, laughter is all they've got left. What an example they are for me.

I've got to start with the village. It's my beginning and my end.

My feelings and Katie's, too, I think, are rather mixed about this trip to Baltimore to see Dr. Jewett. He has been called "the father of the prostatectomy" by doctors I spoke with in Europe.* I haven't mentioned this to Katie but I fully expect Jewett to say, "Get the thing out. You will be stripped of your sexual abilities, perhaps sapped of mental agility. There is a chance that you will have an incontinence of say five percent or twenty percent. Perhaps you will have to go around with a little rubber bag inside your pants for the remainder of your days." I shall have to walk out if that happens. I am not fully recovered from the shock of hearing similar talk after the malignancy was first discovered.

Here I am at age fifty and I know I should have more life ahead of me. But I wonder what Jewett is going to say. This situation is becoming intolerable. The mental replay never seems to stop. Even with all the phone calls and the visits I've made to date to hear doctors' opinions, I have still only the shallowest knowledge of cancer.

It is devastating not to know what is happening inside you or what you can expect. I wish I could take a crash course in cancer medicine. Economics and time most certainly pro-

* The description actually belongs to Dr. Hugh H. Young (1870–1945) with whom Dr. Jewett was associated for many years. Young spent most of his professional life at Johns Hopkins Hospital as head of the department of urological surgery. In 1915 he became director of the Brady Clinic, as it was then known, which had been endowed by Diamond Jim Brady on whom Young had operated. During his career, Dr. Young developed new operating techniques and invented surgical instruments in use to the present time. Among his other talents, he was also founder and editor of the *Journal of Urology*.

hibit that. I've been luckier than most cancer victims so far. So many people would not have had the money to do what I have done in attempting to find the top people. Phone calls alone have been enormously expensive, as have travel costs and consulting fees.

It's rather trite to say that research costs money. I never minded the cost before because I felt if I worked hard enough and well enough, my books would earn back what I, publishers, and the *Reader's Digest*—which has given me tremendous help—had expended. I think I will be very much out-of-pocket on this research even though I am determined to see it through. Still I am lucky to be able to research cancer at all. Hundreds of people do not have the means to explore the options, even if they have the knowledge of how to go about it. This is the greatest tragedy of all. Remembering our dinner conversation of a few evenings ago, I think cancer is probably worse than war for the individual. If everybody in the world had cancer, would any war be more important than the one against it?

⸗ 7 ⸗

IT'S TUESDAY, SEPTEMBER 2, 1970. Katie and Geoff are out dead heading the petunia borders and later they're going to practice golf swings at the club. Katie needs a day out-of-doors, and I hope she and Geoff can manage to have a pleasant afternoon together. We need the boy back in the fold and Katie and I need this day of slender hope with its accompanying gift of the greatest feeling of relief we've experienced in months.

Yesterday's happenings produced this euphoria. I want to record what occurred while it is still fresh in my mind. Because of yesterday we are riding a gentle wave of optimism. It can break at any moment, I suppose, and leave us bobbing without support, but for now we are on a crest—in possession of the most exciting information we have received since the prostatitis first showed up last April.

The man responsible for our mood, the one man I was almost certain would depress it further, is Dr. Hugh J. Jewett.

In the days before our appointment with him yesterday, we tried to figure out the various ways of getting to Baltimore without undue expenditure of travel time. It is not easy to get down to Baltimore and back to Ridgefield in a day if an appointment time is important. One could go by train or by plane, but to be there at 11:00 A.M. we would have needed to stay in Baltimore Sunday night or leave here very early Monday morning, drive into New York, and fly from there. Anne Bardenhagen, my secretary, checked into the travel options and she found it was better to charter a little plane from Danbury Airport nearby which left at our convenience and could place us down in Baltimore a good hour before the appointed time.

Through the Connecticut Air Service, Annie got us a Piper Aztec, a two-engine, comfortable little plane. It was beautiful and hot on the ground yesterday, clear and cool in the air. I found the flight very pleasant. I began to notice just how beautiful this country is. Emotions that had never surfaced began to tug at me. I don't want to leave this earth. Not yet.

We landed around 10:00 A.M., took a taxi to the Johns Hopkins Hospital, found the Brady Urological Institute on the ground floor, announced ourselves, and took seats. After one of the shortest waits we've had to date, we were courteously escorted to Dr. Jewett's office.

I had assumed this renowned man would be forbidding and awesome, but Dr. Jewett is a kind little wren of a man. In a finely tailored brown suit, he rose to meet us almost as though we were old and valued friends. He is slender, balding, blue-eyed, very precise, beautifully mannered. The walls of his office are covered with every kind of parchment and distinction one can imagine. His honors and titles in the field of urology are so numerous that they fill the walls. Still others were neatly placed on a table in the room. Looking at those that were framed, one felt they had not been hung from pride—Dr. Jewett is above pride—but quite possibly they were there because of his courtesy toward the donors, his way of thanking institute and committee members for their kindnesses. Nonetheless, based on what I could see and despite his disarming manner, we were in the presence of a very important man.

In the comfortable surroundings of his office, I started the recital that was by now second nature. Jewett listened intently to the whole story. He read carefully through all the reports. His first comment was that other doctors had noted that the first urologist I'd seen, the doctor who had done the Silverman needle biopsy, had been remarkably accurate in inserting the needle exactly into the tiny cancer area. Dr. Jewett did not find that so remarkable. As he put it, cancer is localized to the nodule in only about 23 percent of patients. In the other 77 percent, it is fairly diffuse.* He thought the first urologist had been lucky rather than accurate. He then took up the slides and asked us if anyone had remarked that those cells had themselves still been making glands.† However, Dr. Jewett told us, on the basis of the gland formation, the tumor might be a slow-growing one.

* At the time of our visit to Dr. Jewett, neither Connie nor I understood the import of what he had said. What he was telling us was that Connie's cancer was not confined. He was among the 77 percent group. Rather than placing an emphasis on the first urologist's accuracy in finding a small, localized spot, Dr. Jewett felt that, because of diffusion, the original specialist had had a good chance of getting cancer cells in any case. To my mind, this was another strike against Connie's chances of a "cure" by means of a radical prostatectomy, for every other specialist except the first thought that diffusion had indeed taken place.
† The malignant cells on the slides had been producing more cells or glands which were discharging secretion possibly into the blood and lymph. This is another indication that at the time of the biopsy diffusion had already occurred.

He then took me to an examining room where an attendant already waited. While I was preparing for the examination, the doctor returned to his office where Katie was waiting. According to her, Dr. Jewett asked if I had told him the entire story of my problem. He explained that he sensed I was much too calm for a man who had been suddenly told that he had an ailment of this kind and he asked again if I had given him all the facts. Kathryn said that to the best of her knowledge I had, but she added that I tended to downgrade fears and illnesses. Thank God! I must be keeping more of my terror to myself than I think I am.

Within a few minutes Dr. Jewett came back into the examining room. Having become somewhat of an expert at being poked and prodded, I knew immediately how good Jewett was at his job. He was minutely precise. His silence seemed to stem from the most intense concentration. When he was finished he asked me to join him and Kathryn in his office when I was ready.

Back in that pleasant room once again I experienced the greatest surprise and confusion I have known since my problems began. Dr. Jewett said gently that the extent of the tumor precluded any possibility of a radical prostatectomy. I didn't have time to react to the word "extent," although I remember it so clearly. Jewett's next sentence was equally startling. Control by such an operation would be less effective, he said, than control by radiation.

I had been certain that Jewett would advocate removal of the prostate. His formidable reputation was built upon the skill of his work in that field. Instead, he gave us an entirely different opinion—one we must now weigh against the three we already have: the radical prostatectomy, hormone therapy, close observation to detect and be able immediately to combat any change in pattern and growth of the malignant cells.

My cancer, Dr. Jewett believed, would be best treated by a technique that uses subnuclear particles fired at diseased tissue by a device called a linear accelerator. I was dumbfounded! I had never even heard of such a treatment, or if I ever had its meaning had been obscure. After all, there was a time when I didn't have cancer. I would not have stored away in my memory the many theories concerning cancer cause and control.

Dr. Jewett went on to explain that extraordinary work was being done through radiation whereby beams from linear accelerators were shot into the cancerous area of the prostate— as well as in other malignant areas of the body—killing off most of the affected cells. He said there were two people he knew who were pioneering radiotherapy in this field. The man he recommended is Dr. Malcolm Bagshaw, professor and director of the Division of Radiation Therapy at Stanford University Hospital in Palo Alto, California. My God! Palo Alto. Three thousand miles away! How long would I be there and what did the radiation consist of?

Dr. Jewett told us that Dr. Bagshaw had ten-year statistics indicating that he had been able to eradicate malignant cells by use of a high-powered linear accelerator. For prostatic cancer, he said, one stands on a kind of turntable and is bombarded with radiating particles as the turntable revolves— and cancer cells are destroyed. The entire procedure sounds eerie and wonderful, more like space medicine than earth treatments.

Katie and I looked at each other. I can read my wife's expressions almost as well as she can mine. In both our minds the thought was the same, I'm sure: What have we got to lose? Let's research it. I turned back to Dr. Jewett and asked him how one got in touch with Bagshaw. Jewett said he would write to him for us. He knew the trip to Palo Alto would be expensive. He did not know how long I would have to be there for treatment, but he did feel this fascinating method would be most effective for my particular case. He felt it might guarantee total success.

"When you say total success—what does that mean? Is it a given number of years or might I get rid of this cancer forever?" Dr. Jewett asked a quiet question of his own, "Well, how would you like many years added to your life?" At that moment and right into today I feel as though they have already been granted.

KATHRYN

That attitude was apparent in a letter Connie wrote to Dr. Jewett that very day. Anne recalls the buoyancy of his mood. "He was eager to thank Dr. Jewett immediately," she remembers. "He opened the door between our two offices and called me in. 'There's one letter that must get off in today's mail,' he said. He began to dictate the minute I opened my notebook."

Dear Dr. Jewett: I am most grateful to you for seeing us yesterday . . . I concede that I am still in shock at discovering that I am a victim of this malignancy . . . But what shocks me most is to discover how much misinformation there is about cancer. . . .

It is frightening to think that I would never have known about Dr. Bagshaw in Palo Alto had I gone along with the first urologist I saw who wanted to subject me to a prostatectomy almost within 48 hours of detecting the carcinoma. That Drs. Neligan, Ward, and Whitmore advised me along the route which led me to you was indeed my good fortune. While nobody knows what my life expectancy may be, your advice gives us something to hang on to. For the first time we do not feel we are grasping at straws.

We will most certainly see Dr. Bagshaw. Dr. Neligan is awaiting your letter and then we will set things in motion. The sooner I can get my mind off all this the better.

I am sending you the first two volumes of my history on the European Theatre of Operations in World War II. The third book may be postponed a bit in view of everything, but hopefully it should emerge next year. Then I have two more volumes to complete. With luck this might be achieved.

Respectfully,

Cornelius Ryan

Connie's letter to Dr. Jewett crisscrossed Jewett's letter and clinical notes to Pat. From the relationships Connie maintained with all the doctors he saw, excepting the first specialist, it is clear that these men were dedicated not only to their work but that they understood full well the importance Connie placed upon his own work. They were in rapport—despite the distances and other opinions which separated them—in giving him the hope and the courage to continue his life and his work. I do not believe or mean to imply that Connie was an exception to the doctors' customary method of dealing with patients. They are dedicated men united, at least, in their fight against cancer. As such, they realized Connie's dedication to his profession, his zest for life, and his determination to do all that he could to help himself. What information they kept from him in the early days of his illness (and there was not much they did not tell him) was largely technical and might have sent him far too early into the deeper research he was to collect about cancer, thereby taking him totally away from his work on *Bridge*. That they were not to succeed in giving him peace of mind was not their fault but that of the cancer and Connie's own investigative pursuits. Even so, as early as September 1970, Dr. Jewett's letter to Pat Neligan held serious overtones of which we were mercifully unaware.

Dear Dr. Neligan: Thank you . . . for your kindness in referring Mr. Ryan for examination. I have studied about 500 cases of radical perineal prostatectomy for cancer done at the Johns Hopkins Hospital. I do not believe much can be gained from the operation when the seminal vesicle is involved. Although I cannot be 100% sure that there has been extension around the lower part of the right vesicle, I strongly suspect that it has taken place. There is, further-more, considerable involvement of the prostate, with very marked induration extending from the base on the right side nearly to the apex, and possibly across the midline to the base of the left lobe . . .

Taking it all in all, I think that high voltage radiation to the prostate, given by Dr. Malcolm Bagshaw at Stanford University, Palo Alto, would be the best thing for Mr. Ryan. The hormonal treatment can be held in reserve, and if spread takes place . . . can be given then. . . . Dr. Bagshaw . . . has had the largest experience of any one in the world in . . . cases of this sort and has followed a good many of them for 10 years or longer.

I hope you will let me know what develops, as I am very much interested in Mr. Ryan's progress.

Sincerely yours,

Hugh J. Jewett

As Dr. Jewett was to write me much later, Connie's tumor had exceeded the boundaries whereby a radical prostatec-tomy could be helpful. Only a nodule surrounded by normal tissue would have been treatable by radical excision, he be-lieved. This "limiting factor," as Dr. Jewett described it, was only beginning to be understood by urologists in the early 1950s and a fifteen-year follow-up of both kinds of cases—the tumor with diffusion and the single nodule circumscribed with healthy tissue—helped to confirm the belief. Since Con-nie's malignancy indicated local extension, Dr. Jewett rec-ommended radiotherapy as Connie's first choice of treat-ment. Neither he, Pat, nor Drs. Ward and Whitmore could know that the findings of the brilliant young radiotherapist, Dr. Malcolm Bagshaw, would alter the outlook once again.

We anxiously waited out the days for word from Dr. Bag-shaw. We did not know if an invitation to Palo Alto would come or when it would come. The doctor's future appointments might stretch ahead for months, making it impossible for him to see Connie soon. Still, we scanned each mail delivery for a letter postmarked California. We rushed toward the telephone each time it rang. We were afraid to get whatever news might come and fearful that none would come at all.

Rather in the manner of making everything tidy before a long trip away, we put together the documents and interviews Connie would need at hand for the first sections of *Bridge*. I turned out scores of pages on *The Betty Tree* (most of which had later to be redone), and we devoted ourselves to family chores. Connie took Geoff for his driver's license and came back pleased that Geoff, who dreads tests, had passed both the written and the driving test with ease. I got school wardrobes ready for the opening of both children's schools on Wednesday, September 16. We saw friends almost nightly, with an ulterior purpose as well as a genuine desire to be with people. If Bagshaw could see Connie in the near future, we hoped to work out a "life as usual" program before such time as Connie might be away for an undetermined stay.

It was that thought as much as any other that caused us to decide that those close to us had to be told what had been happening. We had made a mistake in discussing Connie's illness with one couple. Yet that experience had had its amusing side. Eskimo blood soup and cabbage poultices were the comic relief we could call up whenever we felt overwhelmed by anxiety. But true relief, we came to feel, might possibly be found if we discussed our situation with friends in whose company we had previously spent a great deal of time. I had already found an emotional outlet in being able to talk with Vera Neligan, Jean Safford, and Zelda Gitlin without needing to resort to pretense or guile. Connie, more than I, needed equal opportunity. Besides, we reasoned, we had to trust some people. We had to hope the few we felt should know would keep our confidences.

Accordingly, in those days of waiting to hear from Dr. Bagshaw, we added six more couples to our "need to know" list—certainly more for our relief than for theirs. John and Shirley Tower, Red and Livie Gordon, Margie and Mel Thompson—with whom we had spent the brief vacation in Saint Martin in April when Connie's difficulties first began to surface—were, all six, part of a group of close-knit friends, along with the Saffords and the Neligans. With them all we had gone on vacations, spent numerous evenings together, planned football weekends, golfing excursions, symphony and theater nights. Additionally, we told Myles and Kathleen Eason, theatrical friends, of Australian and British background respectively, who had become, in a rather short time, valued, charming, fun-loving companions. Dan and Louise McKeon were among our closest friends in town, and there was never a week when we did not see them. Pretenses had been especially hard to keep up with them. With the barriers down, we felt easier in our minds. The McKeons, like the others we had confided in, were to be a constant source of support. And last, the time had come when without inflicting our troubles on them we could no longer be at ease with the two people we had known longest in our married life—Ben and Dolly Wright.

Ben's friendship with Connie—like those of many others, among them Joe Ryle, Bill Hearst, Bob Considine, and Herb Caen—dated back to World War II. A day seldom passed without communication between Connie and Ben. They devised lunches and golf games as ruses (or so I had always accused them) to plan still another fishing trip or a visit to European battlegrounds they shared in common.

Dolly Wright and I did not mind their frequent trout or salmon trips, usually in the company of Peter Kriendler. We had long ago become resigned to our roles as fishing widows. But their emotional jaunts to Europe, almost always in the company of other World War II journalists, during which they all covered terrain filled with memories of great feats and absent comrades, bordered on obsession, I thought. They were unwilling to let go of that part of their past. Yet, Dolly and I, along with other correspondents' wives, accepted the inevitable each time Connie and Ben rounded up a group of buddies and set off for Europe and, in particular, for the beaches of Normandy.

There, "the man who invented D Day," as Herb Caen called Connie, always paid his first visit to the dead. He walked beside the steel-gray waters lapping onto the invasion beaches and stood for long moments beside the graves of the men who lay in Allied and German cemeteries in Normandy. I was with Connie once on a research trip when we paid a visit to the American cemetery at St. Laurent-sur-Mer, its row upon row of white crosses overlooking the English Channel. Connie called the memorial ground—172½ acres— "one of the most expensive pieces of real estate the U.S. ever bought." On that trip, we walked through the British cemetery where I came across an inscription that Connie was to use many times in future. Carved into a simple military stone were these words: "Into the great mosaic of history, this priceless piece was set." To Connie, that grieving, poignant message summed up war's futility and waste. So did the sight of the unkempt German cemetery with its black, Celtic-like crosses where, my husband said, other good soldiers too were at rest.

On all his nostalgic trips, there were also visits to the many French friends he had made along the Normandy coast during his research for *The Longest Day*, and then, each time before leaving Normandy, he would go once again to St. Laurent to the graves of the men of his adopted country. "I want to be buried here with them," he told me more than once and long before such a prospect was anything but talk. "Nobody knew their names until I began research for *The Longest Day*. No nation ever gave them any medals—those paratroopers who dropped from the skies, the air and naval personnel involved in D Day, and the infantrymen who stormed ashore in the crucial first three assault waves. I guess I wrote *The*

Longest Day because I never understood why nobody seemed to care about the names of the ordinary men and the civilians involved. If I ever did anything right in my life, I made their names immortal. Someday," he added, "I want to be here with them. Not for a visit. For always."

Ben Wright was deeply aware of Connie's intense emotionalism about the Normandy beaches. He always went on the trips there with Connie. The two men were the prime organizers of what they referred to as "D Day Revisited."

Our relationship with the Wrights was too deep—we saw them too often, there were too many plans Ben might suggest that he and Connie map out for the future—not to tell them what was happening to us. The deception, if we did not tell them of Connie's condition, would be, we knew, too heavy to bear. More so now that there might be a possibility that Connie would be out of touch for some time to come. Still, we often wondered how much worry our confession might cause all our friends to bear.

We took the risk. The time had come when deception and the maintenance of a status quo were no longer possible. By September 16, all six couples had been told of Connie's condition. As he had hoped, we found in them both sympathy and support. An extra dimension of warmth seemed to permeate our relationships almost from the moment we confessed our worries. The pleasure we had always taken in the company of these friends was to remain unchanged. As time went on, because of our early steps in informing these particular people, we would find ourselves the recipients of their most extraordinary help at a most extraordinary time.

Of them all, only Ben and Dolly Wright gave way to deep emotion when they were told. On Saturday, September 12, they came out from New York for a day of golf to be followed by dinner at our house. I cannot remember if we ever ate.

Sitting on the terrace in the late afternoon Connie suddenly said, "I've gone over something again and again in my mind. I've talked with Katie and we've decided we have to level with you."

Startled, Ben looked across at Connie. "Then get it over with, CJ," he said. "But if it's unpleasant I'm going to have another drink first."

"You may want it later," Connie told him. "What I've got to say is short and to the point. I've got cancer. It was confirmed by biopsy in July."

"I— Christ! Let me get some booze," Ben said and headed into the house.

Dolly looked stunned. She stared at Connie for a long time. Finally she asked, "You mean you've known since July and you didn't tell us?"

"I didn't want to tell anybody," Connie said. "I kept hoping it wasn't true."

"Is it sure? Really sure?" Dolly asked, looking from Connie to me.

"We've seen four doctors besides Pat," I told her. "They all agree."

Ben reemerged from the house. There were tears in his eyes and he made no attempt to hide them. He sat down heavily. "I don't think I can take this, Ryan," he said. "And I'm certainly not driving back to New York tonight. I wouldn't be able to sleep at home and I might as well stay awake here. I'm not leaving until you tell me everything."

And Connie did. We sat on into the dusk, Ben and Dolly asking questions, Connie explaining. At one point I remember spending time in the kitchen with Geoff and Vicki, watching them broil hamburgers as I got out the condiments, different for each child, that they required. Suddenly Vicki asked, "Is Daddy telling UB about cancer?" I was too startled to answer immediately. I thought we had managed to keep the worst from her. At that time we had not yet decided exactly how much to tell her. I did not think that Geoff had told her either. Ben was, next to her father, and grandfather, her closest older male friend and companion. She had always called him "UB," short for Uncle Ben. I didn't know how much she knew or what her question meant. Was she puzzled that Connie had not told Ben earlier? Or had she overheard only enough of our own conversations to think that perhaps Connie might be doing an article on cancer for some publication?

"He's telling Ben about cancer, yes," I managed to say.

"But he didn't tell me," Vicki said. "Daddy never told me he had cancer."

I turned to look at her. Vicki can yell loudly with no tears or cry tragically with no sound. She was crying soundlessly, her face wet. I stopped whatever I was doing and put my arms around her. "I knew," she said against my shoulder. "I knew but he never told me." Her body shook. "He won't die. My daddy won't die."

"He won't die, Vicki. He'll be all right. You know Daddy will make everything come out all right." I believed it, too. No matter how anxious the days, how much concern we felt, I knew Connie's strength and determination better than all the doctors. There would be bad times but everything would turn out for the good. It had to. My optimism, like my despair, was quick to come and equally quick to go. It was strong just then, however transient.

"He'll do his best, Vicki," Geoff said as if he'd read my thoughts. "Stop acting like a baby. If there's a way to get well, Dad will find it."

"Of course he will," I told her. Geoff's common sense and support were erratic, but they existed. Vicki, however, was not to be taken in by our words.

"First, you didn't tell me," she said accusingly in a quiet voice, her grief showing in her words and by the flow of tears streaming silently down her face. "Now you say he'll get well. I'm not going to school next week. I'm not ever going to school again. I want to be with Daddy." She buried her head against my body. "I won't let him die. I won't let anybody hurt him. He's mine." She raised her head and stared at me. "Don't you understand?" she asked. "He's mine." The agony in her eyes was unbearable. My own eyes filled with tears. The damnable disease would maim us all. It had already.

I got tissues from the little desk in the kitchen and gently wiped Vicki's face. I hugged her tightly against me and then sat her on a chair and brought her a glass of water. Geoff went stolidly on watching the hamburgers cook.

"You O.K., G?" I asked him, kneeling by Vicki's chair and smoothing back her hair.

He didn't turn around. "I'm O.K.," he said. "She will be, too. You better go on back out."

I didn't want to leave either of them. It seemed at that moment that they had scarcely entered my thoughts in days, except around the fringes of the only thing I truly thought of—cancer. They needed me more than Ben and Dolly. Anything and everything I had done with them for weeks had been purely perfunctory. And while I had been going through the motions of parental care, and the buying of school clothes, and shopping for their meals, they had been going through emotional crises alone. How deep those crises were, I could not even imagine at that time. But I would learn, almost as painfully as they had had to, that cancer is no respecter of "the immediate family." It strikes and scars them all and the scars remain for years.

Vicki's anguish was subsiding. She sat dull-eyed, her face still flushed from tears, and stared at nothing. "I love you, baby," I told her. "Please don't worry. It will turn out all right."

I patted her head. "I'll just be outside if you need me," I told my children, knowing as I walked away that outside was just where I shouldn't be. Not knowing what to do, I did the easy thing that night. I walked away from them and into the adult world where grief, I thought, was handled more discreetly.

But I was wrong again.

Ben had, in my interval in the kitchen, come to no better terms with Connie's illness than had Vicki. I had never seen him crushed by grief, unable to summon emotional command. As I came out to the terrace, Ben rose. "I'll get you a drink, kiddo," he said. "We've heard the whole story. I'm going to get myself another drink, too. You want one, Dolly?" he asked his wife.

Dolly shook her head. "It wouldn't help," she said.

"Don't I know it?" Ben asked. "I've tried to go through practically a whole fifth of Scotch and I can't feel any relief at all."

"Don't tell Pete Kriendler and the others in New York just yet," Connie said. "I intend to beat this thing if there's a way. I'll let them know when things look up."

"If you get the word to go to Palo Alto and aren't around town or in for any dinners or meetings, what am I supposed to tell them?" Ben asked. "What do I answer when somebody says, 'Where's Ryan?' "

Connie smiled. "Tell them I'm rewriting *The Last Battle*," he said.

⸗ 8 ⸗

DR. BAGSHAW'S LETTER in response to the request of Drs. Neligan and Jewett arrived on September 22, 1970. In it, Bagshaw wrote that an appointment had been set up for Connie for Tuesday, October 6, at 8:30 A.M. The letter requested that Connie bring his slides and any films for review. Bagshaw preferred to do a metastatic series and possibly other scans at Stanford University Medical Center. In response to a question in Pat's letter as to how long treatment, if feasible, would take should Connie decide to stay in California, Dr. Bagshaw replied that Connie would "probably be treated as an outpatient during his length of therapy which would be approximately 9 weeks total."*

If Connie opted for treatment in California he would be without the mountains of research, interviews, war diaries, army documents, and other historical files he needed for over two months. It would be physically impossible to move everything he would require for work to some small office or room three thousand miles away for that length of time. It would also be difficult not to arouse suspicions, as Ben had pointed out, on the part of friends and associates about his prolonged absence. *Bridge* could not be the excuse. Its research had long been completed. It was Connie who decided at one of the Neligan-Ryan "combat councils," as we had come to call our meetings, that he would see Dr. Bagshaw, find out all he could about the linear accelerator and how its use might help his condition, and then return home before committing himself to anything.

During September, while waiting to hear from California, Connie saw Dr. Whitmore twice more—on Thursday, September 17, and again on Monday, September 21. He brought Dr. Whitmore up-to-date on his conference with Dr. Jewett and on his plan to see Bagshaw. Whitmore appeared to feel that Bagshaw's technique was a good one, but Connie's impression was that Whitmore was concerned by the idea of radiation, as Connie put it, "being fired into the body even under controlled circumstances." Still, according to Connie's notes, Whitmore said that Bagshaw had ten years of statistics, whereas Whitmore's implant method (the precise placing of

---

* Since Dr. Bagshaw says that the treatment by linear accelerator would have taken 7½ weeks, his letter to Pat must have referred to the additional time it would take to study various tests, X rays, scans, and the like.

radiation seeds into the prostate) had only a three-year history. Largely because of the lengthy records Bagshaw had
compiled, or so Connie felt, Dr. Whitmore did encourage
Connie to make the trip to Palo Alto to discover, after tests
had been made at Stanford, if the Bagshaw method was
practical for Connie. The decision about how and where to
work on *Bridge* would have to be postponed until we knew
more.

Dr. Whitmore's follow-up notes of those two visits stated
that Connie

is still troubled by the fact that his discharge persists . . . and . . . by
soiling of his underclothes."

Connie had said nothing to me in weeks about this, although
the daily laundry, his frequent showers, the purchases of new
undergarments, were all still going on. In some way I must
have rationalized those activities as I had so many other
things. They had become commonplace to me. They were
obviously anything but commonplace to Connie. In his notes
Whitmore also mentioned Connie's plan to see Dr. Bagshaw
and that he had received a copy of Dr. Jewett's notes of our
September 1 visit to Baltimore.

Following his careful plan of close observation, Whitmore
reported no interval changes on abdominal and genital examinations, no bone pain, sciatica, peripheral edema, or
weight loss. He drew a new diagram of the prostate and
wrote:

The gland is generally small. The right lobe is somewhat more
prominent than the left with the ridge of first degree induration
[hardened tissue] along the right lateral border of the gland extending from apex to the base and with very slight smooth thickening
along the right margin of the seminal vesicle . . . prostatic massage
produced abundant secretion which was microscopically loaded
with pus cells.

Under "IMPRESSION" Dr. Whitmore wrote:

Stage C carcinoma of the prostate.* Prostatitis. He will take daily sitz bath and . . . tetracycline [an antibiotic] . . . every 8 hours for 10 days.

CORNELIUS

Friday, October 2, 1970.

The die is cast. I leave in three days for California with very mixed feelings. I hope and I am afraid to hope. Today I went to a conference in New York with Paul [Gitlin] and the representatives of my German publisher. They are excited about the prospect of *Bridge* and anxious to know my target date. So am I. The best and most honest thing I could do was to say that I needed more time to rethink and restudy certain aspects of "Market-Garden." Then I had to explain that Market-Garden was the Allied code name for the drive through Holland to capture the Arnhem bridge and springboard across the Rhine into Germany. The book gets better every time I tell it. If I could only get it down as easily on paper as

---

* Stage and Grade of prostatic cancers are confusing for the simple reason that urologists themselves attach different meanings to them. Not until 1922 did the late Dr. Broders of the Mayo Clinic provide a scale for the urogenital profession to follow. The tumors were divided into Grades I through IV—the first, the least malignant; the last, the most malignant. Grades II and III lay somewhere in between. The Stage of the tumor indicates the actual extent of spread and, like Grade, is separated into four categories—A, B, C, D. In general, according to assessments by Whitmore around 1956, Stage A was a tumor not observed on examination but found by tissue biopsy. Stage B was a tumor with metastases or spread, seemingly confined to the prostate. Stage C was a locally extensive tumor beyond the prostate but, as yet, without sign of spread elsewhere; and Stage D stood for cases that showed clear metastases. Further work is still being done on staging and grading of prostatic tumors. For example, a Stage B I cancer would probably indicate to most urologists a small, isolated nodule, now generally thought to be the only category in which a radical prostatectomy could be effective. Whitmore put no grade on Connie's report at the time he made the notes above, and the American Joint Committee for Cancer Staging and End Results Reporting is not speedy about publishing conclusions. In view of new and changing methods of treatment, perhaps that is just as well. However, I take Dr. Whitmore's evaluation of Monday, September 21, 1970, to mean that Connie's cancer was locally extensive, had gone beyond the prostate itself but had not shown demonstrable spread. He had probably never been a candidate for a radical prostatectomy even at the time of the biopsy on July 23, sixty-one days earlier.

I can talk about it, most of my worries about that aspect of my life would be over.

Later I talked alone with Paul and brought him up-to-date on the medical findings, including the fact that, if Bagshaw thought I was a good candidate for his fascinating linear accelerator treatment, I might be away for some time. He feels that if the treatment can work, I should forget about the book temporarily and go ahead with Bagshaw. Then, maybe I can come home and work the way I know I should. With luck I might even finish the book next year. That thought is incredible in light of the fact that for weeks now I've been feeling I might never last long enough to do it, but first my meeting with Dr. Jewett and now, the prospect of learning more of Bagshaw's treatment methods have almost turned my life around.

Before I began this tape I called Herb Caen in San Francisco. Herb, a columnist for the *San Francisco Chronicle*, is one of my closest friends. His contacts in the Bay Area are so numerous that it would be impossible for me to go to Palo Alto without Herb learning about it. I wanted him to hear it from me. Besides, I can't imagine being in that area at any time without seeing Herb.

All I've told him is that I've got to be in San Francisco, that I want to see him, and would he make a reservation for me at a hotel beginning Monday, October 5? Of course he would, he said. Now all I have to do is get through the weekend. Geoff's gone back to prep school with strict admonitions to keep his nose clean and his grades up. I know the boy can do it, but will he? I've spent a whole summer worrying about myself and still not getting to the bottom of what troubles that lad. Vicki now knows about my condition. Last week before her birthday I asked her what she wanted as a present. She said, "I want you to get well." It damn near broke me up. I'll try my hardest for that little girl. I've never let her down yet and I don't intend to start now. There's got to be a way to win this battle and I intend to find it.

Friday, October 9, 1970.

I am aboard a United Airlines plane headed for home. So much has happened in such a short space of time that I haven't used the tape recorder until now. I haven't wanted to put what I've learned on tape. Not even to this mechanical device do I have any desire to speak about my feelings. I know there is nothing worse than self-pity but that's all I've got left. That, and anger at fate. So I might as well transcribe what I've written in my notebook. It, at least, contains the facts as impersonally as I could jot them down and maybe here, in the plane, amid the usual noise and interference, I can force myself to record what I lacked the courage to do in the quiet of my hotel room in San Francisco. Thankfully, I've got a seat to myself, so there is privacy at least. I want to get the events of these five days on tape before I land in New York because I want to be as calm as possible when I get home. There is no point in going to pieces there again, although I don't know if I can avoid letting Katie and Pat see how much this trip and its findings have affected me. They already know from my phone calls that all the hope I had at the start of this California venture has been crushed once more. I am frankly beginning to wonder what is the use of going on. I suppose the same old cliché applies. I'm going on because I must.

On Monday, October 5, I flew to San Francisco. I brought with me interviews from soldiers now living in the Bay Area in hope that, in the time between hospital visits, I could elaborate on their records and thus keep at least a part of *Bridge* going even as I was delving into the West Coast medical research. I tried to read through their interviews on the trip out and to decide how close each was to the areas in which I would have to be. I could not keep my mind on the interviews. My feelings during that flight were not totally sanguine. If the Bagshaw method was the only one that could be used to eliminate this malignancy, I might be staying in California for weeks. What would that mean to Katie and Vicki at home, to Geoff away at school? What expenses would be involved? Would a new life-style be required? I could not even begin to anticipate the answers. There was no way I could anticipate anything until I saw Dr. Bagshaw.

In San Francisco, I found that Herb had arranged for me to stay at the Mark Hopkins Hotel. Not only had he done his duty well as a friend, he had gone a bit further. The management gave me a suite, beautiful and spacious. I should have lectured Herb about such opulence. If Katie and the children had been along, the suite would have been perfect. But I can think of times when Herb and I would have been happy to catch a few minutes sleep on the ground. I telephoned my old friend as soon as I was settled in and made arrangements to meet him and his wife for dinner

At a new restaurant Herb wanted to check out I told him I had something important to get off my chest. We waited until his charming wife, Maria Theresa, crossed the room to say hello to somebody at another table and then I told Herb about the malignancy. His face changed totally. He immediately ordered us each a double martini. I don't drink martinis as a rule but somehow this one was something more than a drink. It was yet another bond of our friendship.*

Tuesday, the sixth, was the day on which my hopes had now been pinned for thirty-six long days, ever since our conference with Dr. Jewett in Baltimore. In spite of the late hours Herb and I had kept the night before, reliving the war

---

* Kathryn: I sent Herb Connie's references to him and his family. Herb wrote back: "I was touched by Connie's . . . warmth and his incredible memory for details. I remember well and sadly his extreme agitation when he arrived. . . . I had seen him on and off for years, enough to know that he was always in a state of excitement and usually elation. . . . I had never seen him this way . . . and the reason soon became tragically clear. As always he was utterly frank about his condition, his feelings, his pain, his hope—yes, and his lack of hope. And yet he was impeccably thoughtful, never harping . . . on what he was going through, making no demands for sympathy, asking only that we be with him and . . . support him with our friendship. Friendship—the word and the deed and all that friendship entails meant much to him . . . it always had."

and the grand and sad moments since, I was up at 6:00 A.M. and, with a road map of San Francisco and the Northern Peninsula, I attempted to chart my course to Stanford University Medical Center. I had rented a Hertz car the night before, and shortly after 6:30 A.M., I set out to drive the thirty-five miles to see Bagshaw. About an hour later I was in the quiet, beautiful warmth of Palo Alto. The medical center is a magnificent building, much more modern than anything I know of in the East. Inside, I went down through various departments until I came to one ominously marked Radiation Therapy Department. At the receptionist's desk I was told that I was expected, as Bagshaw had written, for an 8:30 A.M. appointment. It was then 8:15 A.M.

There were numerous forms to be filled out and then I was given a folder containing quite a lot of papers and asked to wait in a small, attractive room nearby. Within minutes I was joined by a resident doctor who introduced himself as Roger Miercort. I followed him into an examining room, and, during a physical, I was asked by Dr. Miercort to bring him up to date on my condition. I told him the entire story beginning back in April with the onset of the prostatitis in Saint Martin. From there I briefly described the sequence of events starting with my visits to Pat Neligan, from Neligan to the first urologist, from him to Dr. Joseph Ward. From Ward to Whitmore, from Whitmore to Jewett, back to Whitmore, and now to Bagshaw. Even as I was going through the recital, it began to sound a little like the old Abbott and Costello routine about "Who's on first?"

After the physical and yet another rectal examination, the door opened and Dr. Bagshaw came in. I could not have been more surprised by his appearance. The extent of his reputation is formidable when compared to his youth. He is just forty-five. One wonders how he has accomplished so much in such a short time. By the mid-fifties he was already specializing in radiotherapy and had moved steadily up the ladder in that field. He was on an ad hoc committee for NASA to evaluate astronauts' electron exposure, a member of the advisory committee on radiation therapy for the Los Alamos Meson Physics Facility, and had held positions on radiation study programs and cancer commissions on national and international levels. I didn't find this out at the time. I had looked up Bagshaw before ever leaving home.

None of those facts prepared me for the man himself. Bagshaw, in spite of his rather awesome credentials in his field, is totally without pretensions, earnest, and obviously devoted to his specialty. He was born in Michigan but spent nine years in college and medical school at Wesleyan and Yale universities. His wife, Muriel, I learned, is from Connecticut. She is a pediatrician who is also an expert on the brain functions of the rhesus monkey, the same species used in space research. In our conversation it came out that this serious-minded young man also likes to fly gliders and builds them in his garage. He gave me a very thorough examination including, once again, the dreaded rectal probe. By this time my rear end was beginning to feel as though everybody but a man with a pile driver had had a damn good look at this cancer of mine. After several months of such examinations, I was more than a little sensitive in that area.

After Dr. Bagshaw was finished I was asked to sit in the waiting room. There, I began to feel a morbidity I had not experienced previously. There were other patients waiting in the area. On some, sections of their heads had been shaven, and stenciled on the bald areas were red marks. I learned that these marks were the target points for the linear accelerator beam to cancer of the brain. Fortunately if I was going to be stenciled, my clothes would cover the marks. Notwithstanding, I began to sense the agony, embarrassment, and pain of the people in that room. Marked by red lines or not, I had a kinship with those patients. We shared a ghastly disease—and it was made all the more horrible here by seeing the areas in which cancer could and does strike, leaving human beings without dignity, exposing their vulnerability for everyone to see. The desperate perceptions of our lives, so hard for us to bear, can never truly be understood by those who don't have cancer. Not even by the specialists who work to save us.

I was jotting notes along these lines when Bagshaw came in and asked me to join him in his office. There, we had a very long talk. My slides had by now been examined and, through preliminary testing, the men at Stanford agreed on what all the other specialists had confirmed: I had cancer of the prostate. "But," said Bagshaw, "we feel that you are a perfect case for us here. You are only fifty. By bombarding the area with atomic particles by means of the linear accelerator we can not only reduce but kill off the cancer."

My hopes rose, but I was still concerned about the length of time of the treatment—nine weeks.* Each day I would come to the University Center. I would stand nude on a turntable, embarrassingly exposed to a couple of nurses. But the nine-week program was my greatest concern. I would have to move to Palo Alto for over two months. My problem was whether or not the logistics were feasible, whether or not medically I should do it. I could not possibly move all the research for *Bridge* out there, and what was my family to do in the long weeks I would be away? Psychologically, I was not at all prepared to sit for nine weeks, daily watching the other cancer victims waiting their turn with the linear accelerator as I would await mine. Those pathetic, stricken peo-

---

* The misconception of the treatment time has been explained earlier. Dr. Bagshaw offers a supporting theory. "In the course of a long conversation having to do with explaining the nature of the disease process and the treatment options that are open to the patient, there are often many misconceptions. This seems to be particularly true when a patient has taken an avowed interest in finding out as much as possible about his disease.... This often generates preconceived notions which become increasingly difficult for the patient to deal with.... Connie somehow concluded that our treatment program would have been for nine weeks. In fact, our program is 7 ½ weeks, and while that is only a bit shorter than 9 weeks, if one has a fixed notion that it might be 5 weeks, then perceives that it might be 9 weeks, 9 weeks is apt to be unacceptable because it is twice as long. On the other hand, 7 ½ weeks might have been a more comfortable period of time."

ple! I noticed, by the way, that they seemed either young or quite elderly. I appeared alone in my age group. Bagshaw made that point himself: it was most unusual to find a man of fifty suffering from cancer of the prostate.

The doctor asked me to think over his outline for treatment and then told me that the following day they would begin a series of X rays, including a new kind of test called a lymphangiogram.* The X rays would include a total metastatic series, meaning that the bones would be X-rayed to determine if the cancer had penetrated into the bone marrow. Apparently when and if this occurs, there is little they can do because death is then only a question of time.

Bagshaw explained more about the linear accelerator and how it works. The tumor site is accurately located, graphed, and opaquely marked so that the radiation is given only to the small volume of tissue involved. The bladder is elevated out of the treatment field and the testes are not exposed to radiation. Only the prostate gland lies within the field of the accelerator beam. The patient stands on a turntable which revolves a full 360 degrees, and his position is fixed so that the prostate is at the direct center of the axis of rotation. Usually 150 to 200 rads per day are given until a total dose of 7500 rads is reached.

To me, it sounded like a fascinating procedure, and certainly it seemed the most sophisticated choice I had been given. No surgery was involved. All that was required was that I stand on the turntable while the radiation dose was concentrated to the prostate. Yet, I wondered if I would still run the risk that the cancer might not be killed off. This was a question I felt I had to face and decide on my own. About 1:00 P.M. I drove slowly and thoughtfully back to San Francisco and the Mark Hopkins. I went to my room, stretched

---

* Dr. Bagshaw wrote that Connie was among the first patients to have a lymphangiogram. "It was such a perfect example of a positive test . . . it was subsequently published." See G. H. Fletcher, *Textbook of Radiotherapy* (Philadelphia: Lea & Febiger, 1973).

out on the bed, and thought it all over again. Then I called Pat and Katie and told them both all I had been able to learn.

As a professional, Pat was fascinated by the news. Katie was simply worried about me but willing to go along with whatever I decided. It was the first trip she had not made with me, and, while I am glad she was spared the sight of many of the other patients, I sorely missed not being able to talk this over with her, face to face. I told Pat that Dr. Bagshaw had promised to telephone him and would send him papers on the Bagshaw method so that Pat would understand more of it. Pat wondered about the aftermath of the radiation, what effects such as bleeding, nausea, or diarrhea might occur. But he insisted that I have all the tests Bagshaw proposed before attempting to arrive at a decision.

The following morning, October 7, I again drove out to Stanford, and there began a day of tests unlike any I had ever gone through before. I was X-rayed from head to toe, moving from department to department for each portion of the tests. For the bone scan, a radioactive isotope, strontium 85, was injected in a vein. This isotope is a species of atom used as a tracer in medicine. After the injection, technicians began the bone scan. It involves a machine that moves very slowly back and forth across the body, recording on photographic plates the emission of radioactive waves from the tracer as it makes its way through the body. The plates show whether or not cancer is present or concentrated in any areas of bone. The process was laborious and uncomfortable because one has to lie on one's stomach for as long as an hour without any movement as the bone-scanning device does its work.

The metastatic series was next. Like the bone scan, if the cancer had diffused—spread into organs or tissue beyond the prostate—here was a way they would find it. My feet, head, torso, and legs were X-rayed. I went from one department to another—even to one in which three-dimensional X-ray photographs of my body were taken. These tests seemed to go on forever, and I found myself becoming more depressed by the minute. In part, this was due to my very presence in a world I did not understand; and nuclear medicine experts have neither the time nor, I think, the inclination to bring a layman up-to-date on exactly what they are doing at the moment and why. The processes, so natural to them, are bewildering to a patient. Seeing their concentration I did not want to interrupt their work with questions that would have been not only disruptive but abysmally uneducated.

I signed a hospital form giving permission for the doctors to do the relatively new test called the lymphangiogram. Pat Neligan had recently read about it and he had urged that, because Bagshaw's people were doing this work, I should certainly have it. Independently Dr. Bagshaw had reached the same conclusion, perhaps even before our talk the day before. To my mind, it is an incredible test. Its very name tends to fill one with awe, and while my flagging spirits were not exactly whipping up again, I approached this procedure with intense curiosity, along with my usual apprehension.

To my surprise the site of the operation was my feet. First they were shaved and painted with disinfectant. Novocain was injected and then a surgeon made an incision across the top of both feet. Tiny little catheters were placed through the incisions into the dorsal lymphatics. These small vessels are not unlike thin-walled veins, with valves which carry fluid into the bloodstream by means of lymphs. Fluids that ooze out from the blood vessels into the tissues are sort of sucked up by the lymphatics and taken back to the blood. Unlike blood, the fluid in the lymphatics moves in only one direction—up—going from small capillaries to the main trunk and then to large veins in the body. Lymph nodes are little knots in the cords or chain of lymphatics which filter material to the bloodstream. Nodes can be as small as the head of a pin or larger than a walnut. One of their functions is to keep bacteria out of the bloodstream. But sometimes they misbehave. They can stop cancer cells or, often, they can turn out to be storehouses for cancer. Bagshaw's incredible test would determine what my body's lymphatics and the nodes were up to.

An oily solution called Ethiodol, a compound with an iodine base, was injected through the little catheters to be carried up into the lymphatics system. As the solution moves along, a fluoroscope tracks the slow movement of the oil and its behavior along the way, including its findings of the appearance, size, and placement of the lymph nodes. This incredible test usually takes about two hours. In my case, it went on for five. The time, the pain, the mounting boredom are all very hard to take. Had I not been comforted and attended to throughout that time by an expert technician, I don't know if I could have kept control.

Finally, the test was finished. I had five sutures across the top of one foot and six along the other. The long, fearsome, but fascinating day of tests was over—leaving me with two bandaged feet and the awkward prospect of driving back to San Francisco. I wasn't sure I could manage but I was finally able to get on my loose-fitting brogues and make the trip.

Whether it was fatigue from the tests or a residue of pain, the drive back to San Francisco seemed to produce a deepening despondency in me. By the time I arrived at the Mark Hopkins that depression had turned into something approaching terror. I was so concerned that I left a call for Dr. Miercort, Bagshaw's assistant, in the hope that he would be able to tell me if cancer had invaded the bones. Strangely, despite the ever-present reminder of the lymphangiogram due to my painful feet, I gave that test very little thought. Perhaps I should have. It was to produce the most ominous news of all.

That Wednesday evening I didn't call Katie or Pat. Instead I went to Herb Caen's house and there, with Herb and his family, including his young son, Christopher, I began to feel better. I was among my own kind, back in the world I knew and with people I loved. We had a marvelous evening, so splendid, in fact, that Herb opened a bottle of rare and won-

derful wine. On past trips to Europe with other correspondents to visit battlefields, we had had a standard routine. In
any bistro Bill Hearst would yell "Encore de booze" at a
startled French barman and we would sit discussing "adequate little breakfast wines" with all the pretend snobbish-
ness of the true connoisseur. Herb's bottle was no "little
breakfast wine." Its bouquet and grandeur were superb.
Having associated with battle-wise reporters bent on scoop-
ing one another constantly for so many years, I was both
touched and awed by Herb's bottle. When a reporter gives
away anything, particularly his best wine to a colleague,
there is no greater love in the world.

On Thursday, October 8, I left early for the drive to Palo
Alto. There is no real problem in getting there once one is
familiar with the roads. I was taking this into account because
I could foresee the possibility of spending nine weeks going
back and forth those thirty-odd miles if I opted for Bagshaw's
radiation method. I reached the Medical Center quite early,
went downstairs, and after a small wait, I was called in to
meet with Dr. Bagshaw and Dr. Miercort.

It was then that I learned the disastrous news.

The lymphangiogram had disclosed two nodes, one of
them about eighteen inches away from the prostate on the
right side, the other on the left, which gave every indication
of being what Dr. Bagshaw called "abnormal," meaning that
perhaps they, too, were malignant. God! The fear with which
I heard those words! I hope my face didn't show the terror
that nearly engulfed me.

I listened intently as Dr. Bagshaw explained that this
meant that instead of firing a needle-point type of atomic
particle discharge to areas of the prostate centimeter by centimeter, he would have to open up his lens, in effect, and
eradicate an area running from the abnormal nodes to the

prostate itself. In his opinion I would first require surgery to determine by biopsy if these nodes were malignant. Then would come the radiation, its extent dependent on the biopsy findings. I asked Malcolm what all this really meant. He said, "Well, malignancy in the nodes is really lethal." That was the term he used.

"How much time does that give me?"

"Well, maybe three years if you do nothing," Dr. Bagshaw said. He added that, in his opinion, if the nodes were indeed malignant it meant that I had had cancer for more than two years. I willed myself to stay calm but I don't think I convinced Malcolm.*

He asked me to his house, not far from the University Hospital. Muriel, his wife, is a charming woman, and I enjoyed meeting his children, including a son who appeared to be close to Geoff's age. Malcolm showed me the new sailplane he was building in his garage with which he hoped to capture the championship or whatever it is they have for sailplanes. All of this was psychologically of therapeutic value to me. Malcolm made some very hefty martinis and, as I had done

---

* Of this meeting, Dr. Bagshaw wrote: "I have no doubt this attribution (to me) [Connie's tape of the conversation above and the medical findings] is correct . . . The simple statement as quoted, however, does not tell the whole story. . . . It is true that once a malignancy has been detected in a lymph node, it clarifies the relative aggressiveness of the malignancy and, in all likelihood, the disease will progress to a fatal outcome. . . . What is left out of the statement is that many types of malignancy with appropriate treatment . . . can be cured even though [they have] spread to lymph nodes . . . obviously I was offering Connie a type of treatment which would have addressed the disease in the lymph nodes and which would have been carried out at least with the potential expectation of cure. . . . Also he states that I said he might have 3 years to live if he did nothing. This indicates . . . we were discussing . . . the pros and cons of doing nothing vs. the pros and cons of treating his neoplasm. As I recollect, he had pointed out that he was very busy writing, and rather than take time out for treatment he might wish to simply pursue his writing and let nature take its course. I tried to dissuade him from this approach since, in my view, his cancer, although now deposited in lymph nodes as well as primary in the prostate gland, still had not metastasized throughout his body as far as we could tell. It was my opinion then, and still is, that prostatic cancer at that point in its evolution is still treatable. . . . Connie says that I opined that he had had his cancer for more than two years. Again, I doubt if I was quite that dogmatic. I may have offered two years among a number of possibilities, but I don't know now how one can predict the duration of prostatic cancer when it is discovered sometime along the way in its evolution. I am sure I did not know then how long the cancer had been present."

on my first evening in San Francisco with Herb, I drank one. I needed it more on that evening than I had when I had first arrived in California.

Muriel Bagshaw insisted that I stay to dinner. We had a wonderful evening. Being there with him and his family I had an intense desire to come back to Palo Alto, if only as an onlooker, because I believe Bagshaw is on the threshold of twenty-first-century medicine. His radiation machines may be the answer to many of the problems in treating cancer today. He believes that he can cure people with his extraordinary methods and frankly, I think that is true.*

I left the Bagshaws knowing I had some very serious thinking to do. The lymphangiogram and the findings it unearthed had unsettled me completely. I was floundering in a sea of indecision, but all the time I kept thinking about *Bridge* and how logistically impossible it would be to transport its material to California for even a longer time now than I had first imagined.

Back at the Mark Hopkins, I called Neligan and Kathryn and told them the news, rather baldly, I'm afraid. Each of them tried to be soothing but their voices were giveaways. My "little problem" now sounded very ominous indeed. I told Katie I would see her the following day. The tests were ended. Now I had to go back and think out what to do. I had to find a way to get everything done in a place that was best for me to be. But I think I knew already that I would go back to the East Coast and try whatever Willet Whitmore could come up with. I couldn't pull my family out to California, uprooting them for however much time Malcolm's treatments might now take, and I couldn't work on *Bridge*'s vast material

---

* Connie's evening with the Bagshaws was apparently as pleasant for them as it was helpful for him. As Dr. Bagshaw wrote: "Connie made a very great impression on me . . . We seemed to develop an instant rapport . . . I think by the time we went home . . . I had completely stepped out of the role of physician and was simply a friend offering a port of call in a storm . . . we talked about many things . . . I don't recall that we talked very much about either his disease or his possible treatment . . . We left most of those matters at the hospital . . ."

piecemeal. I had to be surrounded by it and by the ambience of my own home and office. But I still didn't know if I could save my life and I don't think anybody else did either.

My last call, like my first, was to Herb. I told him briefly what had happened and said that I was leaving for home the following morning. It was late but he came around and we had a drink together. We didn't say good-bye. Even if I was a condemned man, and right then the odds were looking higher by the minute, I'd never say good-bye to Herb.

KATHRYN

About 8:00 P.M. on Friday, October 9, 1970, Vicki and I heard the familiar two hoots on the horn—the signal that Connie was home again. This time I didn't wait for him inside the foyer. Vicki and I ran down the front steps, reaching for him before he could step out of the limousine. He embraced us both and then stood up between us, his arms around our waists.

"Nearly forgot this time, Katie," he whispered to me and reached back into the car to bring out his briefcase. He turned to Vicki.

"There wasn't a lot of time this trip to bring surprises," he told her.

"I don't care," she said.

"Well, if you don't care, I'll just forget about it," he teased her. But he handed her his briefcase anyway. "Take it on up to the house." She scampered away, and Connie and I walked slowly up the steps behind the driver carrying the single suitcase. I looked at Connie carefully. I had never seen his face so tired and drawn. His customary energy and zeal were totally missing. There was a pinched look to his face and fine lines etched beneath his eyes that I had never noticed before.

"I should have come with you," I told him. "It was bad, wasn't it?"

"Yep," he said. "Pretty grim. But I met a lot of good people and Herb was a prince. I'll tell you all about it later. I want to call Pat and find out if he can see us tonight. I've got a lot of things to tell you both and I don't want to have to repeat myself."

"All right," I told him. "I'll call Pat and Vera now."

He and Vicki trooped up the stairs to our bedroom where I telephoned the Neligans. We were to come, said Vera, as soon as we could.

"Did they hurt you, Daddy, out there?" Vicki asked.

"No, baby," Connie said, "but my feet hurt a little. I've got to take my shoes off. I wonder if Neligan will object if I wear my slippers over? I'm sure to get some flak from him about my impeccable attire."

He slowly pulled off his shoes and gently massaged his stockinged feet.

"Let me see," I said and pulled off his socks. Across the tops of his feet were two small bandages. Vicki ran a finger tentatively around the dressings. "Poor Daddy. How did you hurt your feet?" she asked.

"It's part of a test the doctors had to do, Vicki. Never mind about it. Aren't you going to look for your surprise?"

Vicki shook her head. "Not until I tell you I've been bad. The school called Mom." Her blue eyes were angry. "I told you I didn't want to go back there. I don't want to be in school if you get sick. I don't care about them. I don't care if they punish me. They're wrong."

"Whoa, wait a minute," Connie said. "Exactly what did you do?"

I answered for her. "It's called 'disruptive behavior on the bus and in the classroom.' On the bus she used some bad language and in English she was writing notes to people and constantly interrupting the teacher, or so I was told."

Connie drew his daughter close. "Why did you do it, Vick?"

With her head against his chest, she looked across at me.

"Mom never asks me that. She just lectures me and yells sometimes."

"We've got enough to worry about," I told her. "You're a big girl now." She had reached fourteen two weeks before. "It's about time you started assuming a little responsibility. Vicki, no one else can study or concentrate with you trying to be at stage center all the time. And your language on the bus was certainly inexcusable. You haven't been raised to behave like that."

"What did you say?" Connie asked.

"Bad words. But it wasn't only me. It's just me they talk about and call Mom about. Other people get away with anything."

"How old are the other kids on the bus?" Connie wanted to know.

"Some of them are little kids, some my age, and some are older. And the bus driver doesn't like me, and if anyone says anything, the driver never checks to see who did it. They all say it's me—all the kids. And the driver reports that I did it. I don't always, Daddy. But I'm the one who always gets blamed."

"Vick, once you do something wrong, it's hard for people not to keep on blaming you, whether it's you at fault or not. Also, if there are smaller children on the bus, I wouldn't think you'd want them to learn bad language from you. I would think you'd want to protect them from those things."

"The little kids all like me, Daddy. You ask anyone. I help them and I'm kind to them. Some of them I like better than I do the kids my own age. I wouldn't hurt them."

"Then don't use bad language. And the next time the school calls and blames you and you give me your word you didn't do or say anything wrong, I'll handle the problem myself. If you're wrong, you're wrong. But if you're being used or blamed for something that isn't your fault, I'll back you all the way. You understand?" Connie asked. "Just don't ever tell me you didn't do something if you did. But when you're innocent, I'll be damned if anybody's going to accuse you and get away with it."

Vicki put her hand in Connie's. "I'll try to be good. Sometimes when I do something wrong, I get scared, 'cause I know they'll call home and so I fight them and say it wasn't me. But this time it was me. I'm sorry," she told him gently.

"O.K.," Connie said, "then we understand each other."

He started to move around her but she stood her ground. "I have to tell you why I did it this week," she said.

Connie waited.

"You were gone and I knew it was to a hospital and I didn't know what they would do to you, and I prayed to God that they wouldn't hurt you and you'd be all right. And Mom said you'd be all right. She promised." Vicki's voice was rising. "One night you called," she said, "and afterwards Mom hung up and she cried and cried. She shut the door to her bathroom but I heard her and I came up and sat on the floor outside the door. Then I called to her and pretty soon she came out and she said everything was all right. But she went downstairs and walked out in the dark and I didn't know what to do.

"The next day I was mad at everybody. All those silly kids and the prissy ones and the stuck-up ones and all the teachers' favorites and I didn't care what they thought about me. Because you were in a hospital and Mom cried when you called and wouldn't talk. I don't care if they like me at school or not. I just care about you and Mom."

Connie sat back down on the bed and pulled our daughter to him. There were tears in his eyes. "If I promise you that I'm doing the best I can in everything, will you try not to worry?"

Vicki put her hands in his. "You worry and so does Mommy, but I'll try to be better so you won't have to worry about that, too," She kissed us both. "I love you guys very much," she said and then, high-spirited once again, she added, "That message comes to you from a person who wishes to remain unknown at this time."

The present Connie had brought the unknown person was perfume, a bottle for her, another kind for me—my favorite— one he had been giving me for years. I wondered with the mental burdens he was carrying how he had ever thought to bring the gifts, much less take time to buy them. He went to shower and shave and I walked downstairs with Vicki. She had the Neligans' telephone number and Alta, our German shepherd, named after Connie's salmon stream, to guard her. I saw her to her room, kissed her good night, and went to freshen up myself. I knew, without as yet being told, that Connie had reached a decision. He had dug steadily into medical research and done the best that he, as a layman, could do in such a short time to understand the various methods that had been proposed to combat his cancer. Whatever his decision was to be, I trusted the instincts and knowledge that caused him to arrive at a judgment as surely as I trusted his writing. The difference was that he could not rewrite this sentence.

Connie took his briefcase to the Neligans. In it were copies of the lymphangiogram films which Dr. Bagshaw had given him before he left California. Pat studied them intently. The expression on his face was impossible to read.

"Tell us what happened from beginning to end," he told Connie, "and don't leave out a damn thing."

Connie drew out his notebook and read from it, beginning with his first visit to Stanford University Medical Center and ending with his last conversation with Dr. Bagshaw. Vera and I listened as intently as Pat, who interrupted only to say, "Yes, yes. Go on," whenever Connie paused for a moment.

When he had finished, Pat tapped the films he had replaced in the large manila envelope Connie had handed him. "I'm concerned about the idea of using radiation now that the nodes are involved," he said. "It would lengthen your stay out there. I don't know what the side effects would be, and I don't know, even if this equipment is as sophisticated as you say, how sure anyone can be that surrounding tissue will not be damaged by radiation."

There was silence and then Connie said, "Cancer in the nodes is lethal, right?" Pat stared at him. "They've found several nodes that are abnormal," Connie said. "Nobody's saying they're cancerous because there's been no biopsy. Well, let's assume they are cancerous. How many others will be in time? And if cancer in the nodes is lethal, how many years have I got? Three? Five? Ten? Six months?" Connie paused. "The diseased ones have got to come out, Pat," he said, "and quite frankly I haven't got the courage to be out in California by myself while Malcolm tries to get them all, plus the prostate, with his linear accelerator. I don't know how severe the aftereffects of radiation are, but I'd rather learn about them here with the people I love than to be by myself. Here, I can at least work on the book. There, without Katie or the kids or you, I really think I'd go to pieces because there'd be nothing but my problem to occupy my mind. I can't take the book there and right now the book is everything to me." He took a sip of the bourbon Vera had placed beside him. "You're getting on the phone to Whitmore. Tell him I'm coming in on Monday to talk all this over. Whatever has to be done is going to be done at Memorial. I feel a little guilty about Malcolm because I really believe in him, but I don't know if even Malcolm could bring this off, now that it's almost a sure bet the lymphatics have been invaded."

"I'd rather have you here," Pat said, "but all along the decision has been up to you. I agree with your reasoning."

"Well, by God, it's the first time then, Neligan," Connie said. "So we go with Whitmore and we get this thing done as soon as we can and then, my lady," he turned to me, "I get this book off the ground." He was pensive, staring into his glass. Then he looked at each of us and smiled. "I have to get the book done," he said. "I took along the addresses of some of the men in California who sent in interviews for *Bridge* and I called a few of them. One was an engineer who'd been with the 82nd Airborne—one of the men who rowed Cook's men across the Waal River to help us take the Nijmegen bridge, just a few kilometers from Arnhem where the big bridge is. I asked him what he thought about that operation. You know, it was one of the most incredible, daring feats any airborne outfit ever brought off, and they suffered terrible casualties. I asked him what went through his mind when he knew he was going to have to make that trip across the river. Know what he said?" Connie riffled through his notebook, and stopped on a page. "He said, 'I figured I was dead as soon as I heard about the order, so I forgot about it and just did the job.' "

Connie looked at Pat. "Let's get on with it, Neligan," he said. "I've got a book to write."

$\stackrel{=}{=} 9 \stackrel{=}{=}$

ON MONDAY, OCTOBER 12, 1970, Connie saw Dr. Willet Whitmore, and a decision was made for him to enter Memorial Hospital on Sunday, October 18, one week later. Strangely, neither Connie nor Whitmore appear to have made many notes of this meeting. From Whitmore I have none at all, and Connie's usual meticulous details are missing both from his tapes and in his notes.

In his appointment book, for the twelfth, he wrote simply,

Saw Whitmore today. Decision on op.

In his tapes he says:

It is decided that I will go into Memorial Sunday, the 18th, for an operation which will consist of the following: an exploration of the entire area; the examination of nodes to see if they are malignant and if so, they'll be taken out; and the implantation of tiny radiation needles or seeds into the prostate itself. This will be done with radioactive iodine (I-125). I wonder if it will be tricky? No matter how one looks at it, this is major surgery and who knows if any of it will work? Anyway, I'm going through with it.

I believe that Dr. Bagshaw's lymphangiogram was probably the deciding factor in determining the speed of scheduling Connie's hospital admittance. The lymphangiogram findings were also, I feel, the basis for Connie's decision to be treated at Memorial, close to home. Normally, Bagshaw's statistics covering a ten-year follow-up on patients treated by the linear accelerator would have weighed more heavily in Connie's mind than Whitmore's three-year statistics using the I-125 implant method. But the node abnormalities disclosed by the lymphangiogram had suddenly made the situation urgent. The suspicious nodes had to be examined— either at Stanford or Memorial—by surgical procedures and quickly. Surgery, all along, had been the one course of treatment that Connie had hoped to avoid. That he had accepted its necessity would seem to stem from Whitmore's opinion that the lymphangiogram films showed that speed was now, indeed, essential; the doctor set the date for Connie's admittance to Memorial only seven days after the October 12 conference.

Sunday afternoon, October 18, 1970, I drove Connie into New York. Close friends had come to stay with Vicki during the day and I had engaged a local, motherly lady to stay with her beginning Monday evening, the nineteenth, the night before Connie was to have the operation, until he was home again.

The drive into town that Sunday was an emotional one for both of us. Connie's tension was building in part, I think, due to his customary reluctance to be anywhere near a hospital. Riding along, he spoke in fits and starts. At one point he said, "I've never felt better. This has got to be some kind of nightmare. If I'm sick, why don't I feel sick?" Still later he asked, "Suppose they muck it up, Katie?" And once, very softly, I heard him say, "I wonder if I'll ever see the land and the hills again." I tried to reassure him, but he was never patient with ignorance and I knew much less than he about his condition, his innermost feelings, and what was involved in the operation.

The admissions office was jammed with patients and relatives and the ambience was anything but cheerful. Connie went to the desk and got his forms, then came back to sit down by me. "I hate this part most," he said. "You're nothing but one piece of rice in a vast rice field, and all the pieces of rice have to be tabulated." I watched as he wrote in the pertinent information and then noticed that he had printed his name as "Ryan, John C." I pointed out what I assumed to be an error. "No," he said. "I don't want publishers or columnists or most people to know. A lot of times reporters check hospitals to see if there's anyone in there who's newsworthy. If anybody gets wind of the fact that I'm in Memorial, the game's up. They'll have me dead before the operation's over. It's a cancer hospital, Katie. Cancer means you're going to die."

"Well, they'd be picking the wrong fellow, this time," I said.

Connie looked at me. "Promise me something," he said.

"Anything."

"Don't ever stop being the way you are. Believe in medicine. Believe I'll get better. Believe we'll get the book done. Whenever I'm down, you keep picking me up."

"But it's true. I do believe you'll lick this thing. Just like you've accomplished everything else you've ever set out to do."

Connie grinned. "If you were talking about anybody else

but me, I'd have my doubts," he said. "But in this case, I do believe you're right."

He finished the forms and then, with a group of other patients and relatives, we were herded onto an elevator. All the patients, armed with folders and papers, got off at one floor. The relatives were let off at other floors as a nurse, clipboard in hand, read out, "Visitors for the following patients ———, floor ———" and then the number. I was the only one left in the elevator when she said, "Ryan, ninth floor." She got off at nine with me and took me to the nurses' station. "This is Mrs. Ryan. Show her to her husband's room."

It was white and rather spacious. The gauzy curtains were clean and blowing from the draft of a partly opened window. The bathroom was rather large, as hospital bathrooms go. There was a desk-bureau combination with a large mirror above, a dark green leatherette chair with footstool to match, a smaller chair upholstered in tan-colored fabric, and a plastic molded chair in yellow. The bed occupied the center of the room, with small tables on each side and a battery of electric outlets and plugs set into the wall above and at each side of the bed. I had plenty of time to study the furnishings; I waited more than an hour for Connie to arrive, using some of the time to unpack from his suitcase pajamas, robe, and slippers which I put beside the bed. His toiletries I put into the bathroom and laid some military books he wanted to study on one of the bedside tables. But there was nothing I could do to make this utilitarian place like home. I wished I had thought to bring flowers or a few photographs to make the place warmer, more acceptable to Connie.

Finally, he came in, coat over his shoulders, carrying his briefcase. "Damn bureaucracy," he said. "In spite of all the records I brought with me, in spite of all the tests I've got, I had to go through all the basic routines again. Do you know how crazy this all is?" He was obviously warming up to a hospital-hatred speech. "The girl who took my weight and height was absolutely unable to do the height. She didn't know how to use the angular measuring stick that runs up in front of the scale. I had to show her how to use the thing. Then there were blood tests and more X rays. By now there must be more X rays of me than Hollywood has film on *Ben Hur*. It's sickening. Let's get the hell out of here and go back home and play some golf."

He didn't even look around the room. Instead he sat down in the leatherette chair and filled out the patient's clothes list. But he did not include the one piece of equipment that not even I was to know about—his tape recorder. I did not see him unpack his briefcase, but I had helped him put in *Bridge* plane and glider statistics, maps of the locations of airfields in England—the departure points for the vast armada of planes and gliders that flew to Holland on Sunday, September 17, 1944—and the big folder holding the location maps of the drop and landing zones for the airborne troops who arrived in Holland that same Sunday, then just over twenty-six years before. He hoped to work on this material during convalescence. But he had obviously packed away more. In all the time he was in the hospital I never saw his tape recorder, although I was often to open drawers at his bedside to get out something for him. Obviously the hospital personnel never saw it either. To this day I do not know where or how he managed to secrete it.

We had agreed during the previous week that now some trusted New York friends should be told that Connie would be in the hospital. He had already entrusted the news to Joe Ryle and Bill and Austine Hearst. After leaving him that Sunday I was to go to Suzie and Charles Gleaves's big brownstone on East Sixty-second and tell them, as well. They were dear friends and, because of our problems during the summer, we had avoided seeing them. Now both Connie and I felt they should be apprised of the news.

I got ready to go to the Gleaveses'. The usual hospital routines were already beginning. Nurses and interns were coming in and out, upset that Connie was adamantly refusing to undress, since, "It is certainly not *my* bedtime," and just as adamantly refusing to hand over his cigarettes. Lacking an ashtray he had already begun to fill a water glass with butts and ashes. I had no desire to witness that battle at its height, and besides I knew that Connie would win it. I kissed him good-bye and told him I'd see him the next evening, Monday, when I planned to move into town for the duration of his hospitalization, staying with Paul and Zelda Gitlin, as we had previously arranged. He nodded, seemingly anxious for me to be gone, and asked me to give his love to the Gleaveses.

On Monday, before returning to New York, I saw Pat and Vera. Pat had been invited by Dr. Whitmore to scrub up for the operation. That, I knew, would be of the greatest relief to Connie. He was always much more tractable if Pat was near, and for this major operation, emotionally and therapeutically it could only be good for him. At the Neligans I borrowed a piece of paper and wrote down something for Pat to give Connie. I did not have *The Longest Day* at hand, but I knew that one of Connie's favorite passages from it concerned the predawn flights on D Day, June 6, 1944, of paratroopers coming over the huge fleet of ships carrying infantry toward the beaches. He had worked on that section of *Day* for nearly a week before it pleased him, and I wanted Pat to hand it to him or read it just before his operation on Tuesday morning, October 20. I wrote from memory: "As the formations flew over, lights blinked down to the ships. They flashed the signal everyone would remember this night—3 dots and a dash. The V for Victory."*

Back at home, packing for my stay in town with the Gitlins, I got a call from Ben and Dolly Wright. Ben had been to the hospital later on Sunday night and felt that Connie was in a

---

* Pat read my message to Connie just before my husband was wheeled into the operating room on Tuesday morning. Although Connie was sedated and drowsy, he said to Pat, "she got it wrong." And then he proceeded to quote from memory, " . . . the men of the invasion fleet heard the roar of planes. Wave after wave passed overhead. . . . Nobody could say a word. And then as the last formation flew over, an amber light blinked down through the clouds on the fleet below. Slowly it flashed out in Morse code three dots and a dash: V for Victory."

better mood than the one in which I had left him. The Wrights were flying to Mexico on Tuesday for a few days. They had wanted to change their plans, but Connie and I dissuaded them. Although he had reported that Connie's mood was up, Ben's seemed to be very low.

"He'll be all right, Ben, don't worry," I told him. "Besides, you won't be gone very long."

"It's not that," Ben said, "it's the room he's in."

"It seemed all right to me."

"You remember when Rex died?" Ben asked. Rex Smith, former public relations head of American Airlines, had been a close friend of both Ben and Connie. Now I suddenly remembered that Rex's fatal cancer had been treated at Memorial, too.

"What about it?"

"Nothing," Ben said. "I guess just seeing Connie there got to me the same as when Rex was in."

"He'll be all right, Ben," I repeated. "He's a lot younger than Rex was and he's strong. He'll make it."

"I'll be back as soon as I can," Ben said. "When you go in tonight, see if they can change his room. I'm going back to see him tomorrow afternoon before we leave. I asked at the nurses' desk about transferring him but they didn't have a bed."

"What's all this about the room?"

Ben's voice was so husky, it was hard to recognize. "It's the same room Rex had, Kathy—904."

⹀ 10 ⹀

CORNELIUS

This is Monday night, October 19, 1970, and I am in Room 904 of Memorial Hospital awaiting the operation scheduled by Dr. Whitmore for 8:30 tomorrow morning. It is difficult to record in this place because people keep coming in and out and I have had to put many things into notebooks and then transfer them onto tape whenever I can get any privacy.

Earlier this evening Paul and Zelda Gitlin were here and we had a great talk while waiting for Katie, who is going to stay in their apartment until the operation is over. Thanks to my "brother" Paul, everything is in order—wills, papers, assignments, and the like have been revised and brought up-to-date. Paul and I have told each other, "Of course, none of this is necessary," but it is. We both know it. I have never been unprepared when I went on a trip in the past and this one is imponderable—more so than any journey I have ever made.

I telephoned Vicki a short while ago. She sounded wistful and near to tears, but the woman who is staying with her assures me that everything will go all right. I wanted to hear Vicki's voice just in case I might be unable to speak with her again, and I also tried to get Geoff at his school, but I had no luck in reaching him. Vicki said, "I love you, Daddy," and, of course, I echoed those sentiments and reminded her to try and keep her promises to be on her best behavior while I am away. It is very difficult to speak to one's child when it might be the last time. There are so many things that ought to be said but they would sound maudlin. What if I don't wake up after tomorrow's operation? What if Geoff, Vicki, and Katie are never again in my world, or I in theirs?

It is difficult to exorcise some thoughts.

Paul and Zelda arrived about five this afternoon and even Ben Wright dropped in earlier, even though he is off to Mexico tomorrow. It is very difficult to preserve calmness and self-assurance with one's friends. But I believe that on the whole I have managed fairly well.

Katie got here about 6:00 P.M., a few minutes after Dr. Whitmore dropped in. I had never seen him in a business suit before. He sat on the bed in my smoke-filled room (the nurses are in a constant state of uproar about my cigarettes), and Katie sat on the other side, holding my hand so tightly that it hurt. Everyone was quite lighthearted, and Whitmore told me that my chum Pat Neligan is getting up at 4:00 A.M. tomorrow to be here throughout the operation. Neligan hates to get up in the mornings so if he's grumpy when I see him at 8:15 or thereabouts, it will probably be because he's been up all night anyway with other patients and then tomorrow, which is his day off, he'll be here with me. I plan to be equally bad-tempered and insult him a few times. That ought to bring him round.

My notebook indicates that there have been batteries of people in and out preparing me for this operation. There were interns who came in and tapped my back and chest to see how my lungs are. Technicians have taken enough of my blood to fill a washbasin. Somebody else sat down and took my medical history all over again. It seems to me that each of these things has been done so many times that somebody ought to put them all into a computer and I would not have to keep on repeating myself. I am really quite sick of it all.

Whitmore has brought in his entire team to see me, I think. Dr. Biss Ray, Dr. Nelson Tyrone, and Dr. James Freel are fellows. They've finished training and are now doing research and further study in genito-urology. Dr. Joel Rosenberg, Dr. Alvin Freeman, and Dr. Paul Heller are, I believe, residents. The radiotherapist who will do the I-125 implants is Dr. Basil Hilaris, Each of these doctors has heard or read my case history, and Whitmore and Hilaris have reviewed the operation with me several times. I've tried to understand it but it is damned difficult for a layman. The anesthesiologist is a Scotsman, Dr. Wrightman, and after he administers the anesthesia, I understand his work will be taken over by a charming lady I've met, Miss Flora Dono.

Today two women therapists came in and their function is to teach me how to breathe. The thought seems absolutely weird but the exercise makes a great deal of sense. My abdomen is going to be opened, which means, I think, that certainly tissue and perhaps some muscles have to be cut. Therefore, the ladies warned, if I cough, sneeze, turn, or move, the postoperative effects will be extremely painful. So I was given a lesson in breathing properly. The chief therapist took my right hand, placed it just below her breast on her diaphragm, and said, "Now feel the way I breathe." These people are totally unaware of the self-consciousness a male patient feels when an attractive lady directs one's hand to a placement just below her bosom. But I kept my mind strictly on the lesson and I think I know how to breathe from my diaphragm. The lady said, "When you wake up in the recovery room I will be there and I will remind you again how to breathe. But remember, there is always the danger of pneumonia after an operation if you cannot clear your lungs. As a result—" She left the sentence unfinished, but I understood and rather speedily took cognizance of everything she told me. The hospital personnel are, all of them, annoyed and alarmed by my cigarette consumption. If my smoking harms other patients I will absolutely somehow abandon cigarettes for the time being, but this little room is my domain and, until the entire administration of the hospital comes down on me, I shall continue to smoke while I can, if patients in adjoining rooms are not in jeopardy.

We may all be jeopardized by something entirely different. While Ben Wright was here this afternoon a large package was delivered to me. I unwrapped it to find one of the largest Steuben boxes I've ever seen. A card attached to the handsome red plush exterior said, "For you, kid, from Gleaves and Suzie." Our friends, Charles and Suzanne Gleaves. I opened it at once and inside was a half gallon of bourbon. I never knew that Steuben made glass like that or hollowed it out for something that could carry so much punch. At all events, it was a perfectly charming gift, and Ben finally managed to get it into the lower bureau drawer but not before I had one small drink. I have always admired Steuben. Now I know their reputation is truly deserved. Jack Daniels, "a rather fine Colonial whiskey," as an English friend of mine once put it, tastes even better when it comes from Steuben's distinguished red box.

Throughout the day a young man has been peering in and, at a frown from me, disappearing with lightning speed. He is a priest. I'm trying to intimidate him by glowering at him. "I'll be around if you need me," he stammers each time I glare at his face framed in the doorway. The man I really want to see is Ed Hogan of St. Ignatius Loyola, the priest who married Kathryn and me. Louise and Dan McKeon, good friends, who know most of the Jesuits at St. Ignatius on upper Park Avenue, have been trying to get in touch with Father Hogan. I don't know if there is any kind of rule or directive here that might discourage his presence if a priest is already available, as the young man on my floor most certainly is, but Ed is a friend, intelligent and amusing, and I'd like to see him. However, he has not appeared and this young man has taken to following on the heels of interns and technicians as they make their rounds. In my case, I believe the boy thinks it's the only way he might make it into my room.

It was not very kind of me but one time when he actually got a foot inside the door, following a girl coming to take yet more blood, I said, "Father, I must tell you right now that you're wasting your time around here because I'm not a Catholic. I am a Buddhist." The poor fellow was absolutely shaken because my admittance form read Catholic for religion. I am somewhat ashamed of myself but these little encounters have been my only source of amusement.

He has the same kind of anxious, protective attitude toward me that Katie has. My little Katie is annoyed with Willet Whitmore. Her antipathy toward him began when I drove myself in to see Dr. Whitmore on a couple of occasions prior to the operation. I did it at his suggestion. I think his reasoning is we can speak more freely and that it is better for me psychologically to be on my own when I visit him. The fault in their present lack of communication is really mine. To anyone who doesn't know us, it is impossible to explain the relationship between my wife and me. We are friends, lovers, parents, and a team of writers who work together. Almost our every moment, except when we are apart on research trips, is with the other. I couldn't and wouldn't live without her, although I suspect there are many times she would like to live apart from me. But I am entwined with her. There is no part of me that she doesn't know about or cannot react to. It is very difficult to explain this to a doctor without sounding like some kind of freak. These tapes are the only part of me I have kept from her, and I do that because I cannot bear to inflict anything more on her. But I should have told Willet some details of our relationship. Since he will now be the primary treatment doctor, he ought to know that Katie is not one of those wives who faint at the sight of blood, go into depths of depression at bad news, or leave decisions up to someone else. She may agree with another's decision, but not until she has expressed her own. She does it rather gently most of the time but her message always gets across. I should have told Willet all of that but I didn't, and Katie has felt that she's been kept from the planning of the most important project in our lives. Together we've decided on the methods of dividing the work on the books, we've come to equal agreements on the additions to our house, the children's schools, our vacations—our lives. We've always done everything together, with disagreements along the way, but still each of us knew what the other thought and was up to. There is one area these days in Katie's life that is secret and apart from me, as my tapes are from her. In the absence of any concrete work of mine on *Bridge*, she has been toiling away on a book of her own. God! Am I proud of her for that! But it has come between us a bit. Right now, however, I am glad that she is getting to the crucial windup and will have that to occupy her mind. Otherwise she might really tell Willet that she's "no fragile woman in some kind of gilded cage" as she put it to me a few nights ago. If I wasn't so obsessed with the operation, its details, its probable outcome, and my future and hers, I would have told him by now that she is intuitive and can pick up vibrations faster than anyone I have ever met. But the operation obsesses me and she already has enough on her mind. If I can get through tomorrow, Pat will help us to understand what the future holds and that will relieve Katie's mind, whatever he says. She only gets upset when she doesn't know the truth or it is deliberately kept from her.

As I understand it, tomorrow morning I am going to have a retroperitoneal exploration, a bilateral pelvic node dissection, and an implant of radioactive I-125 seeds into the prostate. What does it all mean? If I'm clear about it, the docs are going to have a look at the area behind or in back of the peritoneum. Now the peritoneum is a thin, moist membrane that completely encloses the abdominal wall and also surrounds or encases internal organs inside the abdominal cavity. If I understand the operating procedure, an incision will be made low down left of the navel, through connecting tissue to the rectus muscles which are two abdominal muscles, one on either side of the body, that run from the pubic bone to the lower part of the sternum.

The surgeons will explore the lower abdominal field. The peritoneum is a shining, transparent lining that contains cells and networks of capillaries and lymphatics—that last word being something I now understand only too well from my visit to Malcolm Bagshaw in Stanford. Then, again if I am correct, they will cut vertically from the loop of the duodenum (the beginning of the small intestine) to a point near where the aorta divides in the abdominal cavity into what are called the right and the left common iliac arteries. I am under the impression that there is not much room for a surgeon to work in that location. It is quite difficult to get to the retroperitoneal lymph nodes that Malcolm Bagshaw found suspicious on his lymphangiogram.

If the nodes Malcolm is concerned about are excised and biopsies prove them cancerous, then dissection of probably quite a lot of nodes will be made, including dissection of pelvic nodes to discover the areas in which malignancy may have occurred. I can't believe I'm going through this. I can't believe cancer can perhaps be so many places. But if I've had this disease for some time, as Malcolm seems to think, then anything is possible.

After all the surgery is completed, Dr. Basil Hilaris will implant the I-125 seeds into the prostate. The only way I can understand the process is to visualize a small bowl of jelly, crosshatched into tiny areas. The radioactive seeds, each probably not much larger than a grain of sand, are precisely placed or shot into the spaces in the jelly. It sounds to me like a procedure calling for a great deal of expertise. I have been warned to expect to suffer radiation sickness but am told that its onset can be programmed and I can anticipate the dates at which nausea and other side effects will occur.

These impressions of what will happen tomorrow are probably inaccurate in some details since I couldn't record them at the time, but basically I think I am right. Thank God I have not told Katie about any of this. The aftermath will be hard enough for her to bear.

I was watching her this evening as she sat holding tight to my hand. Willet, Paul, and Zelda left together. The Gitlins were to wait by the elevator for Katie. I wish she had gone with them with only a wave or a smile because saying goodbye on the eve of an operation to my Katie was not easy. Besides, what more was left to say? We had decided to research this cancer and the decision on treatment was to be mine, as it has been. But suppose I die during the operation? And worse, suppose it doesn't work for very long? I've told nobody, not even Pat or Willet, that I give myself very little chance of surviving more than a few years at most. But if I don't survive tomorrow, did I say enough to Katie before she left? Sure, I told her I loved her. I said that several times. I tried to be gentle and rather casual, all at the same time. I kept reemphasizing things. And what did my girl do? She minimized the entire thing. "Stop thinking it's serious," she told me. "You've made your choice. You've got excellent doctors. You've done it according to the book, CJ." She held me tight and whispered, "If Dr. Cary Grant Whitmore gives me permission, I'll be over tomorrow as quickly as I can, but Pat's coming in and he'll see me right after they're finished getting you back on the road to health. The road rises up to meet you from here on out, CJ. The wind's at your back, and the good God holds you, as He always has, in the hollow of His hand." My Katie is one hell of a lady.

I'm sure it was because of her and what she said that I finally let down the barriers and invited in the young priest the next time he stuck his head in my door. I really had two women responsible for the priest getting a foothold inside my room. My dependable, wonderful Annie Bardenhagen, secretary and friend (she'll never admit to the last part), gave me some rosary beads before I came in here. The very fact that I took them is a sign of how highly I regard Annie. I would have thanked someone else for the offering and left the beads at home, but Annie gave them to me, and I'd be damned frightened not to have brought them with me. Once or twice in these two days when no one was looking I've taken them out. Tonight after everyone was gone I opened my bedside drawer, saw Annie's beads, and decided that the combination of Katie's trust in me and Annie's trust in Someone higher up was too much to overcome. So I had the priest up to my bedside. Close up, I rather liked him. Also, he wasn't as intimidated as he'd been back by the door.

"You want to hear my confession, right?" I asked him.

Very sensibly, according to his lights, he asked, "Don't you think you should make one?"

"Well, Father," I said, "I may as well confess something. I haven't killed anyone. I haven't started any wars. My sense of guilt is different from yours. Why should I go through all this hocus-pocus just to make you relieved?"

He ignored all I'd said. "Have you sinned?" he asked.

"What is sin?" I asked him.

"Have you sinned against God or God's will?"

"Why should I presume to do anything against God?"

"Have you broken the tenets of the church?"

"Are you speaking of the Buddhists, the Jews, the Protestants, the Catholics?" I asked. "Whose tenets? Who do you have in mind? Frankly, I hope I haven't offended any one of them, but I can't be sure."

Right now, as time drains away before tomorrow's operation, I think I behaved correctly for me, but wrongly for him. What I couldn't explain to this young priest is that I believe the Man Upstairs will deal directly with me and I'll know whenever He's displeased, which, by the looks of it, seems to have been rather often this year.

I had to stop taping because the door opened and two men wearing green operating room garb came in about half an hour ago to deliver to me my greatest indignity to date. Almost wordlessly they shaved me from the chest right down to the pubic hairs. I don't remember when I've felt so humiliated. There's no reason for me to feel that way. It's part of the routine in cases like this, but it made me feel helpless and abused. They were quiet, aloof men. The one who did the most of the shaving was careful and expert. Maybe that's his specialty. I noticed that he used a Wilkinson razor. It came from a sanitized, sealed box, and was thrown in with other disposables as soon as he was finished. They cleaned up the room a bit, including my ashtray-*cum*-water glass, and almost immediately a nurse came in and stood over me while I took pills, apparently for sleep and to ward off infection. I will not do that often again. Take pills. Tonight, perhaps, it is essential. But if I survive tomorrow I shall need a clear head for all the rest of the life that God may grant me. I'm a little drowsy now and perhaps not making much sense. I couldn't tell that young priest about God and me. How could I explain to a youngster that I've known the Gent for a long time? We've been through a war together—my first. His—well, who knows how many? But before the pills work and I go off tonight, I want to say, in case Katie ever has to hear these tapes, that I am not afraid. I may "have a rendezvous with death at some disputed barricade." The second to last word is important: the word "disputed."

Come tomorrow, every instinct, every nerve, every fiber in my body has now got the message, I hope that even in anesthesia my mind will dispute that barricade. I will even dispute the Man Upstairs about it—if I have to.

Part Three
THE ATTACK
October 1970–December 1972

$\stackrel{..}{=} 1 \stackrel{..}{=}$

KATHRYN

I lingered in Connie's hospital doorway, reluctant to leave
him and join Paul and Zelda waiting at the elevators. In that
brief moment with only the two of us facing each other and
no need for pretense, his anxiety, like the fear scents given
off by some animals, permeated the space between us. His
uneasiness regarding the hospital and his concern about the
coming operation seemed almost literally tangible. I believe
he was glad to see me go and terrified that I must. He would
be with strangers now, but they were not Connie's kind of
strangers. At ease in the countries of the world, he found this
territory forbidding and fraught with danger. From across the
room, I said to him, "After the operation tomorrow, wake up
and be well. Then we can go home."

He winked at me mischievously. "That's the best proposition you've made in weeks." He shifted in the bed and
reached for his cigarettes. "Close the door behind you, Katie,
and don't tell the cops I'm in here breaking the law. Come
tomorrow when it's over."

"You know I will."

He nodded and said gently, "Go now, little girl. Go."

In the Gitlins' apartment some twenty blocks away I excused myself early. Paul and Zelda were wonderful, warm

and solicitous, but I had to be alone. Their son, Jon, like Geoff, was away in prep school and I had his room. Zelda, I remember, apologized for a rather sad-looking philodendron that Jon had left behind. He called the plant "Arthur" and had asked his mother to try to bring it back to health. In Jon's room I took charge of Arthur that night. I washed his leaves, stems, and trunk—even the outside of his clay pot. I wanted Arthur to live.

On the eve of battle, Connie once told me, no one really sleeps. He was preparing himself for his battle and a mile away in Jon's room I tried to help him. I willed him to win, just as I knew he was psyching himself up to the same state.

The night was interminable. Every few minutes while ministering to Arthur (who was probably in real danger of being killed by kindness) I looked at the clock. What is CJ doing now? What is he thinking? At 4:00 A.M. I thought of Pat in Ridgefield, probably drinking tea or coffee in the Neligan kitchen before the drive into town. At six, I visualized the nurses in Connie's room going through their preoperative chores. At 6:15 I figured Pat had surely arrived and might even then be with Connie. At 6:30, I heard the low murmur of voices and went out to join Paul and Zelda, thankful that the night was over. They were seated at the table, looking as though they had had no more sleep than I. Their wonderful Mamie, who has been a part of the Gitlin family for years, urged breakfast on me, but I couldn't eat. Instead, I drank orange juice, cool and freshly made, the bits and pieces of fiber clinging to the inside of the crystal glass Mamie set before me. I welcomed the hot coffee which followed, the first of many cups I would drink during that day. Paul, Zelda, and I sat together silently. I think their thoughts were probably similar to mine: what were the doctors going to find? Would Connie remain stable, no matter what the complications, during the operation? And the most critical question of all: would the treatment work?

Testy and on edge, Paul left abruptly to go to the office. It was not yet 7:20 A.M. Zelda and I lingered on at the table, scarcely speaking, and then went to our rooms to bathe and dress. While running water in Jon's bathroom, I came out to look at Arthur. In a strange way it was now fixed in my mind that Arthur's appearance during the hours I waited to hear from Pat would somehow reflect Connie's progress. Arthur was much as I'd left him—clean, his pores opened to the dubious benefits of New York air. There was a gleam of sunlight on the window ledge of Jonny's room. I moved Arthur up to sit in it.

Eight fifteen A.M. The doctors, including Pat, would all be ready now. Connie would be drowsy with preoperation sedatives. At 8:30 I knelt beside Jon's bed and prayed. When I looked up Arthur was streaked by sunlight.

The hours passed. At one time Zelda almost shoved me out the door. "Walk in front of the building," she told me. "If the phone rings I'll call you." I walked, but was back again in minutes. "Sit on the terrace," Zelda said. "You've got to get some air." Instead, I fled to Jonny's room. Arthur was in shadow. It's only the sun moving toward the west, I told myself. Mamie and Zelda tempted me again with coffee but I don't remember that I ate.

At about 3:30 P.M. we were startled by the lobby phone. The doorman informed Zelda that a Dr. Neligan was there to see Mrs. Ryan. I stared at Zelda. "He would have called first if it was good news."

She shook her silky black hair. "No, he probably came straight over as soon as he changed. It's all over, Kathy."

"What's all over?"

"The operation. They've finished. Pat's come to tell us about it." She went out to meet him at the elevator. I sat on a sofa, unable to move.

Pat looked drained but his first words came in a rush: "He's O.K. All right? He came through fine. Understand? He's got a constitution like an ox. But he's sleeping off the biggest hangover he'll ever have. I've been with him and the team around him in the recovery room." Pat stopped long enough for Zelda to take his coat. "It will be awhile before Whitmore calls here. He's got the number and he promised that the minute Connie's brought to his room, no matter what the hour, you can see him. Now," he touched my shoulder, "you got all that through your little pointed head?"

"What about the nodes, Pat? And the implant? Did they do a good job?"

"Whitmore's one of the finest surgeons I've ever watched perform," Pat said. "He has a thorough knowledge of anatomy and a great respect for tissue. It was a pleasure to see him at work. The implant technique is interesting."

"And the nodes, Pat?"

Zelda looked at him. "I suspect you might like some tea or coffee, Dr. Neligan," she said, "and a small drink wouldn't hurt. I can also make you something to eat."

"Thanks, Mrs. Gitlin." She quickly corrected him. "Zelda," he said with a tired smile. "Are you sure it won't be too much trouble?"

"I'll be back in just a few minutes." She paused in the doorway and said, "Actually, I've been boiling water on and off for the past two hours." She went off to the kitchen.

Pat sat down wearily.

"What about CJ, Pat? Will he make it?"

"He's doing fine. I told you that. Be thankful, my girl, that he had such a good surgeon to do the kind of work that was required today. Dr. Whitmore really is splendid at his job."

"Pat, the nodes."

He closed his eyes, his face seemed exceptionally pale. "It's been a long day, Kathy, for everyone concerned. But yes, Bagshaw's lymphangiogram was right. The nodes were positive. So were others Whitmore excised."

Finally I said, "Then what does it mean now, Pat?"

Pat took off his eyeglasses and rubbed his eyes. "I hope it means they got them all," he said. He put his head back against the chair. "The poor fellow," he said, thinking aloud.

"What he's been through today. And for a man who hates hospitals and rules and routines, it's even more remarkable."

"What is?"

Pat grinned. "That he didn't try to direct the operation himself, anesthesia or no anesthesia."

Zelda came back with a big tray and we sat watching Pat as he ate and drank. Color came back into his face. He began to seem a little less tired. But there were subjects he obviously didn't want to talk about and questions I didn't want to ask. If Connie had come through the operation all right, there would be time enough in future Ryan-Neligan "combat councils" to discuss the problems and the outlook. There was no point just then in trying to predict the future. First Connie had to get through the present.

Before he left for the trip back to Connecticut, Pat said, "Don't be anxious if you don't hear from Whitmore for quite a while. Connie will be in the recovery room for several hours yet. You'll see him tonight, but I just can't tell you when."

As I walked to the door with him, I thought the food and drink had helped him less than they had seemed to do at first. There was still a look of shock on Pat's face and in his eyes. For a doctor to watch his best friend being operated on cannot be easy. I hoped that was all that had so subdued his features. I didn't ask. On that day I don't think Pat would have told me. Not even Pat.

On the eve of his operation Connie had put on tape his understanding of the surgical procedures that would be involved in discovering if cancer had invaded the lymphatic system of his body. Before taping, he had had access only to the brief jottings in his notebook, based on what he had understood from the doctors. But, as always, he had been able to depend upon his remarkable memory in filling out his account of what he believed would take place. Lacking medical knowledge, he had described with quite incredible accuracy a layman's view of the procedures and processes which had been involved.

What he could not know on Monday evening, October 19, was that for him, for Dr. Whitmore and his team, and for Connie's close friend, Dr. Neligan, the exploration of the lower abdominal field and the additional surgery which resulted from that exploration would, on Tuesday, October 20, prove to be a voyage of tragic discoveries. Yet, Connie would have wanted truth no matter what the cost. Many another patient would not have tried to discover all the facts about an illness. Had Connie's been a different kind of personality, an instant morbidity would not only have surfaced, as it did back in July 1970, but grown, and perhaps engulfed him, obscuring everything else in his life. But Connie was critically interested in how much time he had left, and knowledge about the findings and future treatment of his condition offered the only hope he would have to plan his life and his work effectively.

Strangely, his research had produced a more dramatic event than even he had anticipated. Even as he lay anesthetized and unaware of what was happening, an unusual liaison was occurring and it had been brought about, in large part, by his dogged investigations. Until Connie's visit to Stanford University Medical Center as Dr. Bagshaw was later to write:

I had not done a lymphangiogram . . . on anyone with such early disease. . . . I think [it] will encourage us to do more lymphangiograms at early stages.

And as Dr. Whitmore wrote to Bagshaw:

Your lymphangiogram really upset our thinking about this patient.

On that October morning doctors in New York were working with the aid of lymphangiogram films developed three thousand miles away by a young radiotherapist who had never before performed the test on a patient with early cancer. The result was a medical cooperation of a kind that, I think, had never been attempted before. If Connie's tenacious determination to research his disease had accomplished nothing else, it had brought the map of Bagshaw's findings to Whitmore whose work would establish its accuracy. Inert and unconscious on the operating table, Connie had become the human bridge connecting the work of these two extraordinary professionals.

In his words describing part of the operation, Dr. Whitmore did

a very limited lower transperitoneal node dissection, removing especially the two large nodes noted on the lymphangiogram.

The nodes were positive. Malignant. Metastases—the dread spreading of cancerous cells—had indeed already taken place.

In skips and jumps, cancer had invaded the lymphatics and infiltrated lymph nodes. Like a demented mass murderer, striking down victims nonselectively, the disease had randomly destroyed the healthy life of the nodes.

In the modified pelvic lymph node dissection that followed Whitmore's first findings, other grossly positive nodes were found. Cancer's invasion of the lymphatic system had clearly commenced. The urgent question was: had the invasion been stopped?

Following the node dissections. Dr. Hilaris's implantation technique was employed. Incisions were made to permit mobility of the prostate and the I-125 seeds—about one-third inch to one-quarter inch long, with the thickness of a straight pin—were put in place. In all, thirty-two seeds were implanted in the right lobe of the prostate, nine in the left lobe—a total of forty-one implants of radioactive iodine which would give off a certain amount of radiation twenty-four hours a day until August 20, 1971, when the energy and activity of the seeds would presumably have run their course.

In this summary of the operation under "Diagnosis" Dr. Whitmore wrote:

Adenocarcinoma of the prostate with early local extension and retroperitoneal and pelvic lymph node metastases.

The verdict was in, the plan, for the time, completed. And the attack to save Connie's life had either been accomplished or had really just begun.

$$\doteq 2 \doteq$$

IN THE RECOVERY ROOM vigilant attendants were watching over Connie. Postoperative notes, supplied by Memorial, attest to his progress:

Patient left OR [operating room] in good condition. Foley bladder drainage—retropubic—low pole."*

At 5:30 P.M. Dr. Breen recorded blood pressure, pulse, respiration, lung and heart sounds. Dr. Freel inked in the estimated amounts of blood loss during the operation and the fluid replacement during surgery. Notes from Rehabilitation read in part:

Patient seen. Still not awake . . . Chest expanding well. We will resume breathing exercises when possible. Catheter draining bloody fluid.

* The Foley catheter is one which is inserted in the urinary tract. A balloon device is attached to one end. The balloon is filled with sterile water which holds the catheter in place until the balloon is emptied.

Dr. Hilaris's notes include a drawing of the implants to the prostate plus the information that:

Final dose calibration will be done after the . . . x-ray studies are completed."*

At 10:00 P.M. Dr. Nelson Tyrone wrote that Connie's temperature was 100 degrees rectally. Blood pressure was stable. Deep breathing was proceeding well.

At 11:15 P.M. the telephone rang at the Gitlins. Dr. Whitmore's voice sounded as bright and energetic as always—even though, I later remembered, Connie's had been but one of his operations that day. In addition to writing up reports and making rounds, his own notes would seem to indicate numerous conferences with teams of doctors not only on the operations he performed that day but on the prognosis of other patients as well.

"Mrs. Ryan," he said, "your husband's been taken up to his room. He came through fine but he's still a little out of things. You know, of course, that visiting hours are long over but I've left word with the doorman that you are to be allowed to go up to see him. I'm sorry to have been so long in telephoning. I know it's been a long wait."

The wait didn't matter anymore. I grabbed my coat and raced for the door, Paul and Zelda following in quick pursuit, telling me I could not go alone. Outdoors the dry day had given way to a soft nighttime rain, making the streets shine and the lights of cars reflect the gleaming roadways.

At the hospital the doorman was expecting me. Paul and

---

* This note relates to the amount of energy the radioactive seeds would be imparting to the prostate and appears to indicate that future X rays would help to determine if any of the seeds had moved and the effectiveness of the energy output in destroying cancer cells in the gland. Each seed had a therapy field of its own. In that small area it would have to put out enough radiation to attempt to kill all the cancer in its own field. It should be mentioned that the implants would lose strength over a period of time, going from full life, to half-life, to quarter-life, etc. They would also cause Connie nausea, vomiting, and weakness from time to time. Dr. Hilaris was able to compute, almost to the hour, the days on which Connie could expect the onset of "radiation sickness" as he termed it; he could thus be mentally prepared for its occurrence.

Zelda sat down in the darkened lobby to wait while I rode—at a snail's pace it seemed—to the ninth floor. My heart was pounding as I headed for 904.

At the door of Connie's room I stopped dead. It appeared to be jammed with people, some in green uniforms, others in white. Tubes, stands, trays, bottles, extra sheets and towels seemed to occupy every area, and then someone in green moved and I saw Connie in the bed. Only his face and arms were visible above the mound of bedding and the welter of hanging bottles suspended from standards that surrounded him. I wanted to cry out against what had been done to him and I wanted to applaud it as well. I was tremendously proud of him. Disliking hospitals as he did, his acceptance of the operation, his knowledge of what it would be like in part, made his courage seem all the more extraordinary.

"Connie," I whispered, edging into the room, "Connie."

His eyes searched the busy figures around his bed. The nurses, technicians, and doctors paid me no notice except that someone motioned me to the end of the bed. Almost behind the Foley catheter and a deep drain which protruded from his body, surrounded by people and mounds of equipment, I looked down at the exposed area of my husband's body, seeing close up the sprouting drain and the catheter. Around this equipment were layers of bandages, some white, some slightly stained, the colors vivid against pale skin. "Connie," I said again.

His eyes were glazed, clouded from anesthesia and the shock of his ordeal. "Kathy?" he asked. "Is that you, Katie?" Suddenly an expression of intense pain distorted his features. "Katie," he gasped, "help me." But the many people in the room were doing that and in a moment the spasm passed. His face cleared. Again he gazed unsteadily at me. "We did it, Katie," he whispered, and then he went to sleep. I stayed on a little longer but I was obviously in the way and only Dr. Whitmore's kindness had made it possible for me to be there at that hour at all.

"May I come in the morning?" I asked one of the figures. Someone nodded but said, "Call first. He'll be very busy tomorrow when he's more fully awake. Call his room and the nurse will know by then when you can come back."

Outside the room I stood for a minute or two. "We didn't do it, love," I said to myself. "You did it all alone."

At the nurses' station I stopped. The people most directly concerned with Connie's immediate welfare were in his room and they were too busy to talk to me except when they had to move around me, tightly pressed as I had been against the end of Connie's bed. But I had to speak to someone on the floor that night. To the nurse behind the desk, I said, "Take care of him. He's the only husband I've got."

As the days proceeded Connie's incredible recuperative strength grew daily. Dr. Whitmore's notes regarding his progress read in part:

Postoperative course was entirely uneventful. Suprapubic drain and the catheter were removed on the first postoperative day. He progressed to a regular diet. He had no urethral or rectal irritation.

Dr. Whitmore was pleased, I feel sure, with Connie's progress. Others were not so satisfied. Although he was cooperating well in his rehabilitation exercises and had been up and out of bed on instruction for a few minutes before 8:00 A.M. on the morning of Wednesday, October 21, the day following surgery, he was once again beginning to assert control over himself. Hospital progress notes record:

Patient complaining of being awakened frequently and is irritable ... less irritable than yesterday but still convinced there is a conspiracy to keep him from sleeping ... Extremely irritable! ... nurse says he's smoking ..."

An interesting follow-up to that report came from one of the physical therapists who wrote:

Patient *is* smoking! Off program.

She had not been able to mend his ways.

Connie's own explanation of that part of the progress report is taken from his notebook:

Miss ——— is responsible for putting the "eager" before "beaver." We have not hit it off. She wants no part of me. That's what she said. "You are smoking a cigarette and I want no part of you." She stormed out of my room. I was so angry that with my stomach still held together by sutures I almost climbed out of bed and chased her down the hall.

As his strength and activity progressed each day, Connie saw more and more of the people to whom he had entrusted our secret. By 5:30 or 6:00 P.M. each evening he was usually holding court, delighting his visitors with stories, particularly of the smoking episode, and teasing his favorite nurses. He was on the phone to Annie in the office at home often during the days, and spoke to Geoff and Vicki, as did I, almost every evening. There was a bright joyousness in the air which radiated from him. He pronounced himself "cured" to all his guests and was eagerly counting the days until his return home to his family and his book. Yet the tapes he made in the hospital contain, in part, a fear he was careful not to communicate to any of us.

CORNELIUS

Not until Wednesday, October 21, did I really come to. The world was still there. The room had stopped revolving. I was alive. Now it is Friday, October 23. I do not remember seeing Whitmore until today. No one had told me what the results of the operation had been. I had to know about the nodes Malcolm had found. Today Whitmore told me that the nodes had been malignant and that he had cut them out. He said that, in all other ways, I was fine. I have a remarkable constitution (his words), and he has made a thorough examination and found everything in working order. But he is very vague about the meaning of the malignancy in the nodes. He is not ready to say what it portends. Do I have three more years? Two more? What? He does not answer those questions directly. One can tell when a doctor is hedging. He sidesteps one's questions and says instead, "I've known people who have lived for thirty years with an illness like this." But that is no answer at all. It is a rather rare statistic. I am thinking about myself and how long *I* am going to live. No matter how, I intend to learn more before I leave here. I've got no desire to come back again.

There is one rather amusing recollection that keeps coming back to me. I remember being in the operating room or maybe just outside it on the morning of the twentieth, more or less surrounded by nurses who were very charming and kind. The men were wearing light green operating gowns with white masks and one of them had his mask askew. It was Pat and he said to me, "What are you doing here? Why aren't you home working?" What a hell of a thing for Neligan to say! I told him I might ask him the same questions and at that point, I must have passed out. It was just as well. He would surely have had a comeback line which I would have spoiled by going to sleep before he could deliver it.

I am still finding bathroom functions next to impossible. The mauling I have received inside has almost totally paralyzed the use of any kind of muscles necessary for voiding. Worse is the pain which, I believe, I am not too successful in hiding. No matter how good Whitmore is, the bulldozing that has taken place inside me is such that the pain at times is unbelievable. The nurses are wonderful in their understanding. I can never say enough about the kindnesses of Nurses Eileen Dwyer, Clara Weisher, and Lucy Reuber. All three are efficient, thoughtful, and, to my mind, perfect examples of what the profession is all about.

Sunday night, October 25, 1970. Katie brought Geoff in today. Vicki did not come although she made me a card. For some reason Geoff appeared to be allowed only to stand in the doorway and talk to me. I've asked about the radiation effects. As far as I am able to understand, the I-125 implants will pose no danger to Katie or, in fact, to anyone who is near me. So why then couldn't Geoff come in? Perhaps the young could be affected. I've got to find out. Geoff appears to be as uneasy around hospitals as I am, poor lad. I'm sure there were many more things he would have preferred to do on a Sunday than to visit me in here. I was very proud of the effort he had obviously made to make me a little more comfortable about his appearance. I wouldn't mind the scruffy look—indeed I rather suspect I had one myself when young—if Geoff didn't have proper clothes. I had none until I began making money for myself and then when Geoff got old enough I wanted the best suits and jackets that could be found for him. He actually wore a jacket and trousers for his visit here, as well as a white shirt and tie. His hair still looks like the devil, but it is clean and he had it off his face and somehow secured neatly at the back of his neck. We kidded each other across the space between my bed and the door. He was obviously making such an effort to please me that I was touched and remorseful about all the times I have upbraided him for his appearance. He can rise to the occasion when he wants to and it warms me very much that he considered this such an occasion.

Katie has lost weight, I think, and she tends to fuss like a mother hen. If I didn't stop her, I think she would be on her hands and knees scrubbing this hospital floor. She seems very nervous and very tired. What I have put all of them through! And how much more, I wonder, will they have to endure because of me? Well, if I have my way, we will be winding down to the end of this problem. I want no more of hospitals. I want to live and be well.

KATHRYN

On Thursday, October 29, 1970, Connie was released from Memorial. It had been twelve days since he had entered the hospital for the fateful two-step operation to excise the malignant lymph nodes and to implant the radioactive seeds into the prostate. For the time, everything possible had been done to halt or kill his cancer.

I had left the Gitlins' affectionate and protective company on Sunday, October 25, and during the days before Connie's release I drove in from Ridgefield to New York to see him. I found him stronger at every visit, keenly anticipating his return home in all aspects but one: his concern about the future of our sexual relationship.

He was now sterile. It was difficult for him to accept the fact. Before the operation, sterility had been simply one of the many side effects he might experience, no matter what the treatment. Then the side effect had become an irreversible reality, a by-product whose impact had suddenly assumed significant importance. Connie felt diminished and humbled. He believed that his sexual desire would wane and this, too, caused him anguish but the anguish was for me.

He did not know if I could accept the possibility of his celibacy. The absence of sexual relationships, if it became total, might, he felt, prove difficult for me to cope with. In the strangest conversation we had ever had, Connie at one point said, "I could never blame you if you did something about it. Just don't ever let me know."

He felt that he was less than whole and he believed that I might think so, too. One of the juices of his life, a part of his maleness, was being burned away by the tiny seeds now implanted in his prostate. The slowing up of sexual drive which had been a medical possibility from the beginning of his research into the modalities of treatment for prostatic cancer was, in the few days before he left the hospital, beginning to assume a reality that he had dealt with only intellectually before. He was finding it hard to cope with and he was desperate about the effect it might have on me.

I explained my feelings to him as best I could. I had not expected that sexual functions could ever again be the same as in the past, nor had they been during that year of worry and concern about Connie's health. But we were committed to each other in work and interests, and, since the diagnosis and all we had learned about how to treat this cancer, I had become reconciled to the gradual phasing-out of the sexual aspect of our lives. What had once been an important part of our marriage had diminished, and I told Connie that, among my priorities, sex had no listing. If it occurred, if it *could* occur, it would be a bonus, treasured and enjoyed all the more for its rarity.

At that time I was still in my early forties. Admittedly, I had given the subject private thought. Any woman would have done so. But my admiration and regard for Connie were strong assets of our marriage. I was proud of my husband and proud to be his wife. He radiated life, enthusiasm, and excitement in ways no one else I knew had ever done. Those qualities fascinated me as they had from the first day I met Connie. I could not see myself seeking temporary liaisons, much less living with the guilt that would have followed. An unfaithful act by me, no matter how discreet, would have smudged and tainted all that we had found together.

Yet, there was a moment when the temptation was strong. My physical desires were unchanged even as Connie's were waning. It would have been easy to satisfy them. I think what held me back most were certain facets of my husband's personality that were highly meaningful to me: his code of honor and ethics, his passion for truth, his sense of self. Had our roles been reversed I think Connie would have remained faithful to me. The rules of conduct by which he lived were deeply ingrained, and he would have adhered to them. I think, too, that my marriage vows, as well as the traits I admired in Connie, kept me from engaging in extramarital sex. I had promised to love and cherish him in *sickness* and in health, clinging only unto him. It is a rather simplistic and possibly old-fashioned philosophy—times change and so do people and there are always reasons for separation or divorce—but when one is lucky, the original fascination remains. I think I loved my husband in his years of sickness more than at any time in our marriage, and the way he handled his illness, the fierce courage with which he fought it, submerged my sexual desires as my pride in him increased. I cherished him too much to be unfaithful to him.

I have mentioned this because other women, younger women, could well have considered the time ahead as barren, the gift and joy of mating too great a treasure to live without. I sympathize strongly with that concept. No one has said it is easy to abstain from sexual pleasure, and each woman, under similar circumstances, has to solve the problem in her own way according to the structure of her marriage. In that, I was fortunate. Our marriage had been built on a variety of interests and activities, including the fact that we worked together professionally. So often the job of one mate seems incomprehensible or downright boring to the other, engrossed with different associates and other work. My husband and I enjoyed working together, bringing to the job those skills and qualities each of us thought we possessed and then deciding which of us was better in the handling of certain facets of the work. But I believe the real glue of our marriage—the bond that never broke—was friendship. We had been, first and always, friends.

My concern about Connie had obliterated nearly everything else from my mind. When he was told he would be released on October 29, I eagerly prepared for his homecoming. Everything was in readiness in our bedroom, his dressing room, and in the office where, in time, he could get on with the work on *Bridge*. I was so occupied with small details that I did not check my diary for that week until the evening before Connie was to come home. Under Thursday, October 29, I had written:

C & K lunch with Mary Luke and her publisher to celebrate pub. date her book.

Mary, a longtime Ridgefield friend, had just completed her second book in what was to become a trilogy of Tudor history. *A Crown for Elizabeth*, the new title, would be in the bookstores that day and, weeks earlier, her publisher had invited Connie and me to lunch with him, Mary, and certain of his staff in honor of the occasion. The plan had been for the three of us to drive into the city together. I felt it was far too late to back out with a lame excuse. On Thursday, the twenty-ninth, I picked up a glowing and excited Mary. On the trip into town I told her what had been happening to us. A little of Mary's glow faded, but not her resolve and determination to help in any way she could. I did not want to spoil this day for her. Connie and I had looked forward to sharing her happiness and the success of her new book, but I felt if Mary would prefer to make excuses for our absence from lunch, that choice should be hers.

The choice Mary made was immediate. She not only wanted me to be at lunch but together we hastily concocted and rather brightly, I think, brought off a cover story for Connie's absence: unexpectedly, he had had to leave for Europe. Lunch went very well, but Mary did not linger afterward. We kissed our hosts, all of us radiating happiness and confidence in the new book's future, and together, Mary and I raced for the garage. In spite of the fact that my news had taken the edge off her happiness, Mary's help was invaluable. She became our chauffeur on that day, waiting outside Memorial while I attended to the chores required to effect Connie's release. Before we could leave a long list of prescriptions had to be filled at the hospital pharmacy. I had to see the cashier and then start bringing down books, papers, and clothes, stashing them in the front seat of the car while Mary—fending off taxis and other private cars—waited serenely at the wheel.

Finally, one of Connie's nurses helped him into a wheelchair and three other nurses, of whom he had become particularly fond, walked out to the car with us. As Connie wrote in his diary:

Poor, dear Mary. The expression on her face on what should have been so totally her day was a mixture of bewilderment and sorrow. I was piled into the back of the car, looking ill I know, and clutching my briefcase (and a bill for something over $3,000 for only basic hospital expenses). Yet Mary never wavered. With Katie and me in the back seat, she drove us back to Ridgefield, chatting happily about the good omens of that day—her book, my recovery. "I'll be your chauffeur from here on, CJ," she said. I told her it was my fervent hope that she would never again have to take on that job.

From the moment he entered the house Connie behaved as though the ordeal of the past twelve days was a dim memory. Victoria had not seen him in the nearly two weeks he had been away. His thinness, the gray sheen of fatigue on his face, momentarily subdued her spirits, but they rose as Connie began to regale her with stories of his hospital stay, including his experience with the physical therapist who had refused all contact with him because he smoked. To my amazement Connie refused to get into pajamas, dressing gown, and slippers. He declared he had had enough of that kind of attire. Brushing aside our wishes to wait upon him, he insisted on having dinner with Vicki and me downstairs. I think he would have spent the night there chatting, delighted to be home, but Pat Neligan stopped by and promptly ordered him up to bed. Connie was stubborn about obeying but eventually, with Pat a close step behind him all the way, he climbed the stairs to our bedroom and, with Pat's help, undressed and got into bed. He was far weaker than he would admit.

Later, after a drink with Connie, Pat came down to talk to me. "Who does he think he is?" Pat inquired irritably. "He's just come out of hospital. Anybody with any sense would know enough to go to bed. He's got to get his strength back gradually. He's gone through a terrible ordeal. Where has the man's reasoning gone to anyway?"

The man's reasoning was that, once released from the hospital, he had every intention of resuming his normal routine immediately. Although he had seen how others needed to recuperate after a hospital stay, Connie did not appear to think that the need for rest and a gradual return to activities applied to him.

On Friday, October 30, he rose early as usual, showered, slowly dressed himself, refusing all help, and, after a light breakfast, painfully negotiated his way to the office. I had tried to cajole him into resting upstairs, but he was anxious to see Annie and to go through the mounds of correspondence that were waiting for him. He worked, despite my pleas and Annie's, the entire day, dictating letters, giving Annie lists of favorite hospital personnel to whom he wished to send copies of his books and in general, clearing his desk of everything but work he would need for *Bridge*. To Annie and me he said not a word about his condition, but in his diary for that Friday he wrote two stark words: "Pain—much."

One of the letters he wrote that day was indicative of the mood he was to convey to almost everyone from that time on. The letter was to his friend Jack Thompson of the *Chicago Tribune*, dubbed "The Beard" or "The Beaver" because of a most elegant Vandyke. Connie once described Jack as "full of strange oaths and bearded like a prophet—the only correspondent I know who has parlayed himself into the purple eminence of the journalist's chapel, all on the formidable strength of this moth-eaten beard."

Jack had had an illustrious career as a correspondent in World War II and had remained, despite distance, among Connie's close friends. They saw each other seldom, except during their visits back to the Normandy beaches. On his first full day at home Connie confided to Jack the story of what had occurred to him since the cancer was discovered in July. After a description of the findings which had led him to Willet Whitmore and Memorial, he wrote:

About the best I can say to you is that I feel as though a half-track has rolled back and forth across my stomach non-stop for several days. I have a neat tattoo of the entire beachhead right across my abdomen. In addition, I have 41 radiation seed implants inside me emitting all sorts of powerful nuclear energy.

I am seriously thinking of setting up a little private practice. Any girls you may know who do not wish to take birth control pills or have a hysterectomy can, for a slight fee, sit on my lap. I guarantee total sterility.*

This is my first day back. I am better than ever. The attack was successful, although I am expecting a counter-attack any moment from all sides, if any more of those nodes are malignant. Notwithstanding, I have surrounded myself by barbed wire, land mines, and several squads of infantry, and we are ready to take on all comers.

Yours in Christ, Connie.

* All I knew about the potency of the radioactive implants came from a standard form called "Recommendations for Persons near Patient with Radioactive Iodine Implants." At the bottom of the printed sheet the words, "No Special Precautions Required," had been typed, and somewhat reassuringly, I also noted on the form that "no special precautions are required for the *spouse* or anyone else who takes care of the patient, if he or she does not expect to have any more children and is not engaged professionally in radiation work." Connie gave me the form. No doctor or radiation officer talked with me at all. Yet someone had obviously talked with Connie and, whether right or wrong, he was under the impression that Vicki and Geoff could not have prolonged physical contact with him. That he was concerned was apparent in remarks such as those contained in his letter to Jack, in his puzzlement about Geoff's lingering in the doorway during our son's visit to the hospital, and in his talk with me about sterility and probable lack of sexual drive. In retrospect, I should have insisted on knowing precisely what dangers, if any, the radiation might impose on the children, and I believe it should be an obligation of doctors and radiotherapists to talk with the family of patients receiving such treatment in order that misconceptions do not arise. Such knowledge imparted by the experts could erase many of the unnecessary burdens that cancer families carry through ignorance and lack of communication with doctors and therapists.

On Saturday, October 31, Alta, our shepherd, barked loudly and I heard a car roar to a stop before the house. I opened the door to see Harold Robbins coming up the steps. We had met Harold first in the early sixties and an affectionate relationship had existed between us for ten years. Harold, writing his fantastically successful novels, always in near seclusion, surfaced only briefly and our paths did not cross often. However, he had come to New York, and Paul Gitlin, his lawyer as well as Connie's, had told him what had been happening to us.

I have often wished that more peope knew the private Harold instead of the public man who, I think, very often adjusts his image to what he believes the many readers of his books expect of him. But the private Harold is quite different, his affections, concern, and interests unknown by his vast audience and by many associates. The roots of his loyalty run deep and his generosity where friends and family are concerned is boundless.

So it was with Harold that Saturday. He came up the steps, ignored our supposedly ferocious dog, and put his arms around me. "Paul told me, Kate," he said. "I had to come. Where is he?"

"Down in the office. I can't get him to rest."

Apparently Connie had heard the car as well as Alta's barking and came up to see who was there. Harold and I watched him as he moved slowly up the stairs and into the foyer. In the bright sunlight his face was ashen against the heavy wool Dutch fishing jacket he had put on earlier in the morning chill. He looked at Harold and suddenly he began to cry—harsh, sobbing sounds that I had never heard from him. The men embraced, Harold patting Connie gently, speaking softly to him, and then leading him down to the living room to one of the big sofas opposite the fireplace. I had started a small fire and the two men sat before it, talking softly and intently. I made tea and brought it on a tray.

"Lord, I'm sorry, Harold," Connie was saying, wiping his

eyes. "It must be the aftermath of the damned anesthetic. I'm so glad to see you. Where did you drop from this time?"

Harold had come in from the Coast and had planned to be back with Grace, his wife, and the children for the weekend. But Paul's news had altered his plans. I have never heard of his spending a night in anyone's house when he is away from home. His locale is the world's hotels, with spacious suites and room service to bring him varieties of ice cream or chocolate. The individuals in his novels may drink, but I have never known Harold to take anything much stronger than tea. Neither are any of his characters expert mathematicians or near-professional chess players. Those traits belong to the world of the private Harold Robbins, the man who was to spend a weekend in a house hardly dedicated to any comfort but Connie's at that time.

Geoff was home for the weekend, I thought. He had brought another boy, one I did not remember having met before, and they had taken over the kitchen. As darkness fell, we three adults sat quietly by the fire. Vicki had gone out Halloweening. I had forgotten the date.

It came back to me in a most unexpected manner. Once again Alta barked loudly and I looked out to see a police car, red lights revolving, in our driveway. The officer was polite but firm. Was my daughter at home? he wanted to know. Vicki had come in some minutes earlier and was in the kitchen with Geoff and his friend.

"My daughter?" I couldn't imagine why he was inquiring about Victoria.

"Yes, ma'am," the officer said. "There's been a complaint. She was seen putting soap all over the windows of a house nearby. The lady is prepared to swear your daughter was involved and she insists that the windows be cleaned immedately. But first, I want to question Victoria."

I glanced toward the sofa. Connie sat rigidly, staring at the officer as if he could not believe what had been said.

"It's all right, Connie," I said and went to get Victoria, just meeting her at the back door. Geoff and his school friend walked in, Vicki and I following their slow steps toward the fire and the sofa on which Harold and Connie sat.

The offense was repeated to a trembling Vicki. She wasn't alone, she told the officer. There'd been others involved, but yes, she had helped to soap the woman's windows. As the conference went on, I called the lady. She was pleasant but certain that Vicki was involved. There might have been others, she said, but she had definitely recognized our daughter. If the windows were cleaned immediately she would be satisfied. I assured her they would be but asked if Vicki was really the only child she'd seen. Again, she repeated that Vicki was the only she had recognized.

At the fireplace Harold was exceeding even his own storytelling abilities. As a polite but by now obviously confused police officer listened, Harold regaled the man with a series of sharp vignettes of his own misbehavior on a seemingly endless succession of long-ago Halloweens. I glanced at Connie. He seemed almost on the verge of collapse, but his eyes followed his daughter as, tearful and defiant, she marched back into the living room with the pail I had given her, detergents, cloths, and cleaning materials laid inside.

Geoff and his friend agreed to go with Vicki, "to make sure the job is done," Geoff said. The three of them disappeared into the darkness while I rushed around turning on outside lights to help them make their way through our woods to the development of fairly new houses where Vicki had perpetrated her crime.

The officer left soon afterward, presumably to check on the progress of the cleanup. Harold accompanied him to the door. "If you don't have anything worse than one little girl soaping windows while the rest of the gang lies low and lets her take the rap, you'll have a fairly quiet evening," Harold said. "But thanks for coming by."

We persuaded Connie to eat a light dinner and, while I cleaned up the kitchen, Harold walked him to our bedroom.

It was late when a still tearful and exhausted Vicki returned with Geoff and his friend.

"She did a good job," Geoff announced. "The windows are probably cleaner now than they were before, but I'd like to get the kids who are as guilty as she was. They all live in that neighborhood and they're all covering for each other."

I put away the pail and threw out the dirty cloths and empty bottles of cleaner. Vicki wanted only to take a shower and go to bed, but I brought up toast and warm cocoa to her. On my arrival back down to the kitchen we had a new guest, one whom I had not heard Alta announce. A tall, quite beautiful girl, older than Geoff and his friend, was sitting at the kitchen table with them. They were smoking, cigarettes, I thought, but the look on Geoff's face was one I'd seen before. He looked glazed, his features somehow out of line. Occasionally he giggled. The girl, I was told, intended to drive Geoff and his friend back to school. "I'll do that," I told them.

"No, we're going now. You stay with Dad," Geoff said.

I thought all three appeared to be weaving as they went out of the kitchen, passing me without a word or a glance. I called to Geoff and tried again to persuade him to let me drive him back.

"You've got enough to do," he said, "and I want to be in school tomorrow."

"Tomorrow's Sunday," I said. "There isn't any school."

"Yeh." He laughed. "So long, Mom. See you around."

I stood in the front doorway watching them down the stairs and in that moment I think I knew what had bothered me about Geoff for months. This was no ordinary growing up. His behavior was erratic and inconsistent, had been for some time, but it all came together in my mind that night. My son, mine and Connie's, was smoking something other than cigarettes.

Vicki went finally to sleep, apologizing again for the trouble she had caused. I couldn't think about that. I couldn't think about anything but Geoff and his new friends and the way I'd let him go off into the night with strangers whose behavior was as baffling and strange as his own. But I couldn't dwell on that for long either. I turned and went up to our bedroom. Harold had gotten Connie into bed and was sitting quietly talking with him. At rest Connie's face seemed less fatigued, but I noticed that he moved beneath the bed-clothes slowly and that lines of pain flickered across his face. There was medication for the pain but he refused to take it. Tea, lemonade, and water were all I could get him to accept.

We sat on into the night. I told Harold a bit about my book *The Betty Tree*, while Connie appeared to drift off into a light sleep. Then he turned in bed and gave a low, drawn-out groan. His eyes flew open wide.

"Oh, God," he gasped. Harold and I were already at his side.

"Get away," he ordered us. "I'm going to the bathroom."

He could not even throw the blanket back. Gently Harold turned it and the sheet aside, Connie swung his legs to the floor, stood up, and would have fallen had we not been there.

"Get away," he said again. "I'm all right." But Harold held him firmly as they walked into his dressing room.

Connie slept in only the briefest catnaps. As Harold and I sat softly talking a faint change in the sky caught my eye. It was nearly dawn. We had spent the night in vigil, Harold helping Connie on his occasional trips to the bathroom, me making seemingly endless pots of tea between conversations random and erratic. At 6:00 A.M. Connie was quiet, easier than he'd been all night. I went down to make some break-fast. Harold came along to help.

"You know something, Kate," he said, "we've got to give him some will to get through this. He's in big pain now, but what he needs is incentive to get back to his book." Harold stood looking out the window at the gray dawn. "I think I know how to do it," he mused, and as it turned out, he did.

Over the course of the next few days Harold commuted between Ridgefield and New York. Somehow he had managed to get Connie interested in the idea of writing a pilot for a TV series, and somehow Connie's enthusiasm was coming back, although not his strength. He went to the office daily, working on correspondence until Harold appeared from New York and then, with Annie—who was as worried as I and unwilling to see Connie's mind diverted further from the book—Connie dictated in considerable detail an outline for a TV pilot. In three weeks' time he would not remember that he had even worked on it, yet it was imaginative and fascinating and it had come from some deep place in his mind still befogged by pain and the aftereffects of his operation.

Connie's determination to carry on life as usual had put a tremendous drain on the precious little energy he possessed. Even without Harold's presence, Annie and I were unable to cajole him into relaxing. His resolve to return to a normalcy he could never regain was pumping, like a severed artery, in every direction. He paid a price for his pride and his fierce hope of putting hospitals behind him forever, a price more sensible souls would not have paid. Abdominal sutures abscessed and Pat Neligan was called in. Even as he berated Connie for his foolishness in working daily, Pat tenderly ministered to him and gave me instructions on how to apply compresses to the wound at intervals. Connie's diary reads:

Saturday, November 7, Neligan very irate that I have not taken a quieter convalescence. I couldn't. The pain was too acute and I could deal with it better on my feet. Have reached conclusion every doctor—including Neligan—should have a major operation. However am on the road to recovery but think the postoperative effects are worse than the surgery itself.

For Connie, in many ways they were. From Friday, October 30, 1970, the day after his arrival home, to Sunday, November 8, Connie's diary records "PAIN" (the capital letters were his). At 8:00 P.M. on Saturday, November 7, hours after Pat's visit during the day, Connie was in such agony that I telephoned Pat once again, helped Connie to the car, and drove him to Pat's office. To Connie, the sight of Pat, even without his ministrations, seemed as beneficial as the medical aid Pat gave him. That evening, for the first time since his arrival home from the hospital, Connie slept through the entire night, only fitfully waking when I applied hot compresses to his abdomen.

During Sunday, November 8, he worked on a plan he had warned Anne and me to keep secret even from Pat. It was the kind of problem-solving, sick or well, that gave Connie no rest until he had resolved it. In this instance, he was obsessed with putting one relatively minor problem to rest. To him, there was nothing minor about it. Ridgefield and New York are both small towns. Rumors spread and one eventually hears them. Connie's research trip to Europe, his flight to California, his hospitalization in New York, had kept him absent from most social events in the country and the city since the latter part of July. He had urged me to attend the cocktail and dinner parties he could not and, by and large, I had—although unwillingly.

Only the small coterie of friends in whom we had confided knew the reason for his absences, and we had spent grateful hours with those trusted few in quiet talk and solitude. But others, uninformed, wondered where my husband was when I showed up alone at many functions. My attitude was hardly cheerful. Connie has said that my emotions too often clearly showed. No doubt I looked and seemed as depressed and anxious as I was. My behavior and Connie's erratic absences soon produced an acceptable answer for the curious. The Ryans, we learned, were on the brink of divorce. That news, spanning the distance from Ridgefield to New York, caused Connie to comment that it was "amazing, despite the size of a place, how small minds conjure and large tongues wag."

Sick as he was, eleven days out of the hospital, a day less than the time he had been in it, Connie was bent on ending, the rumors. He enlisted the unwilling help of Annie, Ben Wright, and me. On Monday, November 9, dreading what Pat would say if he learned about our outing, I drove Connie to New York. The trip was a nightmare for him. Each bump in the road loomed large as a boulder, but he was not to be dissuaded from his mission. Ben met us at a downtown garage and took Connie off to his barber while I hastened to our young friend, Hans, at the hair salon at Elizabeth Arden's. The barber did a magnificent job in grooming Connie's hair but decided to leave on a beard, fearing its removal would expose the gaunt thinness of Connie's face. He had been too ill to shave up to then although, as always, he had been insistent about his daily showers. The beard was very strange and totally at odds with the blondness of Connie's hair. Tricolored, it was red about his lower lip and then blended into black and gray. It was still sparse but, trimmed and sculptured by his barber, it was passable. And if one did not look too closely at his eyes, where I thought pain was all too obvious, I suppose he looked like any other man who had decided to grow a beard which had not yet fully matured.

I met Ben and Connie at his barber's after a quick session of my own with Hans, who accepted my story of an early appointment for which I could not be late, and got me out early. The three of us, following Connie's plan, went to "21" for lunch. We walked slowly until we reached the restaurant and then Connie strode inside, looking as vigorous as always. People we knew stared at us, or so we thought, and looked with amazement at Connie's beard. Peter Kriendler took one look and said, "Where have you been, Uncle Vanya?" He did not embrace Connie as was his custom. I think Peter sensed that something quite extraordinary had happened to his friend. His approach was one of tender gruffness, not the mutual pummeling to which both men were accustomed in their greetings.

Columnists and publishers, movie producers and theater people, women I often lunched with —all seemed to have collected at "21" on that day. Ben and I flanked Connie at the table, bending low to talk as if this were some kind of business conference. In reality, we hoped to screen him from searching glances as well as possible. Somehow we got through the luncheon ordeal and once again Connie rose lightly from his chair and walked steadily from the dining room. I winced at what that effort must have cost him. Yet he maintained his poise until we reached the garage. "Did we pull it off?" Connie inquired. Ben and I thought so, but our memories were mostly of the incredible determination Connie had shown in making the appearance at all.

He was silent in the car going home, sitting upright and bracing himself against the rough road surfaces I could not avoid. About fifteen minutes away from home, he said, "I can hardly remember anything about the luncheon."

"You were utterly fantastic," I said, "and Pat is going to kill you when he finds out about this."

"Katie," he said, as if no other words had been spoken, "everything seems to hurt."

"Why did I ever let you talk me into this?" I asked him.

Feebly, he grinned. "You didn't," he said. "But I want to see which way the tongues wag now. The roving correspondent is again back home with his little wife. The only talk of divorce I'm prepared to hear is if it comes from you."

"Not till hell freezes over."

"Good," Connie said. "Don't let anybody turn off the furnace." He was silent for a moment. Then, "First thing when I get home, the damn beard comes off. It's a lazy way of getting through an illness and it's damn difficult to keep clean." He sighed, "I'm very, very tired," he said. "But happy. Think of all those aching tongues at rest."

On Tuesday, November 10, he was, for the first time, unable to leave his bed. The sutures, undoubtedly jeopardized by his premature trip to town, needed extra care. Connie stayed up in the house for eleven days—the same time interval he had between his hospital trip from New York and his rumor-ending journey back to the city—either in bed or sitting in the bedroom going over work with Annie. His incoming and outgoing telephone calls continued. During each he spoke crisply and lucidly to the caller, as he was always to do, then and in the future, regardless of the intensity of his pain. During those eleven days, he also found the time and the privacy to put down more of his thoughts on tape.

CORNELIUS

Thursday, November 19, 1970. Neligan has changed Whitmore's prescription, Gantrisin, a sulfonamide to clear infection in the urine, I believe. I am now taking NegGram again to clear up the pus which might have occurred there, possibly because of the instrumentation during the operation, possibly because of my foray into New York. In spite of the fact that Neligan is bad-tempered, he thinks I am making a remarkable recovery. The abscesses which formed around some of the sutures have disappeared, in large part due to Katie's constant care in applying compresses to the area. She is in greater need of rest than I. She has become nurse, mother, cook, chauffeur, and God knows what else ever since I became ill. She is tired out and that old nerve pain in her arm, which we hoped had disappeared forever, has come back. She never mentions it, but I see the expression change on her face when she moves her right arm suddenly or has to help me move. I am very concerned about her health, more so than I am my own.

Fragments of memory concerning the hospital keep coming back to me. I remember that when I came to after the operation I thought I had been badly wounded in the war. There appeared to be bottles and tubes all around me, and to my mind these are synonymous with the equipment used by medics in the field.

I have just been listening to myself record. I notice that I am unable to pronounce some words properly. There is a slight slurring of my speech. Why is that? I wonder. Tiredness?

I've thought of one very important subject I want to bring up with Willet when I go in to see him in December. His therapy of doing nothing but observation for a primary cancer of the prostate until it shows change is, in light of what happened to me, a little frightening. What would have occurred had I subscribed to that? In some cases where only a single lesion exists, it is probably a fairly safe procedure, but I still think watching and observing should be done only if a lymphangiogram is made during initial testing. I plan to write soon to Malcolm Bagshaw, telling him most of what I have learned as a result of this operation and also I need to explain to him why I had to refuse his therapy. I still feel a certain amount of guilt about that. The lymphangiogram done by Malcolm's people in Stanford has probably saved my life— for now. Up to the time it was done I thought we were dealing with cancer of the prostate alone. If I had done nothing but have checkups as Willet first suggested, I would never have known that this malignancy was not contained to the prostate. Neligan, I remember, when I telephoned him from San Francisco before Malcolm's long day of tests, insisted that I have the lymphangiogram, and by means of it the cancerous nodes were identified. Whitmore has since said that he would have discovered the malignant nodes anyway and Neligan was inclined to agree with that. But suppose I had simply done nothing but go in for examinations over a period of time? I think I would be far closer to death than I am right now.

I owe my life to four sources: Neligan, and his doggedness in supporting my desire to research every avenue of treatment before committing myself; Malcolm, and the brilliance of his crew at Stanford Medical Center; Dr. Jewett at Johns Hopkins who put me onto Malcolm in the first place; and Whitmore and his team who did the actual work. But I was lucky to find those men and those places. If I had not known how to research I would never have found them, heard their opinions, or learned about their various forms of treatment.

This brings me to a couple of other thoughts. The United States is a country with vast resources, and monies labeled for cancer research. Yet the medical profession as a whole is not abreast of the various modalities of treatment that are available. In many instances there is simply no way that doctors and technicians can familiarize themselves with everything that is going on and still continue their daily work. There should be some sort of method whereby a doctor could dial a number and a computer could tell him immediately what is happening in a particular field. How many lives might be saved or prolonged by such a method! How much easier on the patient's pocketbook if the first doctor he saw could tell him immediately what options he had and where they were to be found!

That reminds me that I must get around to my bills fairly soon. I have not written to Dr. Joseph Ward who was so very kind to me, nor have I paid his bill. The final bill from Stanford is in and, in scanning it, I was certain a mistake had been made. The bill for the lymphangiogram—to my mind, the most important test that has been done in my case—is $45.75. Wouldn't anyone with prostatic cancer pay that amount to find out if the malignancy had invaded the lymphatics? A dinner for two at a fine restaurant costs far more. If this test has in any way helped to prolong my life, it is beyond monetary value. I would pay ten times that amount gladly and still consider it one of the rarest bargains of my life.

Memorial's bill, excluding surgeons and specialists, is $3453.65. I am amazed at all it includes, and looking at the list, I am somewhat astounded that the bill isn't higher. There is, of course, room and board. The little room, 904, was $119 per day. Can most patients afford that? Still, included in the bill are costs for the use of the operating room, for the blood bank, transfusion services, plasma, anesthesia, pathology. And there are other tests and services also in the overall charge: hematology, cytology, diagnostic radiology, bacteriology, urinology, EKG, biochemistry. Even the physical therapists and special-duty nurses are included in the bill. Little enough to save a life, if one gets to the right place and into the hands of the right people.

But I am out of pocket in many other ways: the telephone calls to Europe and throughout Europe, plane fares, hotels, specialists' fees. Since July I have spent close to $7000 for cancer research and treatment. Major medical insurances are essentials for partial payments of hospitalization but they cannot cover the trips and research I undertook. How few people could have afforded to do what I have done! That makes the collation of facts and methods of treatment all the more essential. Every man, woman, and child in the world should have the right to the best and most complete medical information available in order to reduce costs but, more important, in order to save their lives. The horror is that far too often, as I might have done, they will fall into the hands of a doctor using therapy which is already obsolete.

KATHRYN

Dr. Whitmore had sent copies of Connie's discharge summary with its explanation of the operation and the findings to Drs. Neligan, Bagshaw, and Jewett. On November 24, 1970, Dr. Jewett wrote to Dr. Bagshaw:

. . . I am interested to know what made you advise a lymphangiogram. I realize he did have a tumor that was a little too extensive locally for radical operation, but the idea of a lymphangiogram had not occurred to me. The films show that we were right in not advising radical surgery. Perhaps we should do more of these, but I do not see how we can make them a regular part of our work-up in all cases. . . .

Dr. Bagshaw replied in part:

. . . I wish I could answer your question as to why I performed this examination in Mr. Ryan's case. . . . I was quite impressed with the degree of perineural involvement and the somewhat aggressive histopathologic study of the diseased tissue appearance of Mr. Ryan's tumor . . . almost as an afterthought I recommended that we proceed with the lymphangiogram. I was astonished when it turned out to be so classically positive. At this point, I don't think we can say much about its general application although we intend to pursue the use of lymphangiography as a means of predicting therapeutic approach and/or prognosis . . .

And Dr. Whitmore, writing to Dr. Jewett at the time he sent out Connie's discharge summary, observed:

. . . I guess we are going to have to start doing more lymphangiograms on our patients with prostatic cancer but exactly how this should influence our therapeutic recommendations will have to be determined by experience. . . .

Connie's hope for a computerized exact treatment formula would never be easy to realize. Cancer experts would still have to depend upon cases and statistics. As Dr. Whitmore had written, therapeutic recommendations would still have to be made from experience—and only cancer patients could provide specialists with experience. Only individuals and the aggressiveness of each person's cancer could tip the therapeutic balance and determine the course of treatment. As Connie had written in one heavily inked note in his diary, "The guinea pigs are US!"

On November 23, 1970, I drove Connie to New York to see Dr. Basil Hilaris, who had done the I-125 implants during the operation thirty-five days earlier. I waited in the reception lounge while Connie had his conference. He was still weak but, as he put it, "I'm gaining on the thing." He was also angry, and with some reason.

When he left the hospital on Thursday, October 29, a small bracelet was attached to his wrist. It read:

In case of accident or emergency notify the Medical Physics Department, Memorial Hospital, 879–3000, Ext: 333. Patient received 20.4 mCi of I–125 on 20 October, 1970.

Annie had rung the hospital to confirm Connie's appointment with Dr. Hilaris a few days before. She was told there was no such extension as "333." She asked for the Medical Physics Department and, again, the operator was baffled. There was no such department, Annie was told. Finally she asked directly for Dr. Hilaris and got his office. The initial difficulty, Connie found out, was that one digit was missing from the hospital extension number on his bracelet. It read "333." It should have read "3333." That was more than cause for Connie's annoyance but, he told me, the "Medical Physics Department" typed on his bracelet was a code name by which radiation safety services could be quickly obtained. The name did indeed exist and was in use at Memorial, but for some reason the telephone operator Annie got onto had never even heard of it. The bracelet, without that vital fourth 3, was useless. Had Connie required emergency help before he met with Dr. Hilaris, we at home or a stranger on a city street might have encountered an operator's bewilderment.

Connie's conference with Dr. Hilaris considerably bolstered his confidence in his recovery. To date, he had not experienced any effects from the radiation and Dr. Hilaris, Connie said, was pleased with his progress. The effects of the radiation, Connie understood, would be cumulative and possibly reach their peak within two to two and a half weeks' time, presumably somewhere between December 7 and 13. He could expect to feel a chill, similar to that after a somewhat severe sunburn. The chill would pass through his body and seem to center around the bladder. He might expect all or some of the following symptoms: diarrhea, hesitancy in urinating, nausea, a slight elevation in temperature. He felt much better, knowing what he could expect and when he could expect it. And, more important, he decided to get in one more trip before the probable onset of the radiation sickness and his first visit to Dr. Whitmore which was scheduled for December 11. It was a trip I looked forward to as eagerly as did Connie.

On Saturday, November 23, taking as his only medication a bottle of Librium, which Pat had prescribed for him the day before, we left for California. Victoria had once again been taken in by friends, and my father, who had made trips between Iowa and Connecticut ever since the cancer diagnosis was confirmed, had arrived to stay with Geoff. Connie's hospital bills, our mounting concern about our son, schools, and living costs without a book ready for publication, had persuaded us to transfer Geoff to day school. He loved his grandfather and I felt my parent's calmness and wisdom would provide us, for that short time, with a stopgap until I could get back and attempt to get to the bottom of Geoff's problem.

In Los Angeles Harold and Grace Robbins met us at the airport and the four of us drove to a spa. The public Harold would probably not be caught dead in a place that catered to the ill, the dieters, the plain people who came to be made beautiful. The private Harold not only went along with Grace, Connie, and me, but took whirlpool baths and walks with Connie in an effort to help restore my husband's health. And the private Harold talked, for so laconic a man, at length about Connie's work on *Bridge* and how only Connie could make the welter of people, plans and statistics fall into place and the book become a living thing.

We came back to Los Angeles on Thursday, December 4, where Harold, the connoisseur of hotels, had acquired for us a bright and lovely suite with an outside patio at the Beverly Hills Hotel. He put one of his cars at our disposal, but we seldom used it. Harold and Grace were as constantly with us as if they, too, were living at the hotel instead of in their home a short distance away.

Each day of rest in the California sun brought Connie more strength and vitality. Now, for the first time in months, he was eager to get home and go to work. *Bridge* was there awaiting him and it was a rendezvous that by now he was eager to keep.

$$= 3 =$$

ON FRIDAY, DECEMBER 11, 1970, Connie saw Dr. Whitmore for the first time since leaving the hospital. It had been forty-three days since he had seen the doctor and, unlike other times when hospital or clinical visits caused him tension and nervousness, he anticipated this one. He was eager to get as many details as possible about his operation and to have a frank assessment of his health. After months of despair and doubt, he appeared confident. He was looking forward once again—to life.

Dr. Whitmore's "Follow-up and Progress Notes" were thorough:

According to the patient he has had a "rough time" until one week ago. His complaints consisted of variable abdominal pains unasso-ciated with any particular bowel problem. In addition, he has had urinary frequency, urgency and burning with occasional extreme stream difficulty. In the past week, however, his urinary function is essentially back to normal . . . his weight is down to 175 lbs. He had some urinary tract infection which was treated with antimicrobials by Dr. Neligan. . . . He has had variable back pain but no pain requiring analgesics and is currently on no medication whatever.

Dr. Whitmore noted that Connie looked well and that his wound had healed satisfactorily. He did detect some knottiness or slight enlargement in the lymph nodes in the area of the groin, along the upper middle part of the thigh, but had no further comment on them. He diagrammed the prostate and found on digital rectal examination that in size and shape it was relatively unchanged from its contour before the operation.

The outlook seemed brighter than it had in months and Connie's spirits soared. He spent the rest of the month planning for Christmas with his usual enthusiasm, getting out his daily correspondence, attending board meetings he had missed for months. He radiated health and vitality.

"Come the New Year," he told Anne and me, "I'm going to break the back of the book. You girls better be prepared. We've all spent enough time on cancer. It's got to take a back seat from here on. I'll find out at my monthly checkups what the score is and we'll deal with whatever we have to as we go along. But the number one priority is *Bridge*."

We made the rounds of the pre-Christmas parties. The Ryans were back together again and Connie had never looked better. The tongue-wagging in Ridgefield and New York was stilled. Connie announced to everyone that his research trips for the book were over and until its completion he could be found at home.

On Christmas Eve the close friends who knew about our tragic year came for dinner. It was a warming, lovely time spent with people with whom no pretense would ever again be necessary.

It was one of the happiest Christmases and New Year's I remember. The infectious gaiety of Connie's spirit buoyed us all. Swept along by that spirit we looked forward eagerly to the year and the work ahead. As Connie said, *Bridge* was

249

the first priority. Cancer, I believed, was now far down the list.

The stunning speed of Connie's recovery continued, seeming to bear out all our hopes. He began long hours of preparatory work on *Bridge*. He reread the plans of each Allied commander whose men took part in the battle—the September 1944 effort to force open a route through Nazi-occupied Holland by air and land, cross the Rhine, and drive into Germany. He studied German war diaries and the interviews he had held with German tank commanders whose panzer divisions had, by a historic fluke, been in the exact area of the Allied thrust. With Annie, he rechecked long lists of statistics on the numbers of men, machines, and equipment deployed in the massive attack. However traumatic his most recent research had been, the experience seemed to pale as the tragic outcome of Operation Market-Garden, twenty-seven years earlier, began once more to dominate his time.

Even as Connie completed his reevaluation of those events, another Ryan project was ending. In a sudden surge of energy, freed from my fears for Connie's health, I had stepped up the work on *The Betty Tree*. On March 24, 1971, I was at my desk, deep in concentration. Suddenly I was aware that something in my line of vision had been added to the clutter that surrounded me. A double old-fashioned glass, brimful of Scotch, ice, and water, was sitting next to the University of Missouri mug I used to hold my pencils. I stared at the glass uncomprehendingly and then at Connie standing in front of my desk. I had no idea how long he had been there, but the ice in the large glass he had put down had melted considerably.

"You've finished your book, Katie," he said triumphantly. "I could tell it was coming a couple of hours ago."

I stared up at him, then back at the small pile of handwritten sheets on the desk.

"I don't think I have," I told him. "Maybe later. I don't know."

I went back to the page in front of me, reading the last words I had put down. I studied them for some time, and then a sentence which had eluded me, for hours it seemed, fell into place. I wrote it down and saw, to my amazement, that Connie was right. I had come to the end of *The Betty Tree*. It was finished.

I felt suddenly weak and empty. I had become very fond of some of the characters in the novel. They had not always behaved as planned and perhaps I would never have been able to alter them to fit my original concept. Now I had to let them go. They would resolve their own fates, live out their lives without me. The thought made me homesick for them. For a long time I had immersed myself in their problems and they had helped me to forget my own. Now they were gone.

Connie came across from his desk—he had been so uncharacteristically still I had forgotten he was there—and put his arms around me. "I know, " he said as if I had spoken aloud. "But you feel that way whenever we end a book. I'm the one who always wants to celebrate and that's exactly what we're going to do now. I'm taking you out to dinner."

"What time is it?"

"Nearly eight," he said. I must have registered some kind of panic because Connie added, "Don't worry. I helped the kids make their dinner about six thirty. You were coming into the home stretch and I wanted you to cross the finish line. I brought the drink when I came back down but," he shook his head, "it's pretty far gone by now." He picked it up and went across to our little office kitchen where he poured it out. "Come on, Katie," he said, coming back to me and holding out his hand. "Leave the pages for Anne to type in the morning. There are a couple of loyal admirers up at the house who also want to congratulate you. After that it's champagne and dinner. God knows you've earned it."

In the weeks following, just as I was able to begin to take on my share of the work on *Bridge*, a new demand was made on Connie's time. It was one he accepted with pleasure. Victoria had asked her father to help stage her school's production of the musical *Oliver*.

Connie was no stranger to the field. As a sixteen-year-old in Dublin, he had not only mastered the violin, for a time he had had his own orchestra, booking it for dances in Dublin and at nearby country inns. The group was in great demand until, according to Connie's brother Joe, "Mother found out where Con was spending his evenings and that was the end of the Hi-Lo Orchestra." He was also stagestruck and spent many hours, Joe remembers, "hanging about the Abbey," Dublin's famed drama theater, to which he also submitted plays (all of them kindly but emphatically turned down).

Additionally, he learned to tap-dance and, from the time our children could walk, Connie spent hours with Geoff and Vicki, patiently going over dance steps with them, as later he was to teach them photography, fly casting, and trapshooting.

For over a month in the spring of 1971, Connie left the office at 2:30 every weekday afternoon and drove to Vicki's school to work on the choreography, lights, and music for *Oliver*. It may have been the easiest month that teachers had that year with Vicki. We received no word of disruptive behavior or temper outbursts during that time.

Opening night was in early May. To help out, Connie had enlisted the aid of Hans Schroeder and Horst Brettschneider, our young German friends from New York. Each evening of the performance they rushed out from the city to do all the makeup and hairstyles for the cast. After the last performance the young cast presented Connie with a silver plate. They had pooled their allowances to buy it. The engraving on the plate, taken from one of the songs in *Oliver* read: "Consider Yourself One of Us." For once words failed Connie totally and the silver plate received a prominent place among his cherished possessions.

Even as we plunged back into life and work, one priority too long neglected plummeted us back into worry and actual fear. Contrary to all the books and counselors who advise parents to respect their children's privacy, I had invaded Geoff's room and discovered evidence that further convinced me that our son had indeed experimented with more than tobacco. In the office, faced with my findings, he admitted he both had done so and was still doing it. There was a long, stormy session, made more difficult by anger and recrimination.

To Geoff's statement that he was not unique and that far more harmful habits than marijuana were a way of life among his peers, we responded that it was not the path he was going down any longer. Harsh accusations were leveled. Geoff claimed that, at nearly eighteen, we were trying to restrict his life, pick his friends, and keep him penned like a caged animal. I had never heard such bitterness in his voice, but I matched it.

"If you're old enough to run your own life, then maybe you ought to get out of here and do it. See how well things go outside the cage," I told him. "If you think we're supporting a bunch of hopheads and pushers, you're very wrong. Now I want to know where and how you get what you're getting. We're putting an end to this one way or the other."

Geoff sat staring straight ahead. "Well, Geoff," Connie said finally, "do I call the police—or what?"

Geoff's anger flared again. "Do what you want," he said. "I don't care."

"You either give us your word that this is all over now or you leave this house," I told him.

Connie looked at me warningly and shook his head.

"I mean it, Connie," I said. "I don't want him in this house unless he straightens up. Now," I turned to Geoff, trembling with anger, "what's it to be?"

He swore. "What can it be, except to do it your way?" he said.

"You'll stop all this and stop it now?" I pressed.

"Yeh."

I took what I had found in his room and flushed it away in the bathroom.

"Remember what I told you. If I ever find out that you're taking anything ever again, you leave this house. Is that clear?"

He stalked past me and slammed the door so hard the ceiling-high opaque glass panels on either side shuddered violently. I thought they would surely break.

The trauma was not over. Connie's face was ashen when I came back into our workroom. I realized that he had said very little during the scene with Geoff. I'd been too busy shouting to notice until then.

"You'd never send him away," Connie said.

"Oh, wouldn't I?"

"No, because he's my son, too, and I'll make decisions like that."

"Tell me," I said, still filled with sorrow and anger and now, suddenly, with spite, "how much time have *you* spent with him over the past year?" I could have cried out with remorse but the words were spoken.

"That's not fair," Connie said.

"Neither is he. Nothing's fair, Connie. Life isn't fair. I'm tired, worn out. I've got the work here and my book proofs to read and the constant shopping and cooking and driving to his school or Vicki's school for one activity or another. I'm sick of Geoff and his behavior. I'm sick of it all."

"I think I have the list," Connie said. "Actually I think you're frightened about me, the children, both the books. What makes you sick is really very simple."

He was pensive and I waited; the horror of what I'd said seemed to grow inside me.

Finally Connie said, "Maybe you're the one who should

go, Kathryn. Go, before it's too late. Because we don't have the kind of life we used to and we never will again. There aren't any full stops and good new leads. There isn't anything ahead but question marks."

Late that same evening Connie called our friend, Ted Safford, who was also Geoff's physician. Ted came to the house and the three of us discussed the problem. Ted's calmness produced an opposite effect on Connie. Despite his other worries, during the hours since the argument in the office, Connie's concern for Geoff was by then clearly evident, as was his anger.

"Damn it," he told Ted, "I can't have this family upset more than it is. Katie is half out of her mind with worry and exhaustion and Geoff acts like he's not conscious most of the time. How the devil do we straighten this out? I want an end to it, Ted. Now!"

"There isn't anything new about this drug scene," Ted told us. "And the reasons for it vary from one youngster to another. We all expect too much of them from time to time and the pressure imposed gets to be too much for them to bear."

"I've got all the pressure I can take," Connie said. "I can't go through this, too."

"I said there were all kinds of reasons for drug abuse," Ted said. "One of the pressures on Geoff is most certainly the illness you went through last year, and as it intensified so did his desire to make it go away. That might be a big part of his involvement."

"What?" Connie asked. "You've lost me. How could he make it easier for me by getting into drugs?"

"He couldn't help you so he just made your illness go away," Ted said. "He tried to forget it."

Connie put his hands to his face. "Cancer," he said, his voice muffled. "Bloody cancer. It will kill us all."

He pulled his hands away and his eyes were wet with tears. "Well, damn it, I won't let it," he told Ted. "It's not going to ruin anybody else in this family. I'm not going to let it ruin me. I've had it on my mind so long it's distracted me from everything else. No more." He looked at Ted. "If Geoff really got hooked, he'd be worse off than I am. I've got to help my kid get well."

And as the days passed, Geoff, indeed, seemed better. He was more in evidence, still subdued at the table, but eager for us to listen to the music and lyrics he wrote, which now seemed to take up much of his spare time. He was teaching himself to play the guitar and the strain on our ears was often painful, causing everyone at some point or another to beg him to desist. He had always been an avid reader and now he was sharing more of that interest with us, too. His tastes were eclectic. Ray Bradbury, Steinbeck, J. D. Salinger, Chekhov, Hemingway had become his favorite authors, along with Ionesco and Pinter. He wrote a school paper on the theater of the absurd and wrote, produced, directed, and starred in a play which earned him a "Dramatic Achievements" award and the wry comment from his headmaster that "this must surely stand as the most lofty, lonely flight of Ego ever yet attempted."

Additionally, he had delved deeper into one of Connie's passions, photography, and was learning to develop his own pictures, experimenting with color, texture, and tone. He took photographs of individual roses in my garden, going out at dawn to capture each step of a bud's opening and the tiny drops of dew, like tears, that gathered on the petals. The pictures were my birthday present from him in 1971, solemnly presented by him as "probably suitable for framing." As indeed they were.

His birthday, a day before mine, was an occasion of great joy. Seeing his efforts to expand from the tight little world in which he had lived, Connie and I had bought him a small, secondhand car. He was ecstatic. "Why?" he asked. "Can we afford it?"

"We'll manage some way," Connie told him. "Just don't

bang up yourself. You drive carefully and I'll worry about the insurance and the car payments."

"It's a way of saying 'thank you' for coming back," I told him. "Thank you for being you again."

A shadow passed across his face, and then was gone.

$$\doteq 4 \doteq$$

ALL THROUGH THE SPRING AND SUMMER of 1971 Connie had worked steadily on the book. His outline for the first part, composed of one-word reminders that would enable him to recall whole segments of the story, was jotted down on a yellow pad lined up precisely with the right edge of his desk. He was finding the writing agonizingly slow.

"Put down the ideas," I urged him, seeing his daily torment, but he could not work that way and neither could I. Still, of the two of us, he was the greater perfectionist. Each labored-over sheet was handed to me for editing, then taken back by him for reediting, and over to me once more. By the time Anne received a page only her expert eyes could read it and make a clean copy of it.

It was dogged, wearying work. Beset by family problems and the ever-present shadow of the cancer we prayed had been wiped out for good, he had written only forty-seven pages of the book by August 20.

Yet to his doctors he seemed "the picture of health," as Dr. Whitmore noted on one visit. But, Whitmore added,

. . . mental attitude is the problem.

In further elaboration he wrote:

Although he denies preoccupation with his illness, the fact is that he has been unable to do productive work on his book. . . . He claims that his slow progress . . . is the consequence of inability to concentrate although he is not knowingly diverting "thinking time" to his neoplasm. I wonder if a tranquilizer would help.

Not even to his doctors would Connie admit that a more placid family life might have worked better for him than a tranquilizer. Except for his single talk with Ted, he did not confide to anyone, as far as I know, the fears and worries he had about his family as well as the all too evident ones about his book. Even in his tapes and notebooks there is no mention of any other difficulties. He was never again to record any serious details of his children's lives. Their problems were, to him, completely private, and he protected their privacy and mine even from the doctors who could best help him to overcome his mental worries. In good times or bad, his family was sacrosanct. His pride would not let it be otherwise.

On July 6, a day before Connie's midsummer visit to Dr. Whitmore, he saw Dr. Guy Van Syckle, a specialist in radiology, practicing in Connecticut. At Pat's instigation Dr. Van Syckle had last done a series of X rays on Connie in January 1971. At that time he had found nothing unexpected, given the nature of the operation Connie had undergone the previous October. But on July 6, Dr. Van Syckle encountered an abnormal change. Films tracking an intravenous injection of a radioactive substance to determine normal kidney collection and drainage (an IVP) revealed disquieting news. Connie's right kidney had ceased to function.

Unrelated but equally grim events were soon to engulf us. As the months passed Connie worked steadily, but his efforts seemed futile to him. Page after page of handwritten copy was discarded as he tried to bring his book to life. And meanwhile other dramas, frightening and unexpected, surfaced with shocking suddenness.

Around 11:00 A.M. on October 15, I felt intense, heavy pressure throughout my chest and a numb ache pulsed along my left arm. Within minutes I was as drenched as if I had been thrown into a pool. I could not take a deep breath. The pressure, numbness, and sweating continued.

Connie, engrossed in work, was unaware of what was happening. Finally, taking careful short breaths, I got his attention. He took one look at me and called Ted Safford, his eyes never leaving me as he described my symptoms. Ted's instructions were brief: Connie was to take me immediately to the emergency entrance of Norwalk Hospital, about fifteen miles away.

I was reluctant to go. Whatever was happening would surely pass. Connie swept aside my arguments. In brilliant fall sunshine he drove me to the hospital. There, an emergency team was waiting. Before I could step from the car, attendants swiftly moved me to a rolling cart and wheeled me speedily to the Coronary Care Unit.

I lost all track of time. When I came to, I was in bed wired to a cardiac monitor, an oxygen apparatus in my nostrils, and an IV infusion dripping slowly through a plastic tube inserted in a vein in my arm. Connie was sitting on a chair beside me, a lost, desperate expression on his face.

"I'll do anything to get attention," I said drowsily. I felt extremely tired.

"Hush," Connie said. "Don't talk. Rest."

And I did.

Some time later I woke to see both Ted and Pat in the room.

"Is Connie all right?" I asked, trying to sit up. I had forgotten where I was. Seeing them I thought that cancer had struck once more.

Ted gently eased me down. "He'll be better when he can stop worrying about you," he said.

I knew then where I was. "I'm fine," I said. "I can go now."

Ted shook his head. "Not tonight."

"Where's Connie?"

"Where he's been most of the day," Pat answered. "Stalking up and down outside, making a nuisance of himself, bothering people. Do you think you can get him to go home?"

"I'll try. Promise to tell him everything is all right."

Connie was brought back to the room. He glared at Pat and Ted and sat down, obviously prepared to stay.

"I feel fine, just tired," I told him. "Please go home. Don't let Geoff and Vicki worry."

"I have been home. I took them out for hamburgers. They're all right."

"You've got a full day's work tomorrow," I told him. "You need rest and I'll feel better if Geoff and Vicki aren't alone."

Connie looked at Pat and Ted. They nodded. Reluctantly he got up. "If anything happens to her—" He leaned forward and put his hands alongside my face, then smoothed back my hair.

"Take it easy, Katie." He kissed my cheek.

"You, too." I told him. "Promise?"

He nodded, turned abruptly, and left the room. Pat followed him out.

The threatened heart attack did not apparently go any further. Ted Safford and heart specialists, after a battery of tests, could only say that I had had "an undiagnosed chest pain" possibly triggered by exhaustion. Within ten days I was home. During my hospital stay Connie had come by daily, sometimes bringing Geoff and Vicki. Each time he looked distressed and worried. My illness had absorbed his time and thoughts and, once again, his work on his book had suffered.

At home everything was organized. Connie had arranged for the same good-hearted woman who had stayed with Vicki when he had been hospitalized to do the cooking for a time. Good friends shopped or brought in food. Others came for brief but welcome visits, and two of them, Billie Newell and Jean Deems, filled the house with fresh flowers. But it was Connie who carried trays to me, ran my baths, and spent his evenings entertaining me with stories.

For a time I often slept as much as fourteen hours a day. Ted reiterated that work and worry had put me over the border between plain tiredness and total exhaustion. He urged a slow convalescence, but I had a feeling Connie's mind would not be easy until he saw me up and about again. Against Ted's advice, I resumed limited activities, and on November 20, I went with Connie for nearly an hour to a formal party at the Neligans, getting scowls from both my host and Ted. But Connie was happy.

Solicitous and protective, he would not let me cook or clean and limited my time in the office to an hour or two in the morning and the same in the afternoon. He found temporary cleaning ladies and even a woman who was a genius at the ironing board—a skill I had never mastered and never would. Left to my own devices, I always sent the laundry out.

These temporary luxuries reminded me of the days when we had had the services of an English couple for two years during work on *The Last Battle,* when both of us were often away on research trips at the same time. I relived the enjoyment of a house I hadn't cleaned, meals I hadn't cooked, and the knowledge that someone else would run the errands.

But money was going out far faster than it was coming in, and finally I convinced my husband that I was both fit and well. Not well enough to do the ironing, maybe, but in other ways recovered. On December 1, I spent my first full working day reading proofs of *The Betty Tree* with my New York editor. My final work on the novel was, at last, completed.

And then, once more our family toppled backward into crises. The evening of December 9 was rainy and unseasonably warm. Dinner over, I was in the bath. I was still tired. Five to six hours seemed my limit for work and then exhaustion would set in again. An hour's rest might gain me an extra hour of work if I paced myself carefully but I felt drained afterward and usually went to bed early. That was my plan that Thursday evening when Connie knocked at my bathroom door. He came in, his face stricken.

"Kate," he said, "some kid just now called here for Geoff. I got him on the intercom and stayed on the phone to make sure he'd picked it up. Before I could get off, this fellow told Geoff he had the stuff and asked if Geoff could get the seventy-five by tomorrow." Connie paused. "Geoff said he thought he could. Katie, you don't think—?"

I stepped out of the tub and reached for my robe. Connie helped me into it. "Lord," he said, "it all happened so quickly. Maybe it's not what I think."

But it was.

Geoff didn't attempt to lie. Connie was distraught. He wanted peace and no more illnesses—not his, nor mine, nor Geoff's.

"Get out," I told my only son.

"I never stopped, Mom. It just seemed that way to you," Geoff said. "Buying me the car was a big mistake. You can't buy me what I want."

I saw Vicki appear suddenly in the foyer leading to our bedroom. She was in a rage. "Don't blame him!" she screamed. "It's my fault. The kid who called him goes to my school, not his. I'm the one who told Geoff about him."

"What's his name?" I asked her coldly.

She shook her head.

"It doesn't matter at the moment." I turned to Geoff. "You remember what I told you if this ever happened again?"

He nodded.

"Then take whatever you need and get out."

Vicki began to scream again—long, howling noises that seemed to go on endlessly. "Stop it!" I yelled at her.

"It's not his fault!" she yelled back. "I told you that. It's not his fault!"

"We're not discussing this tonight," Connie said. "Not one of us is up to it."

Geoff walked out of our bedroom and down the stairs.

Connie sat Vicki down on the bedroom sofa and knelt beside her. "Tell me who he is—the one who called," he said.

She did.

Connie was on the phone immediately. He dialed information and got three last-name listings in the area Vicki had told him the boy lived in. Vicki didn't know the father's name. But Connie found it on his second call. He told the boy's father what had occurred. The man flatly denied that his son could be involved in any way.

"Let me talk to the boy," Connie said. "Please." The man hung up.

"He's lying, Daddy," Vicki said.

"Maybe he doesn't know. Just like other parents."

"But I know. So do half the kids at school. You can't blame Geoff. It's my fault."

"But Geoff promised he was through with that," I said.

Connie wasn't listening. He was on the phone again to the police in the town where the boy lived. They had no record of him in their list of juvenile offenders.

None of us heard Geoff leave.

He had gone silently, taking nothing but the clothes he stood in. His car keys were on his desk, the car in the garage. The rain was falling gently but steadily. He'll get drenched,

I thought, and shivered myself, standing barefoot with Connie and Vicki on the wet blacktop, staring into the garage.

We came back up to the house. Vicki left us at the stairs to go to her room. She turned to me, her face wet with rain. "You made him go," she said. "You're to blame, not him. He never was."

She went into her room and slammed the door. Staring at it, I could hear Connie banging other doors in his dressing room. I climbed the stairs as though each tread were a mountain, and sat down on the bed. My dear God! I thought. I *was* right, wasn't I? I warned him.

Connie came out of the dressing room. He had changed his clothes and was wearing a light Windbreaker over a sweater and corduroy pants.

He looked down at me. "Our only son is gone. Is there anything more you'd like to destroy tonight?"

I couldn't answer. I was thinking of Geoff out in the rain and of Connie and the long, slow, steady climb he had made back to health. I was remembering the days he'd labored in the office, the play he'd helped produce at Vicki's school, the tenderness and love with which he had surrounded me since my illness and always before. I knew the love he felt for our children and now he was angry and frightened.

He started down the stairs to the foyer. I ran after him. "Where are you going?"

Connie didn't answer. From the hall closet he took out two high-powered flashlights and slung his heavy raincoat over his arm. He walked on down the hall into the children's suite of rooms and opened Vicki's door. I stood in the foyer watching. He came out, a piece of paper in his hands. He held it out to me.

"Don't worry," it read, in Vicki's neat writing. "I'll be all right. Don't worry."

I looked from it to Connie and started past him.

He took my arm. "Don't bother looking," he said. "She's gone, too."

He headed for the stairs leading down to the lowest floor and to the garages. Then he stopped and stared at me.

"Are you satisfied, Kathryn?" he asked. "Is this really what you want? They're both gone."

He turned and ran down the stairs. I followed him out into the rain again. "I'll get dressed and take another car. We can both look."

He came back to where I stood, picked me up, and carried me to the back door. He opened it and set me down inside. With the rain, it was impossible to tell if one or both of us were crying.

"Go up and change. Dry your hair. You'll catch cold."

He freed my arms from around his neck.

"How long will you be?" I asked him.

"Until I find them."

"Maybe one of them will call."

"No. They won't."

"Will you call *me*?" I asked.

"If any place is open."

"Find a place."

"Go up to bed."

"I can't," I said. "I can't go to bed."

"Then just stay inside."

He left me and went out into the softly falling rain that had swallowed up our children.

A little after 5:00 A.M. on Friday, December 10, Connie telephoned. His voice was bleak. "Nothing," he said tersely. "I'm heading back."

"Where are you?"

"Outside Danbury. I've still got some back roads to check. They're not in any of the motels or diners or roadhouses in this area and I've been through the main roads all the way to Westport."

"Come straight back, Connie, you're exhaus—" The phone went dead.

At 6:30 it rang again. A teacher at Geoff's school told me Geoff had shown up at his house a few hours earlier and had been put to bed. His voice was guarded and I sensed, or thought I did, his hostility to the kind of parent who would order out her own child on a rainy night, or any other for that matter.

I told him that Connie had been searching for Geoff all night—it was obvious that Vicki was not with her brother— and the man asked that we telephone him at his office around nine.

To my mind, then and now, the schools were as responsible, if guilt had to be placed, as I was. But that was hardly the point.

Later, close on eight, I heard noises coming from the kitchen. Connie, still in his Windbreaker, was brewing coffee. I sat down and told him about Geoff. Geoff was safe.

He stared at me wearily. "And Vicki?" he asked.

A few minutes before Connie made his call to Geoff's benefactor, I called Vicki's school. The reason she hadn't been on the bus that morning was that I'd forgotten to let the school know she'd stayed overnight at a friend's house, I said.

"But she wasn't feeling too well," I added. "Did she come in today?" My heart was beating so hard I thought my entire body was shaking.

But Vicki was at school. Slumped against the kitchen desk, weak with relief, I waited while someone went to get her. Her voice was neutral but she seemed in control of herself. She was all right, just tired, she said. She didn't mean to worry us. She promised to come home on the bus that night. She had something to take care of during the noon recess.

"Vicki, don't go near that boy," I said, suddenly attuned.

"It'll be all right, Mom. You and Daddy please try to rest."

"Vicki, it's under control. Geoff's at school. He went to one of the teacher's. He's all right."

"Thank God," she said tremblingly, then added, "I'm going to see the nurse now. I think I have a cold."

"Where were you last night?"

No answer.

"Please, Vicki," I begged. "I've got to know. I love you. Please."

Her voice was very low, guarded from the secretaries in the school office. "I hitchhiked to within almost a mile of school and then I walked. I slept out in the woods and came inside when the others did."

"I'll come and get you right now."

"No." She was firm. "I'll get an aspirin or something from the nurse. They've already given me a scolding because my clothes look so mussed. I can't afford to miss today. Don't worry anymore. I'll come home tonight," and she hung up.

Even as my call to Vicki was ending, Connie was speaking on the other line to the teacher at Geoff's school. The man was sympathetic to our problem and, equally, to Geoff's. He advised that for the time it would be better for Geoff to stay in a school dormitory where, I believed, this trouble had begun in the first place. But no one else was willing to accept any blame for what had been happening to our son. We and we alone were the culprits—the bad guys who had finally driven him from home. By implication the teacher made it clear that any fault lay in the environment in which Geoff had been raised.

I thought a great deal about that environment and remembered the words of the pediatrician the children had had in New York. Once, when I was feeling guilty about the long hours I spent on my job in the city and was wondering about the effect my absence and Connie's research trips were having on the children's psyches, the pediatrician said, "Well, they never had any other parents, did they?" He explained. "To them, your routine is normal. They have nothing to compare it to except what they are told by other youngsters about their home lives. But how many mothers might be better parents if they worked, instead of spending every day with their children? How many fathers might find more enlightening, interesting things to do with their youngsters if those activities were unusual instead of a dutiful weekend chore?

"Your children," he told me, "are in some ways better adjusted and more precocious, which is not a bad thing, than most of my patients whose parents are always on the scene. The time you and your husband give to your children is solely theirs. It is not fragmented by resentful parents to whom children are often a constant reminder of duties and responsibilities."

Certainly part of what he had said was true. Geoff and Vicki had known no other way of life—and we had thought it was a good one. I remembered the times we four had taken vacations geared around activities we enjoyed in common. We had seen plays and ballets together, gone to the Philharmonic and to every museum in the city—and later we would talk about our varying tastes in art and music, excitedly interrupting one another to give our individual views. We had flown about the country and to Europe with our children before either of them was four years old.

Connie had taken Geoff on a two-month research trip to Europe one year, putting the then twelve-year-old in charge of travel details, teaching him the ins and outs of hotel check-ins and departures, customs forms, and railway border crossings so that he would not be a stranger to the world his father inhabited.

All readers, we had taken pleasure in one another's favorite authors and had spent hours together talking about books, their content and construction. There had been the mutual fun of swimming, tennis, and golf lessons and the kidding about "Mom's" obvious lack of expertise in all three sports. We had never believed in banishing the children from parties or formal dinners at home. As a result they had met and dined with many of the historic figures Connie wrote about and worked with. Wernher von Braun had given Geoff the first space helmet I ever saw. Queen Juliana of the Netherlands had walked with him around the lake behind her palace. John Kennedy had always remembered their given names.

I felt defensive then and even now about the attitude of schools and teachers who place all blame on parents for children's misbehavior. They know as little of us as we know of them. Was home environment at fault in the days when we had all lived in France during the filming of *The Longest Day* and Geoff and Vicki had gone to school with French children, picking up the language and comically imitating my bad accent? Were they stunted, diminished, wronged by that experience in a foreign country? They had returned to the United States achievers, readers, doers, but, teachers im-implied, we had failed our children; their problems were all our making. The pediatrician's words seemed more appropriate than ever: "But they never had any other parents, did they?"

Our love for them and theirs for us had not changed. The problem was that they had moved outside the family circle into a kind of world we had not known was coming.

A week after Geoff left home, the school asked me to bring some of his possessions there. Upon arrival, someone directed me to a dormitory where I was to put down the boxes, suitcases, hanging clothes in a hall. I made a series of trips to the car. Finished, I asked someone where I might find Geoff. He stared at me coldly. "How would I know?" he asked and walked off.

Teachers and advisers seemed all to be occupied. Slowly, I walked back to the car. Geoff was standing beside it. I looked at him and began to cry.

"I never meant it to be like this," I said.

"It doesn't matter."

"When will we see you again?"

"I don't know," he said, and then, "I'm glad you did what you did. I don't ever want to go back there again."

"My God, Geoff! It's your home."

"No, Mom, it's yours," he said. "Your house. Your family. Your life-style. I don't want it."

"That's not true. You're not thinking straight."

He was silent.

"Will you come home for Christmas?" I asked. "Please, Geoff."

"We'll see. Better go now, Mom. Take care." He opened the car door for me. "Thanks for bringing my things. I didn't know what time you'd get here. I was over in another dorm and didn't see you drive up. I would have carried in my stuff. You shouldn't have."

"I'd like to load everything back in the car and you, too. Geoff, if this is where the temptation is, don't stay. We'll find another school."

"They're all alike. Besides it's my senior year. If you've paid the tuition, I want to graduate. I couldn't get into someplace else at midterm." He shut the car door. Quickly I rolled down the window.

"Will you please come home for Christmas?" It was just ten days away.

He thought a minute. "What time's dinner?"

"One? I'll come and get you."

"No. I'll be there." He put his elbows on the car. "You know," he said, "I never thought you'd do it but I'm glad you did." Quickly he leaned over and kissed my cheek. "Hey, Mom, stop crying. I love you."

He turned abruptly and walked toward his dorm.

"Geoff," I called after him. "I love you."

Without turning he waved, and went inside the building.

Christmas Day was warm and filled with sunlight. We three had gone to midnight services and come home to the pile of presents under the tree. Without Geoff they seemed like just so much decoration. We wouldn't open them until Geoff was with us.

From noon on Vicki and I took turns looking out the kitchen window down the sunny driveway, lined with bare trees. We could not keep from staring at that driveway.

Connie had been often remote and withdrawn since Geoff left. He brushed aside my queries as to how he felt, but there were many nights he paced the floor and days when he sat for long periods in the office staring out at nothing, his thoughts far away. None of us at home were happy and all three of us were waiting on that Christmas Day for a boy who might have decided not to come.

Suddenly, in the kitchen, Vicki shouted, "I see him!" and ran out of the room and up the driveway to meet her brother. I watched from the window. Geoff had on a colorful cape, like a serape, slung across one shoulder, and a blue pillow-case tied to a stick across the other. In the middle of the long drive, brother and sister embraced. Unable to wait any longer, I dashed up the stairs, calling "Connie, he's here," and met my children coming toward the house. I threw my arms about them both, smothering each with kisses mixed with tears.

Once inside our bright, handsome house, Geoff's mood changed, as if the house was haunted with memories he chose not to remember but could not dispel.

An impatient Vicki began distributing the presents. Except for the first two or three, Geoff did not open his. He sat, like a foreign visitor, baffled by the customs of the natives. Finally, the place strewn with gift wrappings, he untied the pillowcase. In it was a present for each of us which he had made himself—necklaces for Vicki and me; a bookmark, I think, for his father; and another shawl—similar in its rainbow colors to the one he was wearing—for Vicki.

He had hitchhiked to the house, he told us, starting early. Rides had been few and far between. He had walked the last mile and a quarter from a main highway up the steep country road that led to our house. Thinking of that journey, seeing the presents he had made, I realized only then that he had been without pocket money for some time. The same thought struck Connie. But Geoff refused the offer.

"I have friends," he told us. "I get by."

We did not talk about it further.

At the table we made a strange contrast. Festive dinners had always been eaten in festive dress. Geoff, his long hair falling to his shoulders, a hand-strung necklace bright against a faded blue shirt, jeans frayed at the knees and bottoms, seemed like a stranger from another world. Call it counter-culture, subculture, youth revolt, his appearance clearly expressed the distances between us. I thought of the cashmere sweaters, tailored twill trousers, fine cotton shirts, and gleaming shoes that I had packed to take to him at school and of others, still unopened, in his pile of presents.

When, where, how, and why had it happened? On what otherwise remarkable day had we lost our son and never known it?

Connie looked ill and very pale; Geoff and I were not very talkative. Only Vicki kept our Christmas dinner from degenerating into silence.

In the late afternoon Paul Slade, our friend from *Paris Match,* drove out from the city. I had not expected him and would have welcomed him much earlier. It might have relieved some of our tensions. Connie, I was to learn later, had talked with Paul that week. He had just finished a series of photographic essays for *Match* on youth and drugs. His experiences had shocked even his normally unshockable nature, but he had learned the language of the drug culture and he could talk to youngsters on their terms, in their tongue. He had come, at Connie's invitation, to see Geoff. They had always liked each other and both were happy to be reunited.

Shortly after dusk Paul offered to drive Geoff back to school. Again Geoff refused money from Connie and most of his presents were left behind. Vicki, Connie, and I sat together in the living room, silent and sad, feeling again the absence of Geoff.

Connie suddenly got up and made the two of us a drink, took one swallow of his, and disappeared up to his bathroom almost immediately. He was unable to keep the liquor down. I heard his shower running and, some minutes later, he came back down in dressing gown, pajamas, and slippers. And we sat on, the record changer playing softly through the stack of Christmas carols I had put on earlier. It didn't seem like Christmas.

Shortly after 11:00 P.M., Paul returned. I made him some tea, his constant beverage, and he told us startling news. His horror stories of what he had learned on his recent assignment had made an impression on Geoff, but Paul guessed our son's mind had been made up long before. In Paul's presence Geoff had taken out some packets like those I had found at home, and, as I had done on that day in our office, had flushed them down the toilet.

"I've got to tell you," Paul said, "he didn't do it for you. He did it for himself. He isn't into the heavy stuff, he never was. My guess is he got involved because everybody else was into something and that kind of peer pressure is tough to resist. You get all sorts of flak if you don't go along. One more thing," Paul said. "This will be hard. He wants to see you now and then but he doesn't want to live here.

"There's a boy at school who went through Geoff's problem, far more seriously, I gather, and came out the other side. His parents will take Geoff in to live with them. That way he's not under pressure from you and he's not under pressure from his former friends who got him into this.

"But don't expect him home unless he wants to come and don't expect his attitude to change right away. He told me he's made the first decision he ever had a chance to make for himself. That's what he resents most. You two made the decisions and he had to fit into them whether he wanted to or not. School, clothes, activities—he says he never had any choices."

Stunned by Paul's revelations, we were silent. Finally Connie said, "I don't want him living with another family."

"CJ," Paul said, "I tell you straight. You got no choice. He feels intimidated here. Your personality overpowers him. Kathy's neatness and compulsive orderliness bug him. He wants to find out who *he* is. Someday, not now, he may want to know who you are—as people, not the parents who made every decision for him."

"He really won't come home?" I asked. "This is his home."

Paul shook his head. "Not now. No way, baby. I'm sorry. But there it is."

Three days later Geoff telephoned and asked if he could bring a friend to dinner. The boy was handsome, clean, polite. He listened without comment as Geoff told us his plans. He was moving to the boy's house. The parents had sent along a letter telling us about themselves, their household, and the family crisis they, too, had met and thankfully survived. Geoff planned, with our agreement to continue his tuition, to finish school and, hopefully, later go to college.

But, he told us, he did not want to live again at home, not now, possibly never. And then he sprung the most surprising news of all: he had voluntarily enrolled in a drug rehabilitation program to learn more about how others met and solved the pressures of their lives. His evenings would be spent at the center with counselors and in therapy sessions and he would work on the grounds and in the kitchen of the place. He was, in short, beginning a new life—apart from us—in an intensive effort to find himself and his place in the world.

"It's my decision," he said finally. "And that's the way it's got to be."

And that is the way it was. The four of us had come through two unsettling years. For Geoff and Vicki the time had, apparently, been even longer. Now, at eighteen, Geoff was taking charge of his own life, one he chose to live away from us. Hurt and saddened, we were also proud of him. He had no intention of drifting through life. He had decided to try to master it and, as he said, he had to do it on his own.

We still asked ourselves the questions parents always do: where and when did we go wrong?

He would eventually have left the nest. It was the manner of his going that was hard to take. Geoff had begun his attack on life at the very time that we were struggling to maintain our own.

On Wednesday, December 29, 1971, a day after Geoff's visit, Connie wrote a letter to his friend Norman Cousins, who had recently resigned from *Saturday Review* and was planning to round up funds for a new magazine. In part, Connie wrote:

God knows trying to start a new magazine is a hazardous undertaking at best . . . I don't know what you have in mind but if I can help in any way, please let me know. My resources are a lot slimmer than people believe. Still . . . let me know what's happening.

I'm trying to finish the third volume on the war which I'm calling "A Bridge Too Far." All in all, with the state of the country and the various vicissitudes that have hit me and my family within the last 12 months, I shall be glad to see the end of 1971.

Bear up, old friend. In the end loyalty and integrity to one's faith and ideals are really all that matter.

⸗ 5 ⸗

CORNELIUS

Today is Saturday, January 15, 1972. I have been sitting here
in the office most of the day and I am becoming a little desperate. The book is not moving. If I remain bogged down
much longer without so much as a new sentence on paper, I
will be totally frustrated. There is a communications break-
down between my mind and my hand. The facts that have to
be introduced at this stage are absolutely crucial to the
reader's understanding of the situation leading up to Operation Market-Garden. Yet, while I am fully aware of them, and
their importance, I am unable to write them in a coherent
sequence. The thoughts pour but the writing trickles.

Is it me or the book that's stalling out? I have got to get
some straight answers about my health. What is the point in
torturing myself about how to get through this section of the
book if I don't last long enough to write it all? I think if I
could put cancer behind me I could come to grips with the
book research. As it is, I am on a treadmill going noplace.

The monotony of not being able to write is terrible. But the
constant fear of cancer which inhibits my ability to work is
becoming unbearable.

It even invades my sleep. The other night I sat bolt upright
in bed. I heard Neligan say that the operation hadn't worked.
It was seconds before I realized I'd had a nightmare. Yet,
given the nature of cancer, the dream may be the reality.

Three days ago, on January 12, I saw Whitmore. He was reassuring. The prostate is smaller, tough and burned out by the radiation implants. Willet said he could feel some of the seeds. There was some pus in the urine which Gantrisin is supposed to clear up. That is about the extent of what I learned.* Whitmore asked me to come back in two months. Will the day ever come when he says, "Give me a call in a year or two"?

I think not. Because the truth is that I'm in a holding pattern and sooner or later I'll be making a descent. I am absolutely convinced that this disease will show up someplace else. From all I've read about the subject it would be a medical rarity if it did not, particularly since the lymph nodes were involved. It is apparent that medical science simply does not know what cancer is or what causes it to strike. There are a great many educated guesses but no absolutes. All the specialists can do right now is try to contain it once it is discovered. If it metastasizes, the patient has the dubious pleasure of playing guinea pig while the doctors experiment with various combinations of therapy.

The tricky thing is that a form of treatment may work for one patient, at least for a time, and be quite useless when applied to another. I think cancer is as individual as the person it inhabits. At this point it would be sheer blind luck, not medical know-how, that produced the right therapy for each patient or one therapy for all.

I have been reading a book called *End Results in Cancer*. Could any title be more oppressive? It is a little tome filled with records and statistics about the kinds of cancers there

---

* What Connie did not learn is that for the first time Dr. Whitmore noted: "Abdomen—liver edge felt at costal margins, soft, non-tender. S and K [spleen and kidney] not felt." This was the first indication that the liver was enlarged and succeeding blood chemistries indicated increasing liver involvement. Again on May 3, 1972, Dr. Whitmore wrote: ". . . liver felt about 2 fingerbreadths below the costal margin, small and non-tender. S and K not felt."

are and how long it takes particular age groups to die from each one. Actually, the graphs reflect "survival rates," but one sees immediately that victims are merely bench marks that measure cancer's destructive power. The chartists herd people into one category or another: "Rectum," "Lung," "Stomach," "Prostate," and show the number of cases treated by surgery, radiation, chemotherapy, and hormones, and the survival rate by treatment and stage. The median survival time for my age group with cancer of the prostate is 5.5 years. That means I have a 50/50 chance of living that long after diagnosis.

I wish I had never acquired this book.

KATHRYN

Connie's demons were confined to tape. Outwardly, he seemed more cheerful with each passing day. While his work on the book was slow, it was constant. He had never written speedily. There were too many facts to check and accuracy was his passion.

Two events in early 1972 did, however, sadden him visibly. Geoff's continued absence from home, although he dropped in regularly, was a grief we shared but seldom voiced. During those visits, Connie would be silently attentive to Geoff's accounts of his new life. We were coming to know a different Geoff, a stranger beneath the familiar facade. His attitude was often hostile, softening slowly as the evening went by. The meetings were difficult for all of us. His newfound independence did not appear to make him more tolerant of us and it was difficult to find much common ground for talk. Connie was often pensive for long periods following a visit from Geoff. Despite our differences, I think, at every appearance, he hoped to hear our son say he was back for good.

In early February, our close friend and nearest neighbor Jessie Royce Landis died. With Roycie and her husband,

General "Jeff" Seitz, we had shared many warm and happy evenings. Roycie's infectious laughter, her beauty, her presence, honed by her years as an actress, brought a special joy to everyone who knew her. Her death from cancer affected Connie deeply. And, as did all their other friends, we spent many hours with Jeff Seitz trying to ease his days and weeks of sorrow. One does not succeed at this, no matter how sincere the effort.

The general had a standing invitation to dinner at our house and often walked through his woods and ours to spend an evening in talk that he and Connie equally enjoyed. Together they refought many of the battles of World War II until, late at night, Connie would take a flashlight and walk back home with Jeff as they wound up a conversation.

We saw more and more friends as Connie's health seemed steadily to improve. Dick and Jean Deems came out often from the city to their jewel-box country house for weekends. Will and Austine Hearst were out as well, and we saw them as frequently as their busy schedules would allow; and George and Billie Newell, living a few miles away, joined us frequently for dinners. Those evenings were like rewards after a week of work.

With the Newells we went on a Caribbean cruise in mid-March, taking Vicki, who was on spring vacation and, we discovered, on permanent leave from childhood. Connie had taken a large suite on the ship plus another stateroom adjoining ours for Victoria. The Newells were at the top of the corridor and it seemed as if every college in the East was represented in between. By the time we cleared Ambrose Lightship, Vicki seemed to know all the boys by name. Billie and I were hard-pressed to keep the group in sight. The favorite late-night hangout was the ship's lounge, where an all-Italian band managed to juggle rock, ballads, and the bossa nova with varying degrees of success. For Billie and me, the lounge became a second home—one that George, immersed in the latest novels, and Connie, working on material for *Bridge,* were only too pleased to avoid. "Our little girl," as Billie called Victoria, could be found most any evening singing with the band while we bridged the generation gap and tried to camouflage our roles as chaperones.

On that voyage I noticed immediately that Connie, who had always loved to dance, avoided it almost completely. Soon after dinner each evening he excused himself and went to our stateroom. I would find him later, either lightly dozing or immersed in work. Our lives aboard settled into a routine: lunch and bridge, dinner together, then the Newells and I watched whatever festivities were scheduled in the ballroom, and finally, Billie and I would count down the wee hours of the morning in the ship's lounge, one eye on Vicki and the other on the clock.

Often Connie was still up and working when we returned. He was well aware that our young duckling had become a swan. Sometimes in his sleep, he would mumble "Vicki" and then sit up, panic on his face as on the night our children both left home, and get out of bed to reassure himself that she was in her room. For Vicki, the cruise was the highlight of the year. Young, with the first blush of beauty beginning to show, she was becoming aware of herself and of the impact she was making away from school and family ties. But the experiences with Geoff had made us wary and we kept close watch on her. At times our children seemed older and more worldly than we had ever been.

As we neared midpoint on the cruise Connie told me what I had suspected and was stubbornly determined not to recognize: his health had subtly slipped a notch or two. He could not pinpoint pain. A general malaise, he said, like a creeping weakness, was draining his vitality.

"It's why I haven't wanted to dance, Katie," he said. "I don't want to spoil your fun but it hurts to move to rhythm."

"Where does it hurt?"

"I don't know," he said. "It's just pain—not localized. Just there."

He continued his evenings at sea working as often as possible on the book. He would not let me stay and help. "This part is rough," he told me. "I've just got to break through on my own."

Still, he joined us for every excursion onshore, investigating the ports where we docked, going on shopping excursions, and delighting in our one-night stop at Saint Martin where the Thompsons, Towers, and Saffords were in residence at Margery's and Mel's and came to meet our tender when it arrived one day near noon.

That was a day of picnicking, swimming, and talk at the Thompsons' where, two years earlier, the outward symptoms of Connie's illness had surfaced. There was no talk of that. We were all together, enjoying life and friendship, joking about another evening on the island when Connie, trying out Morse code learned years before, had inadvertently caused a departing cruise ship to stop dead in the water, a radio room man thinking Connie's blinking lights were some kind of signal to the vessel. He never knew exactly what it was he had sent.

Connie had seen Dr. Whitmore three days prior to the cruise and had another appointment scheduled for five days after the voyage was ended. On March 15 before we sailed, Dr. Whitmore's notes state that:

Approximately one month ago he developed sudden severe pain over the lower sacral area unassociated with any change in bowel habits . . . no blood or mucous in the stools . . . pain has diminished . . . tends to be worse at night than during the day.

Connie had told only Pat and Dr. Whitmore of this new pain. Obsessed by his book, his hope to somehow preserve his family, and his grim determination not to be pitied, he had kept it secret, except for that brief mention of it to me on the ship.

But, even before the March 15 appointment with Whitmore, Pat had known of Connie's "malaise." He had sent

Connie to Dr. Van Syckle who, on February 25, found "an area of radiolucency in the left sacral wing."* It could be insignificant, unrelated to cancer. The change was of doubtful importance, yet Dr. Van Syckle took no chances. Under "IMPRESSION" he wrote:

1. Possible metastatic involvement, left sacral wing.
2. Normal coccyx.

On Wednesday, April 5, five days after our cruise, Connie saw Dr. Whitmore. And again Connie told me nothing. But Dr. Whitmore's notes read:

No change in pain. It has been variable in the morning . . . It is neither better nor worse and is quite erratic in occurrence but it remains. . . . He is obviously very apprehensive about the implications of his pain. He specifically asked about his blood tests and I told him that there was some elevation in his acid phosphatase.† Decision was made for him to empirically take diethylstilbestrol‡ 1 mg. daily for one month and return at the end of that time for repeat acid and alk. phosphatases.

Connie must have known immediately the import of that visit to Dr. Whitmore, and he may have known Dr. Van Syckle's impression of his condition back in February. But he did not confide his suspicions to either notebook or tape. He bought but did not take the diethylstilbestrol. He knew full well what it was—and what it meant. The removal of malignant lymph nodes and the I-125 implants in the prostate

---

* Connie's first bone scan was done by Dr. Bagshaw's team at Stanford University Medical Center. After the October 1970 operation, Pat and Dr. Whitmore arranged for Dr. Van Syckle in Connecticut to do most scans. The arrangement saved time for everyone. Connie would take Dr. Van Syckle's films to Memorial on his visits to Whitmore. Dr. Van Syckle's interpretations of scans and X rays were sent to Pat who, in turn, passed them along to Dr. Whitmore. As time went on bone scans were done in Memorial as well.
† The level of acid phosphatase in the blood rises when cancer is present. The norm is 2.5 and can go up to 4.0. By April 1972, connie's tests were showing an elevation considerably above the norm, somewhere in the region of 7.29, as I was to discover much later.
‡ Diethylstilbestrol or DES, as it is now commonly known, is a synthetic estrogen.

had failed to kill all the cancer. He was heading into another phase of treatment. To him, Dr. Whitmore's words to us on Connie's first visit some twenty months earlier must, by then, have been all too clear: if the time ever came that the cancer began to reassert itself, the doctor had said:

Hormones . . . would arrest [the cancer] to a degree . . . But I think if your condition came to that, the cancer would override the beneficial effects of the hormones in the end.

The pain he was experiencing did not stop Connie from once again working on a play at Vicki's school. That year it was *The King and I*, and Hans and Horst were called upon by Connie for even greater effects than they had expended the year before. They did the hairstyles for the small pupils from the lower school who would play the king's children, drawing their hair into tiny topknots, darkening their skins, making up their eyes. Victoria had the role of Tuptim. Her pale hair was darkened for each performance, and after it she washed the soot away, only to apply it again the next afternoon. Connie was everywhere around the stage as always. He choreographed the show but the actual steps were taught by someone else. He did not admit to anyone that they were too painful to attempt.

We gave rather hurried dinner parties each night of the performance. Among the guests were friends from the city whom Connie had cajoled into coming to see the play. After each night's performance, people drove back to the house. At home, keyed up and surrounded by friends, Connie was as exuberant as the young actors. The fears he must have had of a new attack of cancer were deeply hidden from us all. Eyes bright, motions quick and nervous, he appeared to be everywhere at once. And usually was. He had loved his daughter in the Tuptim role. For the first time it was evident that he felt she had a potential for the stage which he, himself, had once aspired to. Vicki, as Billie Newell and I were well aware, had arrived at that decision independently. For

Vicki—even before our spring cruise—plays, music, and drama were not just schoolgirl pastimes. Daily, they occupied more and more of her free hours. In time, the theater would become her chosen profession.

On a soft, late, spring evening in 1972 Geoff came home again to live with us. He had telephoned ahead, as he always did, to see if his visit was convenient—never knowing that we always made the time available, regardless of what had been previously planned. Our evenings with Geoff, during the months he had been away, had not given us much real insight into the changes he was going through. He had been encouraged, it appeared, to display hostility often—if he felt it—in his "encounters" with us. "Encounters" is a very difficult word for parents to accept as a definition of their association with their own children.

But the attitude of the counselors at the center he attended was apparently based on bringing out a personality which we were told we had suppressed. In sometimes vitriolic language Geoff informed us that his problems had been largely due to us. The therapy group, the center's director, the counselors, he told us, all agreed. He was, however, "strong" by then. If we could accept him as an individual, not restricting or impeding his freedom, he wanted to come home.

He did not ask what our problems were, or inquire about his father's health or about the progress of the book which, if finished, could help safeguard not just us but him as well. Everything connected with his life, including his new "independence," was being paid for—as had been the case throughout his life—by his father's work. These things apparently did not occur to him. But they were very real to us. Medical bills were now continuous items in our budget. If *Bridge,* because of Connie's health, could not be finished, the publishers' advances on it would have to be repaid somehow. *The Longest Day* and *The Last Battle* royalties, had, with the passage of time, diminished greatly. Yet, until or unless *Bridge* was completed, those royalties were all we had to live on. But to any mention of money, Geoff, who had lived with its benefits all his life, said that money was all we ever thought about.

Indeed, he was not far wrong. Still, he came back home.

Each day he drove to school and most nights he went to the rehabilitation center. No rules of ours were applicable to him. The center gave him rules and values, codes and ethics. His zeal and dedication were extraordinary, but I often wondered if they could have been accomplished in less selfish ways. At a time when worry about his livelihood and ours was overwhelming, I asked myself: where was that single grain of charity for parents? The center did not dispense charity for parents. Back at home, yet not back, Geoff led his own life, seldom joining in or seemingly concerned with ours.

≕ 6 ≕

SHORTLY AFTER GEOFF came home to live, Connie was scheduled for a 9:00 A.M. bone scan. That time the appointment was at Memorial. Thanks to some fortuitous break in traffic and, again, a vacancy at the small garage next to the hospital, we were there a full fifteen minutes ahead of time.

By now Connie knew the corridors and turnings of Sloan-Kettering and Memorial as well as if he had spent all his working years there. We went directly to the radioactive isotope department. To our astonishment the waiting room was filled with patients. None of them had seen any hospital personnel about.

Connie, notebook and pencil in hand, started down the line. "What time is your appointment?" he asked each person. "What time did you arrive?" Finally he came to a child-like young woman in a wheelchair, accompanied by an elderly woman who turned out to be an aunt. They spoke little English, and my rusty Spanish was almost more hindrance than help. The girl's dark eyes were beautiful, prominent in the wasted face. Her hands, long-fingered, clutched the arms of the wheelchair. Her aunt—the sole surviving relative, if my understanding was correct—stood anxiously beside her.

The two, we learned, had left their home in East Harlem a little after 5:00 A.M., traveling by subway, then down long blocks to reach the hospital. They had arrived by 6:00 A.M. For over three hours they had waited for someone to come and do the bone scan. Both women looked exhausted. The girl in the wheelchair seemed as fragile as a feather borne on the wind. Her huge, expressive eyes went from me to Connie.

Suddenly he looked up from his notes.

"Katie, every one of these people here today are welfare patients. They were told to come in for bone scans and so they came. I'm the only one with a definite time and appointment." He looked at his watch. "It's now nine forty-seven." He wrote it down. "No one's turned up to take me in for my nine o'clock appointment and what about them?" He gestured toward the line of people. "Christ," he said, "it's bad enough to have the bloody disease. But to treat them like this—"

He knelt in front of the tiny figure in the wheelchair. "Ask her, Katie, if she'd like something—juice, tea, coffee—" I translated. Her eyes stayed fixed on Connie. Shyly she declined. "Tell her I'm going to have something," Connie persisted. "She and her aunt must join me." Again, I did the best I could, and this time she agreed.

The aunt, whose English was far better than my Spanish, was reluctant to leave, afraid they'd lose their place in line. She said that other ambulatory patients had moved ahead of her niece.

As she was speaking, a man came into the room. "Mr. Ryan?" he called. "Mr. Ryan."

Connie rose from beside the girl's wheelchair. Deliberately he looked at his watch. The man said, "I know, sir, we're running late."

"Yes," Connie said, "you sure as hell are. These people are all ahead of me."

The man looked blankly at Connie. "Sir, I am sorry for the delay. But we are ready for you now."

"We're all in line here," Connie said. "You take these people first."

"They will be seen," the man said.

"Damn right," Connie said, "and now." He pulled out his notebook. "This young lady was here first—shortly after six A.M. And this lady next. Then this gentleman." He looked up—not at the technician—but at the line of men and women. "Go by turns," he told them. "I've got your arrival times. I'm last, aren't I, Katie?"

"No one else has come in," I said, "but him."

"Mr. Ryan—" the man began and stopped.

Connie was moving toward him. "Let's get going, Buster, shall we?"

He turned again and came back to his young friend in the wheelchair. He pushed her forward. The hospital employee stood stock-still watching. "Come," Connie said to him in a low voice that I knew meant his patience was at an end, "you're late enough as it is."

Meticulously he ticked off each patient in the room, giving them numbers. Tiredly, wearily, they sat down but I don't think they were frightened any longer. I have already said that there is an affinity among cancer patients and their families. It is not a question of who can afford to pay and who cannot. It is a question of human dignity, and on that day Connie returned to them a value some of them perhaps had felt was lost forever. He helped them be people again—not victims.

"It will probably take two to three hours—maybe longer—for the results of your tests," he said to the group. "Don't stay here all that time. Go walk around, sit in the park across the way, go back home and rest. You don't have to spend a whole day on a bone scan. If you've not had breakfast, have it after your test is over." He stopped abruptly and was silent for a moment.

"What I'm trying to tell you is—don't be afraid. Not of hospitals or attendants or anybody. You're you—not a statistic. Be yourselves, damn it. Don't be afraid."

He was in the midst of an Irish story, groups clustered about him, when the dark-eyed girl came out. The next patient went in and then another. "The place is finally coming to life," Connie said, and smiles broke out on faces that had not smiled all that morning.

He came back to the girl and her aunt and bent down again in front of her wheelchair. "What would you like most of all to eat?" he asked her as gently as if she were the child she seemed.

"Ice cream." She knew those English words.

"I'll be back, Katie," Connie said and darted out the door. He returned some minutes later with an ice-cream cone, a little the worse for its time in transit. The girl reached out for it and then, impulsively she took his hand and kissed it.

"Get her out in the sun and air," Connie said, gesturing to me to speak to the aunt.

Her flood of Spanish was too much for me to understand and then the aunt said haltingly in English, "Señor, each day we pray for you. It is all we can give."

I tried to reply in kind but Connie's kiss on her cheek was far more appropriate. They left, the girl half turned in her wheelchair to look back at Connie. Her eyes never left his face until she and her aunt rounded a corridor and were out of sight.

After the other patients, Connie went in for his bone scan. When it was over, he suggested we go to the Plaza and have breakfast—although by then it was considerably past lunchtime. We talked about the book as he ate heartily, and later we walked back to the hospital to see if anything more was required by the lab. Nothing was. Sadly, they had all they needed. Connie was never to see the report of the findings that Dr. Whitmore received. In essence, in the right hip, in the head of the left thighbone, and in scattered areas in the chest vertebrae and rib cage, cancer had struck again, spreading its deadly cells in Connie's bones.

About ten days later, I went along when Connie kept his scheduled appointment with Willet Whitmore. As gently as possible Dr. Whitmore gave us the awful news. Of that examination and meeting he wrote in part:

Pain has been variable and was considerably improved by a trial on butazolidin instituted by Dr. Neligan. However, he does have sciatica intermittently and he does have numbing discomfort in the perianal area ... Dr. Golbey reports that bone scan shows increased uptake of radioactivity in multiple sites and we have agreed to start him on estrogen therapy.

On examination he looks well ... prostatic area is mildly enlarged and indurated. The right lobe somewhat more prominent than the left and slightly more irregular. There is ill defined fibrotic thickening over the entire bladder base area more marked in the area of the right seminal vesicle.

Situation discussed with the patient and his wife. Think one can conclusively say on the basis of his pain, the elevated acid phos. 7.29 and findings on bone scan it seems little doubt that he has

disseminated metastatic prostatic cancer. Accordingly, I would recommend institution of diethylstilbestrol 1 mg. daily p.o. (by mouth)
with reevaluation in six weeks.

A few weeks earlier Connie had told Bob and Peter Kriendler and Jerry Berns about his malignancy. As time had
passed his need to be honest and at ease with his friends had
caused him to draw more of them into his confidence.

Two days after our visit to Whitmore he wrote Bob Kriendler:

Bob, under the circumstances I am not sure whether I'll be able to
attend the Leatherneck Ball but if my name can help on the committee, go ahead and use it.

I need hardly tell you that Wednesday's body blow, which I told
you about on the phone, has left Kathy and me in semi-shock. I am
not going to become morbid about it or in the least way depressed.
At least I know the truth and dire as the news was I have a sneaking
suspicion that you, Pete, and I and our wives will be sitting somewhere 20 years from now laughing about all our ailments and the
prognoses of all our various doctors.

As always, my love to you and Florence.*

Perhaps Connie had been dealt so many body blows by
then that he was attuned to shock. As he had written Bob, he
did not outwardly show depression. He kept on working
daily, now taking the estrogen pill faithfully, but he appeared
to treat it much as he would a vitamin pill.

Over the next few months we saw friends often, Connie
played golf occasionally, and after Geoff's graduation from
prep school in June and the news of his acceptance by the
University of Missouri, where he planned to major in journalism, Geoff and his father made two short fishing trips together. He was extremely proud of Geoff, who had gotten a
summer job with the Parks and Recreation Department in a

* Bob Kriendler died on August 15, 1974, during his convalescence following open
heart surgery.

nearby town, was working long hours, saving money, and seemed happier and healthier than he had been in months.

With Vicki, and Ben and Dolly Wright, we drove to June and John Watkins's home, in Providence, Rhode Island, and then to Newport to watch the start of the Bermuda races from John's boat. Connie occasionally took over the steering, amused as his uneasy passengers grumbled about his helmsmanship and ducked the water sprays that were reduced to a minimum as soon as John again took the wheel.

With Ben and Peter Kriendler, Connie took a four-day fishing trip to Canada, and he spent time having Geoff's secondhand car tuned and fitted for the drive Geoff made to Missouri. Worried because he had not made such a long trip before, we asked Geoff to call us en route; he did so faithfully, reporting on the countryside and the motels where he stopped, his enthusiasm noticeably greater as he neared his destination and then was finally settled on campus. His college life had begun and his resolve and inner strength were growing.

Connie continued his regular visits to Dr. Whitmore, who noted:

gradual resolution of his low back pain . . . is working more effectively now than in many months . . . looks and feels generally well . . . has had no sciatica or peripheral edema . . . appetite good, weight increasing . . . Gl function excellent . . . no urinary symptoms . . . no inguinal adenopathy . . . no masses or tenderness . . . peripheral pulses are good . . .

The estrogen therapy appeared to be working. Perhaps this second line of attack against the cancer would be sustained. The question was: for how long?

CORNELIUS

This is Saturday, September 30, 1972. Last night about 8:30 Katie and I finished Part II of the book. This has been the most complicated writing I have ever done. I think it was not until I began to describe General Horrocks's briefing to XXX Corps in the little theater in Leopoldsburg that I began to feel the full power and awesomeness of Market-Garden. I can never remember feeling so elated before. I couldn't write fast enough, so I dictated that entire section to Katie, who took it down on the typewriter. There is nothing quite like knowing your material and then finding it come spilling out faster than you can put it down. I was actually afraid I'd miss something, because my mind was racing even as I was trying to capture the color and crowds and spirit of that briefing.

After the Horrocks section was done and Kathryn had inserted all the pertinent quotes from the interviews with men who attended that meeting, it seemed almost childishly easy to segue to England and pick up the stories of the airborne men waiting for the big day. Katie and I had only one argument about this entire section and it turns out that her thought was the best one. She had come across a British 1st Airborne interview, which was verified by several others. It told of the men in a sergeants' mess chalking up the hours until departure on a big mirror over a fireplace. She wanted to use it as the device to mark the hours as the men sweated out the wait. I didn't think it would work, but it has, beautifully. She wrote the last paragraph of Part II, which is so simple that it's absolutely correct and gives just the tone of tense expectancy that was needed. The last message on the mirror was "2 hours to go . . . no cancellation."

Now, starting Monday, patient little Annie has got to go over with me the numbers of aircraft involved and the fields and directions of the airborne attack. We've already been over it dozens of times, but I come up with one set of figures and Anne gets another, and this time we've got to agree.

When we can put in the kind of work we've done the past two or three weeks, I don't have time to think about my personal health. I don't even care about it. Nothing is as important as the satisfaction I'm feeling at the moment. This can be a magnificent book. I know it can.

It's only when I hit a real snag that I find my mind wandering to cancer. Mentally I keep checking out my body. Nothing really hurts, or at least not for very long. I seem to have a lot of movable pains which appear and disappear, but nothing is localized. I don't think I feel as well as I did a few months back but that may be due to the fact that the book finally seems to be picking up steam. I am trying very deliberately to keep a positive attitude and not turn inward, or to attempt to second-guess what may happen next. Because I think I know what will happen. The estrogen will hold for a while and then something else will go wrong. I've learned enough to know that this is a last-ditch fight. If the estrogen fails, I don't think there's much more that can be done, except perhaps more radiation.

I have been praying lately, something I don't think I consciously did for years. I want the time to finish this book. There is so little else I can do for Katie and the kids. It is very hard to accept the fact that my sexual desires are now nonexistent and harder, still, to know that manhood is eroding away each time I take a female hormone. If I didn't have the book and the family, I don't think I would have taken the estrogen at all after Willet told me the cancer had invaded the bones. If I'd been alone, with no commitments, I would have allowed the disease to take over. But I will fight it as long as I can because I have a great deal to live for and it would be a form of suicide if I didn't do everything in my power to stay well as long as possible.

I have not mentioned on these tapes before that some time ago Kathryn had Geoff remove all the ammunition for my guns. My mood must have been pretty black for her to think that I would end my life that way. I just don't believe that anyone has the right to take his own life. It is a gift and when one gets cancer one realizes just how precious life really is. I don't expect to go hunting again soon but I would like to know what Geoff did with the ammunition. I don't even know how Katie got the key to the case unless she took it off my key chain and got it back before I noticed it was gone.

How difficult and tedious this illness must be for my family. I've tried to carry on as many excursions and pastimes with Geoff and Vicki as possible. I want to share outings with them as I've always done because there'll come a time when I won't be able to and I want them to remember me as an active and interested father. I have prayed that when this thing finally eats me up, it goes about it very fast. I don't want my children's last thoughts of me—or Katie's—to be of some querulous invalid. As long as I am able I will live as active a life as possible and then I hope the good God doesn't let me linger.

Katie is starting to hit the promotion trail for her book. I think she is anxious about how well she'll do in radio and TV interviews and it is doubly hard for her since she's so occupied with *Bridge.*

Half the really excellent ideas for promoting the book have come from Marilyn Evins. We've known David and Marilyn for years and, as so often happens, we lost touch. A few weeks back Marilyn and Katie got together and then all four of us had dinner and it was one of the best reunions I've ever had.

I told them about our problems. Marilyn is as sentimental as she is generous and loving and she damn near broke up at the news. Dave maintains his calm and quiet mien and it is a joy, as it always was, to have the companionship once again of these two friends. Young Matt, their son, has grown from the infant I remembered into a young man. Time goes quickly. I'm poignantly aware of that.

KATHRYN

Nineteen seventy-two seemed to leap toward its end. Connie had obtained the services of a fine publicist, Abby Hirsch, who held my quaking hand through most of the interviews I gave about *The Betty Tree*. But Connie was right: my mind was seldom on it, although the book was important to me, as every book is to its author. I found myself more often thinking about Connie working in the office than about the forthcoming radio, TV, and newspaper interviews Abby or one of her staff propelled me to. Each time I arrived back home a page or two of Connie's work was on my desk for editing. He was working steadily, taking his estrogen, and overseeing even the household details while I was away. I saw among the papers on his desk that he had acquired material on estrogen therapy and had marked the possible side effects with red ink.

I read them: possible erections but no ejaculate; breast tenderness and enlargement; female hair pattern; smaller testes. In the same red ink, Connie had written along the margin, "Oh, Christ! No!"

It seemed so tragically unfair that he should have to contemplate such alien changes at a time when he was struggling to write the best book of his career. He needed desperately to marshal his emotions, thoughts, and ebbing strength for that. He had suffered so much in mind and body, bearing that suffering silently, fighting his way out of each new wave of depression. But the humiliating aspects of his malignancy, as much as the pain, were eroding his pride even as he stubbornly fought to keep his self-respect.

That agony, I think, is one of the more exquisite torments of having cancer. Not even loved ones can help much. Only the patient can come to terms with the changing body, the weakened limbs, the mind that acknowledges that the struggle is probably useless.

Connie was not ready to admit defeat, no matter how one-sided the battle. His enormous willpower was his strongest ally. It actually appeared to grow even as his body wasted and softened.

Near year's end, two events gave Connie a great deal of pleasure. One was the autographing party Bill Fine, then president of Bonwit Teller in New York, held for me. The store's staff had created a gardenlike setting on the second floor and the publisher had sent over stacks of books. Advertisements and invitations were sent out and large placards in the store directed shoppers to the area. Marilyn Evins, Lyn Revson, and a host of their friends dropped by. Jean Deems and Susan Fine brought in others and Abby did everything but kidnap shoppers from every floor of the store, urging them to attend the party and buy *The Betty Tree*.

Harold Robbins was in town and, with Connie and Paul Gitlin, came to watch the proceedings. Seeing my rather grim and nervous face, Harold began to whisper bits of dubious advice to me, so outrageous that they cut the tension and I relaxed. The smiles on Paul's and Connie's faces were cheering and supporting. But one of the most touching moments for me that day was when Jon Gitlin, Paul and Zelda's son, came by to purchase a book and have me autograph it. He stood beside me in the late afternoon as the crowds waned and was as much a comfort to me as his father, Connie, and Harold had been earlier. It was a satisfying day, made all the better by the new friends I made and the old ones who had come to bolster me. The great gift, Connie said, is having friends. All else aside, in that respect we were richly blessed.

In early December Connie announced that we were giving an enormous Christmas party which, with our finances, we could not afford. But Connie would not be dissuaded. With his mania for perfection, he stopped work in the office and spent hours with me going over the menu, decorations, and guest list. The last included, as Victoria said, "the entire world with one or two exceptions."

House & Garden, where I had first worked when I came to New York after college, sent an editor and a cameraman to photograph the party and the house. Some of my happiest years before my marriage had been spent at Condé Nast Publications and some of my oldest personal friends in New York were still with its magazines.

Jay Pinchbeck, whose family owns a nursery and greenhouses, brought a crew of workers and spent long hours each day and almost up to party time, putting lights on two huge trees—one placed on the big terrace outside the living room, the other sweeping a fourteen-foot-high ceiling indoors. Tiny lights were nestled among the bare branches of the dogwoods on the front lawn, and Jay's contributions to my ideas for flowers and evergreens had turned each room into a garden.

The day of the party my friend Polly Forcelli and some six or seven women brought in the food. We had decided on a Dickensian Christmas. We couldn't afford the food any more than the party but Connie was working on his pet theory that "when you're broke, that's the time to go out and buy a Rolls." My menu and Polly's cooking had produced a groaning board of food that looked too beautiful to eat but that nonetheless disappeared quite effortlessly at dinner, served at tables for eight and ten scattered all over the house.

Gino Bob Polverari and Pat Vozzo, festive in red jackets, were our bartenders, working without letup to take care of the dozens of people toasting the season.

But the highlights of the party were two secrets Connie had specially engineered for me. He had managed to get the Salvation Army band to come to play the Christmas carols, and he had sent Geoff extra money to have a tuxedo made in St. Louis before he flew home for the holidays.

Connie had dressed early and was in and out of the children's quarters an hour before the party. From our bedroom I could hear some scurrying sounds from there and, occasionally, a quickly stifled laugh.

Shortly before the first guests were due to arrive, someone knocked on my dressing room door.

"Madam," I heard Connie say, "does it please you to inspect the troops?"

I walked into our bedroom and saw the most precious people in my life lined up before me. Connie and my father were flanked by Geoff and Vicki—all of them glowing in their party finery.

Standing beside my father, Geoff was dressed as I had never seen him—in evening clothes tailored to perfection. He wore them as easily as if he had done so for years. His hair was brushed back, trimmed and layered. I had forgotten what fine features he had, having seldom seen them in the past few years through his long locks. He winked at me but otherwise maintained a military bearing.

Alongside her grandfather, Vicki looked poised and elegant in a soft silk shirt and long rustling skirt. Her white-blond hair fell below her shoulders, framing her face. My silver-haired father stood beside her, proud and ramrod straight—and there was Connie, unable to keep from smiling at my astonishment and obvious delight. He was impeccable, as always, his tall, slender body erect and self-assured. His handsome face bore no signs of pain or illness. He was simply as he had always been—my dearly beloved Connie—his special magnetism surrounding him like an aura.

Speechless, I stared at my beautiful family. Connie broke ranks and came to me, giving me his silk handkerchief.

"Are you crying because we're pretty or we're not?" he asked.

I had not realized that I was crying.

"Because I love you all," I told him. I looked at the others. "Geoff, you're gorgeous. All of you are just incredibly beautiful."

Geoff joined his father and kissed me on the cheek. "Dad thought you'd like us," he said, gesturing toward his own evening clothes.

"I can't believe it," I told him, bemused by them all.

Later, during the party I watched Connie, moving among his guests, laughing and talking. I remembered that dark day two and a half years earlier when we had first gotten the report that the lesion in his prostate was malignant. I had thought it couldn't be. No one so vital, so charged with energy and life could be sick. He had changed hardly at all since then. How could he look so well and be so ill? Stopping constantly to speak with guests, I was also praying silently and desperately for my husband's life.

The huge tree which Jay Pinchbeck had trimmed with hundreds of lights had not been lit, and was hidden in the darkness of the terrace. Stage-managing the evening as he had choreographed Vicki's plays, Connie had slipped outside to await the arrival of the Salvation Army band. The group had been singing and playing all day in towns throughout the area and were weary, but they came. Connie led them through the darkness to the steps of the terrace. We, inside, heard the first pure, clear notes of a trumpet playing "Joy to the World" and the vast crowd of guests fell silent. At that moment, outside on the terrace, Connie plugged in the lights of the giant tree. It stood out in breathtaking beauty. Geoff rushed to open the double terrace doors and the Salvation Army band came in, their uniforms and music evoking memories in all of us, I suspect, of the wonder and majesty of Christmases past.

For over forty-five minutes the entire house party sang the ancient carols, sharing the printed lyrics or—like my father, Geoff, and Vicki—recalling them from memory. Across the room I caught a glimpse of Zelda Gitlin and Marilyn Evins. There were tears in their eyes as they sang, looking at the band and at Connie standing in our family group beside the Salvation Army players, their dark serge uniforms a humble contrast to the bright swirl of chiffon dresses and the glossy darkness of dinner jackets.

Looking at the faces of our guests I thought that Connie had, indeed, brought off a minor miracle. He had made us children again as we each remembered some magic, warm, and loving celebration years before.

In the early morning hours our house guests, David and Marilyn Evins, went wearily to their room. Polly and her helpers had washed and put the party fare away. The house smelled of flowers and pinecones and on the terrace the great tree remained still lighted. From our bedroom we could look down through panels of glass and see it glowing like a stained-glass window in the soft December dark. Geoff and Vicki, still keyed up, sat with us in their party clothes. Connie dimmed the bedroom lights and the four of us, once more a family, talked quietly together.

"It's been the best party ever," Vicki announced.

"Except that Mom's still in shock at seeing me dressed up," Geoff kidded me. "Dad was on the phone to me almost every day. I had to make two trips to St. Louis for fittings."

"It was worth it," I told him. "You're gorgeous."

"Who was the prettiest lady tonight?" Vicki asked.

"Your mother," Connie said.

I put my head on his shoulder. His arm held me gently against him. "You need your eyes checked," I said drowsily. "There were several great beauties all around you. *Women's Wear Daily* and *Town & Country* can't be wrong. Half the faces here tonight are as well known as movie stars."

"They're not you, Henrietta," Connie said.

"Henrietta? Who's she?"

"You," Connie grinned. "I decided to give you another name for Christmas."

"Thanks, but I'll keep the ones I've got. How did you happen to pick on that?"

"It's my secret," Connie said. "I'll never tell you." And he never did.

Soon, Geoff stood up and stretched. I realized suddenly that he was now as tall as his father. "Well, you guys, here's a college man going to bed. Hey, Vick, ever see a college man going to bed?" He grinned at the double entendre.

Vicki came over to the bed and kissed us. "It was just so beautiful and everyone loved the Salvation Army band. Thank you. I love you."

Geoff bent down and kissed me. "I'm so proud of you and all you've done," I told him. And he clowned again, "But, Mom, I didn't know you cared."

He rested a hand on Connie's shoulder. "Thanks for everything, Dad. Good night, you two. Sleep well."

Our young adults trooped downstairs. We sat propped against the pillows, looking out at the tree.

I caught Connie's hand and held it.

"What are you thinking about, Katie?"

"I wish we could stop the clock. Tonight, particularly this last hour with the children, is the happiest time I can remember."

"That's good," Connie said.

"What are you thinking about?" I asked.

His eyes were fixed on the terrace, velvety black from a light mist. "I'm wondering if the photographs I took of the tree turned out well. Sometime you ought to have a Christmas card made up with the tree on the cover. Be sure to give the photographer credit."

"Are we sending out separate cards next year?"

"Sometime you may want to use the tree. I've got a good message for you to have printed inside." He paused and then continued, "The greatest lead ever written for a story is 'Today in this town a Saviour was born.' Have that printed on the card."

"I'm to send the card alone?"

Very softly Connie said, "Katie, there are lots of things you'll have to do alone."

And suddenly I knew why he had insisted on the party.

Part Four
THE BATTLE
January 1973–October 1974

÷ 1 ÷

MEMORIAL HOSPITAL

2–21–73 . . . In late January while he was still convalescing an episode of flu he had migratory pain in his back and legs. In the past week he has had left anterior thigh pain associated with a marked sense of weakness in his legs but without numbness or paresthesias [tingling]. He has had no other symptoms to suggest relapse . . . He has taken his estrogen faithfully. Pain has been sufficiently severe to require percodan for relief.

. . . he . . . ambulates with great difficulty due to pain and weakness in his left anterior thigh. His complexion is slightly sallow . . . Neck—no adenopathy [enlargement]. Breasts show moderate gynecomastia [abnormal enlargement of mammary glands in the male]. Abdomen—LSK not felt. No masses or tenderness. Groins negative . . . Genitalia—there has been a good estrogen effect in the form of testes atrophy and of female pubic hair pattern . . . the prostate is generally small and flat . . . Extremities—no edema.

IMPRESSION: *Carcinoma of the prostate clinical stage D in probable estrogen relapse.**

* The italics are mine.

Situation discussed frankly with the patient and his wife. Do not see any point in further X-rays at this time.*

Blood chemistries done today prior to examination and he was started on Provera 50 mg. t.i.d. He will discontinue the estrogen . . . Return in one month or prn [when necessary]. If the pain persists after 2–3 weeks of provera therapy, focal irradiation could be considered but I have advised both the patient and his wife that therapeutic decisions in this setting are basically dependent upon symptomatic developments.

Dr. Whitmore

CORNELIUS

This is Saturday, February 24, 1973.

For nearly ten months I have been on estrogen therapy. I have suspected for almost a month now that the estrogen was no longer working. Three days ago Willet Whitmore confirmed my fears. Cancer has overridden the treatment once again. All along, I think I knew that my luck was too good to be true. My legs, where the pain is mostly concentrated, feel as if they are made of rubber. At times I am almost afraid to stand in case they cannot support me. Pat Neligan has given me Percodan for the pain but it is a narcotic and I use it rarely and then only at night.

I am afraid to take pain-killers during the day. I need an absolutely clear mind in order to work on the book. I am finding that the more intensely I concentrate on Market-Garden, the less pain I feel. It is only when I get up after sitting a long time at the desk, that I am aware of how intense it really is. Along about 4:00 P.M. it seems to gather itself and sometimes it hits me so hard I want to cry out. It is almost

---

* In December 1972, Dr. Guy Van Syckle's films showed widespread skeletal metastases. It is his detailed report to which Dr. Whitmore is referring. If Connie knew what the films revealed he did not mention them.

impossible to do any useful work on the book between four and seven so, instead of attempting to write any longer, I read through the chronology cards and check myself to be sure that I have not left out anything essential.

I will have to start coming down to the office earlier than 6:00 A.M. in order to make up some of the three hours of writing I lose in the late afternoon.

The British and American anecdotes are absolutely superb, just as good as the interviews we got for the previous books. I continue to be constantly amazed by the courage of men in battle. And by their humor in the midst of catastrophe. There is a desperateness, I suppose, in courage and in wartime humor. I have seldom encountered a soldier who thought he had been courageous and I would tend to discount a man who said he was. I rather think that courage is man's unplanned positive reaction to what appears to him to be a last-ditch situation. I believe courage is at its peak when one has run out of hope. A soldier figures he has nothing to lose because subconsciously he has arrived at the conclusion that he has no future.

Yesterday I was working on the 101st Airborne drop. The troop planes had run into intense flak and yet the pilots held to their courses in order to deliver the paratroopers to their drop zones. Planes caught fire and crashed as men in other formations watched their comrades go down in flames.

As I was writing about the tragedies that occurred during the drop, Katie brought over three interviews that showed the other side of the picture: a fatalistic humor that men developed. One particularly interested me. One private, as his plane came in low through enemy fire to approach the drop zone, saw Dutch civilians holding up their fingers in the V-for-victory sign. "Hey," the soldier yelled to his buddies, "they're giving us two to one we don't make it."

The odds against me are far higher than that but I can appreciate that macabre humor. Sometimes all a man can do in such circumstances is make a joke.

The new pill Willet put me on as of last Wednesday is called Provera. It's a steroid hormone, different from the estrogen therapy. I think it, too, will cause changes in my appearance. What it will do to cancer is anybody's guess.

The estrogen effects have been subtle compared to what I think I can now expect. I was mortified at the thought that the estrogen might cause me to develop noticeable breasts. I tried to joke about it, but the thought of having a bosom did appall me. When enormous worries—like those about the cancer itself—become overwhelming, I suppose the mind fastens on some ridiculous but related fear to relieve the burden of the crucial one. But I am now even more concerned about growing breasts. With the high dosage of this new hormone, which aids the development of mammary glands, maybe I *should* think about going out to buy a bra.

I wish I could get the hell out, go away where no one knows me, and finish the book. But I need Katie and Annie and I need Pat and Willet to keep me alive so it can be finished. *Bridge* has got to be what I am not: a testament to the endurance of man.

Ever since my legs began to give out, I've been telling people that I sprained my ankle. I can't even be truthful with close friends, although, of course, Neligan knows. Thank God I've got Pat to talk to. I know I interrupt him a lot with phone calls, but I feel better afterward. Today I called up and when I got him I asked, "Is this the Reverend Father Neligan?" And before I could go any further, Neligan started yelling. "For Pete's sake I'm busy. What do you want? What are you doing? Why aren't you working on your book?" He sputters like a machine gun. I didn't answer any of his questions. I said something quite rude and hung up. He called back immediately and we went through the conversation in reverse.

I'm going to get a sign made that says, Beware of the Doctor, and post it right at his driveway. It would serve him right.

Katie and I have been seeing a lot of friends lately but I am finding that the leg pain limits my evening hours. It is all I can do to hold out until 10:30 or 11:00 P.M. When the outward signs of Provera begin to show I'm going to dread social encounters, but I can't have Katie living twenty-four hours a day with me without some kind of respite. I keep thinking of how my illness is affecting her. She has lost a great deal of weight and is working far too hard. I am terrified that all of our worries may become too much for her. Yet, I cannot get her to ease up. She still talks so optimistically that sometimes I want to shake her, and yet it is her optimism and her belief that we can polish off the book that keeps me going.

I have been thinking a great deal recently about Ireland. Mother's letters indicate that she is not in good health. I would like to fly over and see her and my brothers but I am afraid of becoming overly emotional. It is really impossible to have Mother here. We are both busy constantly in the office and that would leave her stranded in the house, far more isolated than she is now. And yet I long to see her. But I don't want her to see me the way I will become.

From the time I first left Dublin years ago Mother has never written me a letter that was not filled with love and her belief that I could accomplish anything I wanted. She has also been a go-between—pleading cases of support and aid for my brothers—and I have sometimes told her harshly that I have given to the limit. Her faith in my abilities to conjure rabbits out of hats, to produce money for the Irish family, has not diminished from the first day I sent money home from England—nearly thirty-five years ago—up to the present time.

It is a curious Irish trait that the parental family feels itself entitled to a portion of the success of one of its members, regardless of that member's changing responsibilities. From time to time I have supported my brothers in various enterprises and it is ironic that the only letters, with two exceptions, I recall ever having received from them have been when they wrote to ask for something. Once I had provided it, silence reigned until something once again was needed.

Mother, quite the contrary, seems to be the only one who feels a responsibility for thanking me, although she never fails to tell me that she is certain no more requests will be forthcoming. But they have been and at times, against my better judgment and Kathryn's ire, I have done what I could to advance their ventures. Now, the well has run dry. I should have refused to shell out years ago, except for Mother. But in Irish families one grows up with a sense of obligation and continues to have it far longer than is either wise or prudent.

The other day I came across a candid photograph of Mother and Father. How young they were! That was my first impression. Then I began to study the picture. Shabby tweeds are elegant when one has the money to dress any way one likes. Still, my father wore his like a lord of a manor. Mother was quite beautiful. She has always been. In the photograph she is smiling up at Father and their arms are linked. They were not able to share much happiness together but obviously that moment was one of the rare and better ones.

Now Mother's better moments seem to come when Katie writes her, as she does nearly once a month. Mother's letters back are full of love, good advice, and incredible optimism. Of the new book, she wrote, "I feel with all Con's experience that the words shall flow from his pen. He is daily in my prayers and I know he shall overcome all his difficulties. I am anxiously awaiting the book."

Dear Lady, so am I.

KATHRYN

On Wednesday, March 14, 1973, a little less than a month after Dr. Whitmore told us that the estrogen therapy appeared to have ended its effectiveness, Connie went again to Memorial for a checkup. The steroid hormone, Provera, in the massive doses Connie was taking, had begun to shove up his weight but other problems were somewhat eased. Dr. Whitmore found that:

Breast sensitivity has disappeared since he stopped estrogen. Has noted brittle nails. . . . Nocturia 0–1X but has noted slight increase in voiding pattern during the day without stream difficulty, burning or hematuria. Denies significant pain. Occasional twinges of discomfort in his left anterior thigh. No peripheral edema or sciatica. Has taken no medication for pain. Has been working productively. No intolerance to provera.

Looks well. Neck—no nodes. Breasts—residual gynecomastia but without tenderness. Abdominal exam. negative. Groins negative. Pubic and axillary hair normal . . . Prostate . . . without definite interval change. There is really more induration in the seminal vesicle area bilaterally than there is in the prostate itself. Gland is not significantly enlarged.

. . . Continue provera.

Two weeks later, after hours of long work in the office, Connie and I flew down to the Thompsons' in Saint Martin with John and Shirley Tower. Connie was working better than he had at any time since his illness. Despite his fears, his rather rapid weight gain was not too noticeable and none of the other symptoms he dreaded had, as yet, begun to surface. He was greatly pleased by one aspect of the new treatment: his chest had not expanded; it was nearly back to normal.

The work on the book had made us both desperately tired and Connie's stamina was limited. Yet, almost up to the minute of our departure for Saint Martin, Connie vacillated about going. He had "a head of steam," as he put it, and he was fearful that the time away would slow him down. He packed the growing manuscript and research material to study on the island.

On the way to the airport he became nauseous and complained of pain in his legs. Jerry Lewis, who operates a chauffeuring service, was driving us to JFK. During the ride Connie suddenly asked Jerry to pull in at the next gasoline station he came to. There, he was in the men's room so long that Jerry went to check on him. He came back to the car leaning on Jerry, looking pale and sick. "I don't know whether I should go to Memorial or Saint Martin," Connie said—but we continued to the airport. By the time we arrived at the terminal Connie's nausea and pain seemed to have vanished. The respite was not to last for long.

On Saturday, March 31—just three days after our arrival—he became frighteningly ill. Unlike the symptoms he had experienced on the way to the airport, there was no warning before this attack. Like a vise, pain suddenly gripped him. It was so intense he could not speak. Not even the Percodan he had brought, along with the Provera, helped relieve him. Sweating, pale, and twitching, as spasm after spasm raked his body, he bit his lips until the blood came, fighting against the pain in a ghastly kind of silence.

The ordeal is best described in a letter I wrote on April 12 to Geoff at Missouri:

"We arrived home last night from St. Martin. Dad became suddenly very ill there. He was in agony and at times seemed hardly conscious. Mel and Margery, John and Shirley and I decided we must try to get him back home. Mel and Margie were on the road constantly, hunting down airport managers while I waited for 3 hours to try to get a call through to the States to Pat.* I learned he was out of town. Mary Chapin, Pat's nurse, got in touch with Ted and within hours I had a cable from him telling me to stay put and to contact Dr. Leonard Short, a neighbor of the Thompsons.

* Flights to and from the island were infrequent and heavily booked in advance. Also, during the time the Thompsons were trying to get us out on an emergency basis Connie seemed so critical that we were worried as to whether he would be able to stand the trip, should reservations become available.

Dr. Short could not have been more supportive. He came twice a day every day and I think just knowing he was close by was a relief to Dad. The doctor made several trips by air to other islands to get some medicines which seemed to help. He would not take any payment for his care of Dad.

The island is quite primitive—no telephones or electricity except in scattered areas or in the Dutch and French capitals. The home-owners on the French side are true pioneers who forged their way through jungle to build absolutely beautiful houses overlooking the Caribbean. They are a close-knit bunch and they came by one's and two's every day because, even though they didn't know Dad, he was sick and they wanted to help.

This trip has been a classic example of what the word "friends" means. No people could have been more steadfast, loyal, and lov-ing than the Thompsons and the Towers. They read the manuscript which we had taken down to work on and their enthusiasm gave Dad as big a boost as Dr. Short's ministrations.

Whenever your father could get a few moments' ease from pain, everyone told him how great the book was and how important it was that he get it finished.

Every morning the household was up by 7:30 and the Towers and Thompsons cooked huge breakfasts for us all. Margie and Shirley always put a flower on Dad's tray and usually John Tower would take it in to him and sit by the bed to see that he ate. Then we'd get his bed freshened up. I showered with him because he was too weak to stand by himself and I was terrified he would fall if left alone. Then I helped him into fresh clothes and back to bed. I did his laundry and even gave him a haircut.

I didn't want to spoil the others' vacation and insisted they go off and leave me to cope around the house which worked out fine. But none of them were ever gone for long. They wanted to be near him. In our bedroom Mel and John fixed all the shutters so that Dad got the sea breeze but not the brightness of the sun. He would doze off and then one of us, looking in on him, would find him awake and everyone would troop back into the bedroom to bolster his spirits.

We rearranged Margie's sofa in the living room and John and Mel often half-carried Dad out to it where, for an hour or so in the early evening, he could look out to sea and watch the yachts and little boats. Margie has a hanging saucer on the terrace and little birds called banana twits which seem to eat nothing but sugar gather there by groups. John took care to keep the bowl filled and Dad studied the birds for days. He should now be an authority on their habits.

About four days ago he rallied, and refusing everyone's plea to take life easy, swam with John for the last three days of our stay for half an hour or so. He said the buoyancy of the water soaked away his pain. Then he would come back to sleep almost around the clock.

The flight back with John and Shirley was tiring and, driving home, even the smallest bump in the roadway seemed to cause Dad pain. This morning he called Pat Neligan and is now, as usual, sitting at the desk, so it's back to the helmets and combat boots just when I was beginning to get the calluses off.

I cannot stress enough how wonderful the Thompsons and the Towers were. Now that we are back home perhaps we will know exactly what went wrong these past weeks. Pat tells Dad his collapse was due, in part, to intense strain, worry, long hours of work and too many pressures. Anyway, just keep praying, if you ever do, that there is and will be a way out of this illness.

Love from us all. I've got to climb back into my foxhole. Dad's ready to hit the dusty road again.

Whatever had happened to Connie in Saint Martin was, as far as Pat was concerned, far too critical to ignore. He was on the phone to Connie several times a day and usually dropped in at night, exhausted from his own hectic schedule. Connie's leg pains, which had seemed to ebb during our final days on the island, had again increased in intensity. Yet, now that he was working again, he stubbornly refused to take Percodan for relief. Daily the pain continued. It no longer racked him from late afternoon and through the night. By then it was a constant presence he fought doggedly against, even as he turned out more handwritten pages daily than he had ever done before.

Clearly Connie could not go on suffering as he was much longer. Pat reached the conclusion that it was vital that Dr. Whitmore see Connie as quickly as possible. He placed call after call to Whitmore's office, listening with mounting concern as the number rang and rang. Memorial's operators were unable to help, despite Pat's insistence that an emergency existed. All they could do was to continue to ring the extension number that no one ever answered. I had friends who knew other doctors at Memorial. Perhaps those men might be able to get in touch with Dr. Whitmore or, at least, know his whereabouts. In desperation I asked my friends to help us out. Their efforts were no more successful than Pat's had been.

On Saturday, April 21, Pat's pent-up anger exploded. In our office he called Memorial's admitting office and told them to have a bed for Connie on the following day—Easter Sunday. Meanwhile Marilyn Evins and Austine Hearst were each still trying to reach doctors and administrators whom they knew. It seemed, as Austine said, that everyone was away for the Easter holidays. Almost up to the time we left for the hospital on that warm Easter afternoon, Pat in Ridgefield and Marilyn and Austine in New York were still trying to find some way of alerting Dr. Whitmore's department that I was bringing Connie in.

Connie had seemed almost unaware of our frantic efforts. But he had agreed with Pat that he should go into the hospital. His capitulation was a sure sign that Connie knew his health was slipping. At any other time a hospital would be the last place he would willingly agree to go.

I was fortunate once more in obtaining the services of the woman who had looked after Vicki in the past. Even if I did not stay many nights in the city, I wanted to be near Connie and with him whenever possible without worrying that Vicki would be on her own.

When it came time for us to leave for the hospital, Connie's progress down the long, wide steps from our front door to the driveway was agonizing. He seemed suddenly too weak to go anyplace. His pain was very obvious. At the car Vicki and I had to help him move first one leg, then the other, into the car. He looked anxiously at Vicki as she bent to kiss him.

"I can't do the play this year," he said. It was *Half a Sixpence* and had been in rehearsal for several weeks. Connie had attended no more than twice. "You'll work hard, won't you?"

She nodded solemnly.

"I'm sorry to let you down," Connie told her. "Just give it all you've got, and tell the others to do the same."

We drove out of the driveway. I gave the family signal—two hoots on the horn—and Connie waved until our daughter was out of sight.

The admitting procedure at the hospital had not changed much in two and a half years, except that this time Dr. Whitmore did not know that Connie was coming. Failing to reach him, Pat had given me a letter to present at the admitting office and had called to alert clerks there of Connie's arrival. The room was crowded as families and patients filled out forms. Then, patients were taken off for various tests and family members settled down to long waits until these preliminaries were over.

I remember a group of us sitting in a long row of upholstered chairs under white fluorescent lights while outside the warm brightness of Easter Sunday flooded the city streets. The fresh air, the warmth, the cadence of the Easter throngs did not touch us in the hospital. We, the families and our cancer victims, were severed from that outside world. In sterile, artificial brightness we sat sheeplike, far away in thought.

Eventually, patients began to trickle back and among them I saw Connie. They all had been divested of their clothing for their tests and each man and woman wore only shoes and a green cotton smock. Until that moment I had not realized the extent to which Connie had undergone physical change. As he stood there in the scant and clinical hospital garb, the effects of the drug therapy were pitifully apparent. He limped down the hall, a sheaf of papers in his hand, his stomach seeming to bulge out against the gown. His face was puffy, his legs like fragile sticks below a torso suddenly grotesque.

I watched him searching the rows of people and for a moment I sat rooted to my chair. I was utterly shocked by how he looked. Far worse, I was embarrassed by his appearance. For one frantic moment I did not want to get out of the chair and go to meet this ludicrous, overbalanced stranger, or even admit I knew him. And then the feeling passed as quickly as it had come and I walked out to meet him, filled with self-loathing for my initial reaction.

But Connie was not easily taken in. He had seen or sensed my antipathy, brief as it was. "Don't walk with me, Katie," he said. "We've got to get dressed again and then I have to find out where they're going to put me." He moved painfully away, leaving me more ashamed than I have ever been in my life. For the first time since Connie's illness I had failed him. In the trials that cancer imposes on the victim's family, I had flunked a most important test. For one brief second, the sight of him had repulsed me and he had seen my revulsion.

I was composed again and so was Connie when he came out dressed, his briefcase in his hand. Once again he looked himself, but I was by then aware of the outward changes in his body. I put them out of my mind. They would never be important to me again. I took hold of his hand and together we walked to the elevator. At the fifth floor, the attendant called out "Ryan" and we got off the crowded car. There was but one bed available on the entire floor, we were told, and we followed the nurse down the hall and into Room 508.

No matter what one reads or hears of overcrowded hospitals, nothing ever prepares one for the sight. In a room occupied by seven other men, Connie was led to an empty bed. It was the only uncluttered area in the ward. The rest of the room was a tangled mass of bottles, tubes, and catheters, sprouting out of shriveled, sallow bodies. The smells of sickness were overpowering. Moist and cloying, they permeated us and our clothing immediately. Two windows, raised by only a few inches, let in dim light. I had a wild thought that even had the windows been open wide, the outdoor air and sun would have refused to come inside that place.

In the bed next to where we stood a gray-haired man lay dozing, his mouth open, his crumpled white gown damp and stained. Little driblets ran from the corners of his mouth and gathered in the deep hollow of his throat beneath a prominent Adam's apple. Directly across the way a figure was sitting sideways hunched over the bed, head down, staring at the floor. One leg hung over the side of the bed. The other had been amputated above the knee. With one hand he endlessly stroked the bandaged stump. Farther down, a woman and two children sat beside the bedside of an emaciated man. It was impossible to tell how old he might have been. His face seemed flat, almost featureless, except for the prominence of his nose which, alone, had not caved in to cancer. On his bedside table was a small cake and a handful of presents in white tissue paper. The children stared at the figure in the bed as if they did not know him. The woman coaxed the wasted form to open its eyes and look at the cake. Her voice, falsely bright, carried across the room and then ceased. She put her hands to her face, shaking her head slowly back and forth, the children mute and wide-eyed beside her.

The nurse showed Connie where to put his clothes and pulled out a gown from the bedside table. He ignored it. "I can't stay here," he said. "Come on, Kathryn. We're going home."

We went back the way we had come, past the lines of silent figures wasting steadily away.

In the corridor the nurse stopped us. She reminded Connie that he had arrived as an emergency patient, that he could not leave the hospital, and that he would be seen to. He shook his head. The nurse became exasperated. Connie became angry. I sided with him. I knew he could not go back into that ward. I was furious about the overcrowded room, the suffering I had just seen, the lack of dignity accorded the dying. The dilemma confronting us was one that we three could not solve. The nurse did not know Connie or his aversion to hospitals. She knew nothing of his previous cancer history or of the dramatic week of endless phone calls which had brought us to her floor that day. Equally, we did not know her problems and, selfishly, I, at least, did not care about them. I knew only that Connie would be worse by morning, his personality and sense of self severely damaged, if he went back into that room.

He had no intention of going back. He threw his briefcase down on an upholstered bench in the corridor. "I'll sleep here," he said, "but I will not set foot in that room again." The nurse informed us if he did not obey she would be forced to call a doctor. She could not understand why we both began to laugh. We had been trying to find a doctor for a week. The threat of one actually materializing seemed hysterically funny. We sat down on the bench. The angry, bewildered nurse walked back to her station.

Eventually another nurse appeared to tell me visiting hours were over. "I'm not a visitor," I said. "I'm staging a sit-in." She stared at me. "Why don't you call a doctor?" I suggested. Abruptly she turned and left us.

Meanwhile Pat, at home, had not ceased his search for Dr. Whitmore. We knew no other doctors in the genito-urinary department and all the other specialists Austine and Marilyn knew were still apparently away as well. In those days, each doctor seemed to have but one extension and, to my knowledge, busy department heads, like Whitmore, saw outpatients only on specific days—in Dr. Whitmore's case, it was usually on a Wednesday. Unless the caller had an extension number, switchboard operators were of no help—as the missing digit on the hospital bracelet Connie had been given in 1970 had made all too clear. One could be transferred to administration only to encounter the same dilemma. If the doctor's extension did not answer, no other means of contacting him was ever suggested, at least to me. Probably because he was, himself, a doctor, Pat got lucky. My own notes for that Easter read:

Running battles all day . . . Whitmore called Pat at 10 p.m.

My memory of those later evenings hours is virtually nonexistent. At some point Connie insisted that I leave for the Evinses', where I had planned to spend the night, and walked with me to the elevator. He told me he intended to remain in the corridor. Arriving at the Evinses' apartment, I found Marilyn on one phone and David on the other, each still trying to track down a doctor friend who might be able to help. I must have called Pat late in the evening to learn that he and Dr. Whitmore had been in touch. I did not speak to Connie again until 9:00 A.M. on Monday, April 23, according to my notebook. To that reference I added,

Kaiser in. Not much else.*

But Connie's notebook for that date has one cryptic line:

* The reference is to a genito-urinary fellow.

Moved to 523.

When I arrived back at the hospital, having spent a sleepless night at the Evinses', I found Connie alone in a minuscule room that someone told me had once been used for storage.

$$\stackrel{=}{=} 2 \stackrel{=}{=}$$

KATHRYN

The intricate work-ups to determine the cause of Connie's relapse and how best to treat it had already begun. The initial admission examination on Easter had shown his blood pressure to be 144/94, not critically high but by no means normal. His temperature was slightly elevated: 99.4; his pulse was 88. For the first time in eleven months the words "liver palpable" were recorded, "two fingerbreadths below the costal margin." The finding could suggest liver enlargement or a change in the organ's position, brought about by a number of reasons which could be quite normal or spell trouble.

There were strong indications that hormone therapy had been no match for the disease that was coursing through Connie's body. It had not held out for long against deadly cells extensively invading the pelvis and femora. The traveling hit-and-run pains in Connie's spine and legs, the bladder spasms, the return of the "prostatitis feeling," seemed all too clear. He was being consumed by cancer. Only his will to live was untouched, unbreakable as always.

The young doctors did not know the man inside the cancer. Their jobs lay elsewhere. His body was providing them with learning. That is the subtle cruelty inherent in cancer medicine. What the doctors would come to know of Connie's cancer might help them to treat some future victim more successfully. Meanwhile they bypassed Cornelius the man even as they logged his past and present medical history and compared his erratic blood chemistries with the norm.

Nothing about Connie was ever merely average. Tragically, neither were his laboratory tests. His hemoglobin showed a reading of 10.2 gm; normal is in the range of 14–18. His hemacrit (the reading taken after a centrifuge has separated solids from plasmas in the blood) was 30 percent. The average is often referred to "as plus or minus 5 on either side of 47%." A red blood count should range between 4.2–6.2 million. Connie's was down to 3.3 million. Only his white blood count was respectable: 9.7, with normal platelets and differential. He was anemic by every standard of the first three counts, but apparently his white cells could fight infection.

He failed to meet other biochemistry standards, in some instances, spectacularly. Against a calcium norm of 8.5–11 mg, he registered 12.2. Hypercalcemia—an excessive amount of calcium in the blood—was to persist and his calcium levels would rise even higher. He did much better in the phosphorus count: 3.7, within the normal limits of 2.5–4.5; and his uric acid count was 8, as opposed to a normal range of 3.0–6.0 mg—elevated but not, as yet, unduly alarming.

But in other findings, biochemists saw more serious signs. Urea nitrogen, BUN on most blood chemistry charts, was 31—some 11 mg above the highest normal number. That reading indicated possible renal problems. Dr. Guy Van Syckle had discovered on July 6, 1971, that the right kidney was not functioning. Now, the left might be involved.

Alkaline phosphatase—essential in bone calcification and

present also in the kidneys, plasma, and intestines—was extremely elevated. Its average was between 30–85. Connie's was a soaring 254. That reading told the biochemists of probable involvement of the liver, which excretes the enzyme. LDH, another enzyme found in certain body tissues and serum, has a chemical norm of 100–225. Connie's was 328, possibly reflecting tissue change.

Transaminase (SGOT on many laboratory charts) is another enzyme highly concentrated in the liver and the cardiac muscle. Tissue injury can leak the enzyme into the bloodstream and measurement of the levels in the serum gives a clue to heart or liver damage. The norm of the serum in the blood is 10–15. Connie's was 57.

Probably the most telltale test of all for a patient with prostatic cancer is the level of acid phosphatase in the blood. This enzyme is present in the kidney, semen, serum, and the prostate gland. When acid phosphatase is elevated, the prostate is usually the culprit. The normal count is around 2.5 to 4.0. Connie's count had risen from a reading of 7.29 on May 3, 1972, to levels, during this second Memorial hospitalization, that would soar right off the charts.

Beginning on Monday, April 23, other tests were made. An IVP again showed no visualization of the right upper urinary tract, although the left kidney, despite the high urea nitrogen count, was functioning normally. Bone films taken on Tuesday revealed extensive osteolytic and blastic metastases.* These findings and the high level of calcium in the blood showed, as Dr. Whitmore wrote,

relapse following an initial response to estrogen therapy.

The massive doses of estrogen and then Provera had begun to change Connie's features like the painting of Dorian Gray.

* When cancer spreads to the bone, two forms of damage are commonly seen on the X rays. Blastic metastases refers to an increase in density of cancer cells in the bones. On film, such areas show up white, almost like calcium formations. Osteolytic metastases vary in shade from gray to black on X rays, and tend to indicate much more danger of bone collapse.

But Connie's situation was the reverse of that literary character's. Under the external changes and the masses of evidence that seemed to indicate he should not be alive at all, the real Connie existed, stout of heart as ever. He was a challenge young doctors might find puzzling, for the clinical Connie and the fundamental man were Siamese twins now totally severed. Medicine could practice on the ailing body but could not penetrate and did not try the door beyond which all that Connie was, had been, and would become, existed.

The batteries of tests went on for three days as doctors, therapists, neurologists, and clinicians worked to resolve and relieve the sciatica and perineal rectal pains that Connie felt were building in intensity. Worse, too, were the bladder spasms, the constant urgency to void and the searing flash of pain that came with each attempt.

Alarmed by his own condition and the setback imposed on his writing, Connie found new cause for concern—the patient in the room adjoining his. Her name was Ann* and, like Connie, she was no stranger to the hospital. She was dying of lung cancer, gasping agonizingly for breath and screaming out against the pain that narcotics could seldom control for even an hour.

Like me, her husband was seldom absent from the hospital. Bill was a tall and gentle man whose nerves were frayed by his continual concern for Ann's life. The couple had a fifteen-year-old daughter, Beth, who came once with her father to the hospital. "Once too often," Bill said grimly. Against his better judgment, at the urging of relatives, he had brought Beth in to see her mother. But the wasted, half-demented

* The name I have used is not the patient's true one, nor are those of her husband and daughter.

woman in the bed was not the mother Beth knew and, terrified, she fled for refuge to the waiting room.

Connie's concern for Ann grew daily. As her condition worsened, her screams and desperate rasping breaths could sometimes be heard halfway down the corridor. At times Bill was unable to watch his wife's anguish and came next door to Connie's room for a brief respite, although he was never able to escape the awful sounds of her suffering. Occasionally Ann would rally and the harsh screams and soggy breath sounds would ebb. At such times she would recognize Bill as he sat beside her, covering her hands with his. At those times, too, Connie would sometimes limp next door to stand beside Ann's bed and comfort her. Her eyes would go from Bill to him and she would manage a faint smile. "My dear men," she would whisper before pain once more took control and reason away.

Bill and I often did each other's shopping. He bought Connie shaving cream and magazines and papers. I took in sandwiches and tea to him during his long vigils at Ann's side, and once I bought a little bracelet for him to take to Beth. He told Connie that he had been advised that nothing more could be done for Ann except the positive measures in effect to help sustain her life a little longer. But there was no hope that she would leave the hospital alive. To case the end Bill had brought in special nurses to give round-the-clock care, but his expenses were overwhelming and each day Ann's fight for life was harder for him to bear. Still, he tried to cling to hope a little longer, despite the diagnosis.

On Wednesday, April 25, our concerns turned inward once again. To determine the causes of Connie's continued voiding difficulties and racking urethral muscle spasms, Dr. Whitmore decided to perform a delicate operation Thursday morning, the twenty-sixth. By means of a narrow viewing instrument, inserted through the tubelike urethral opening in the penis, Whitmore could examine the bladder and urethra. He found thickening in the bladder neck and stricture (or narrowing) of the urethra, which discharges urine from the bladder out. The urethra was dilated to open up the passage more. Then, using a painstaking surgical technique called TUR (transurethral resection) Dr. Whitmore, working through the incredibly small confines of the urethral opening, carefully carved away some of the fibrous thickening of the bladder neck and prostate. As he skillfully pared away the tissue which was impeding free flow of urine, the minute chips he excised were submitted to pathology. In time Connie would have far fewer spasms and voiding would become a different kind of problem. Instead of hesitancy and scant results, he would experience some intermittent incontinency.

The report on the tiny shavings Dr. Whitmore sent to pathology revealed the kind of news to which we would never become accustomed. "The Clinical Diagnosis" read:

Ca of Prostate . . . Adenocarcinoma, Grade III.

That evening, with Connie resting fitfully, I drove home. At the hospital Bill was keeping vigil between Ann's room and Connie's. Because of her critical state he was apparently able to spend more time there than normal visiting hours allowed. Before leaving the hospital I had talked with Vicki, assuring her that Daddy was doing well after the operation and, reassured, she returned to school for the dress rehearsal of the play. *Half a Sixpence* opened the following night. I had totally forgotten about it.

Arriving home, Mary Luke and Helene Merrick cajoled me into having dinner at a nearby restaurant. For me, it was an evening out of another world, almost out of another time. My thoughts and efforts, ever since our March trip to Saint Martin, had been directed solely to concern for Connie. For the first time in a month I relaxed that night. The soft lights, the everyday ordinariness of people at dinner, the companion-

ship of these two close women friends, were the best therapy
I could have had.

Friday, April 27, was rainy and chilly. I drove back to town,
knowing I would have to return to Connecticut that evening
for the opening of Vicki's play. Matthew Evins (Marilyn's
and David's son) and a friend of his were going back with me
to see the play and spend the weekend. I had forgotten that,
too, until Vicki reminded me. I arranged for Matt and his
friend to meet me at the hospital in the late afternoon. I
wanted to spend as much time with Connie as I could.

As was invariably to be my luck, I had missed Dr. Whitmore's visit to Connie. Like many another doctor, he came
by to see his patients quite early or quite late. Those schedules make it difficult for family members to see the doctor,
ask him questions, or get hard facts. This is, I think, particularly true when one is dealing with staff doctors in a hospital.
There are no regular daily office hours, no receptionists or
nurses to relay messages. Only by happenstance does one
encounter the headman. For a patient's family this can be
totally frustrating. It often produces fears that have no basis
in fact. Or it may produce just the opposite result: when a
new plan is decided on, those nearest to the patient are not
apprised of it and they are totally unprepared to help their
sick ones adjust emotionally to the news. I was about to encounter that kind of problem.

As I stepped out of the elevator, Ann's labored breathing
could be heard all down the hall. I had stopped at a little
flower shop to buy bunches of daffodils for Ann and Connie
and for the patients in 508, the eight-bed ward where Connie
had been taken on Easter afternoon. The ward was, by then,
a regular stop for me.

Bill met me at Ann's door and relieved me of the flowers.

"No point in taking them in there," he nodded toward Ann's room. "She hasn't known me since late yesterday. She just screams between those gasps. I don't think the oxygen or the narcotics or anything else are doing any good at all now." His face was haggard. "Kathy," he said, "I swear I wish she could just die. That isn't Ann in there. Ann's already gone. I can't spend my life here. I've got to be with Beth and I've got to go to work by Monday. I've used up my vacation, my sick leave, and any goof-off time for good. I have to make a living and a home for Beth."

He handed me back a bunch of daffodils. "I'll take the others into 508," he said. "You go see Connie."

"How is he?"

I had discovered early on that one gets more sensitive reactions from another cancer victim's relative than from any of the specialists and experts.

"He was restless last night after you went to the country. His doctor came in today. They talked." Bill paused. "Connie's real upset about something."

He was indeed. The reasons are clear from a portion of Dr. Whitmore's notes:

... because of the somewhat migratory and variable nature of this pain, it was elected empirically to start him on chemotherapy with a combination of 5 F-U and cytoxan. Modest dosage was recommended because of the chronic nature of his illness and the possibility of extensive marrow involvement ... *

Connie was lying in the bed staring vacantly at the ceiling. I bent over and kissed his cheek. "Hi, Henrietta," he said listlessly and went back to his examination of the ceiling. I

---

* 5 F-U is Fluorouracil, an anticancer drug, used to kill cancer cells which have rapidly divided and spread. Cytoxan is an anti-neoplastic drug used to slow down or impede new abnormal tissue formation. In bone marrow normal cells duplicate and repeat quickly like cancer cells. Since bone scans had revealed metastases in multiple bone sites, danger existed that the chemotherapeutic agents could attack normal cells even as they went to work against the cancer cells. Thus, the "modest dosage" for Connie's first chemotherapy treatments. The strength of various anticancer drugs and their combinations can often only be determined by trial and error—and hope that normal cells will escape extensive damage.

put the daffodils in a vase of fresh water and placed them on the table by his bed. The agonizing noises from Ann's room, even with the doors closed, came through clearly. Connie did not appear to hear them.

"They're putting me on chemotherapy," he said suddenly. "Katie, this must be a pretty hopeless case. God knows they've tried everything else."

"You're far from hopeless," I said.

He turned to grin at me. "I know that and you do but you couldn't get a doctor to agree." He paused, then said, "I'm not exactly relishing the thought of toxic chemicals in my bloodstream. Jessica and Rupert would never approve. What I need is a hefty, nourishing bowl of Eskimo blood soup."

"Or a cabbage poultice," I said.

Connie laughed and then again turned serious. "This proposed treatment worries me," he said. "I suppose I could always refuse it."

He had read up on chemotherapy some months earlier when he was acquiring books, papers, and pamphlets to familiarize himself with his illness. He had once discussed the therapy with me and his attitude at that time was not dissimilar to that he showed on Friday, April 27.

Chemotherapy had, in only a few years' time, emerged from the backwaters of the laboratory to the forefront in the war to kill off cancer which had spread beyond the primary site or posed a danger of metastasizing. A combination of chemical reagents, introduced into the cancer victim's bloodstream, has a toxic effect on cancer cells. The treatment was still too new to predict its success over a long period or to know if it might be effective against all forms of cancer. But, even without years of performance statistics, it had been found to shrink tumors and kill off malignant cells ranging far beyond the original site.

The drawback was that chemotherapy could also damage healthy organs and tissues even as it demolished cancer cells. Like other forms of therapy it did not promise a cure for all cancer victims and its side effects could be far more drastic than those of other treatments. There was a fear, too, that in destroying cancer, chemotherapy might also do away with the body's natural immune response.

The trick was to obtain a combination of toxic chemicals in proper dosages that could effectively aid the individual victim. There was no standard formula for everyone. Too much or too little of various chemical substances combined together could prove as devastating a killer as cancer itself. Connie's blood studies and bone scans would have to be heavily monitored to detect if chemotherapy was going after healthy tissue as well as diseased cells.

In light of all Connie had read, his uneasiness was not difficult to understand. Still, there was a chance the treatment would work, and I urged him to look at it optimistically.

Because of the two-night run of Vicki's school play and the presence of young houseguests, I would not be able to see Connie again until Sunday. I stayed with him as long as possible on that Friday before going down to meet Matthew and his friend who, I found, had waited nearly two hours for me in the hospital lobby. When I left him Connie had seemed cheerful and had asked me to deliver to Victoria an assortment of messages pertaining to the performance of the play.

He had apparently played a role himself entirely for my benefit. Memorial nurses' notes for both that Friday evening and the following day contain these entries:

Very depressed and verbal . . . about chemotherapy . . . Patient appears somewhat apprehensive as to his prognosis.

The silence on the fifth floor when I reached it Sunday afternoon was alarming. Hurrying down the corridor I saw that Ann's door was wide open, the bed stripped, all hospital apparatus removed. As soon as I entered Connie's room he

330

said, "Ann died." I sat down on the bed beside him. "I've got a lot of pain in my left shoulder and the left side of my neck," he said. "It's something new. They've given me medication for the pain a couple of times. Oh, Katie," he said without a pause, "did you know that she was only thirty-six? Poor little Beth," he said. "Poor Bill."

Bill had left a note for me. It read:

Dear Kathy. At least it's over. I'm glad for that. Connie took Ann's passing very hard. Look after him. My prayers are with you. Bill.

On Monday, April 30, Connie had a battery of tests and X rays. His shoulder, neck, and pelvic pain had increased; and a tremor in his right wrist which he had had for months seemed worse. On the plus side he was voiding more easily since the TUR and the bladder spasms were almost nonexistent.

At 5:00 P.M. he was given the first course of chemotherapy—750 mg of 5 F-U and 50 mg of Cytoxan. He would take the Cytoxan by mouth twice daily.

The chemotherapy appeared to have some serious side effects that surfaced on the day following each of the treatments, which were spaced about one week apart. On the days after chemotherapy Connie would be weak and severely depressed, and his coordination seemed out of balance. His spirits would lift gradually but the periods of silence and withdrawal were painful to watch. They were totally alien to Connie's nature.

Because of his continuing pelvic pain, radiation therapists reviewed his charts and X rays. Their report, on Friday, May 4:

... we consider, at present that the patient is not a candidate for R.T. Pain is not so severe and not well localized. We would give R.T. when the pain is not controllable.

That time would come but not until Connie would admit that pain had exhausted his reserves and that he could not hold out against it any longer.

I think now that in those late April and early May days of 1973 Connie was attempting to come to terms with cancer. As he had said once on his tapes, he had believed all along that the malignancy would kill him. Still, he planned to give the disease a run for its money. Each new setback made him more determined to finish his book. It had become an obsession. To write, he was prepared to accept any and every treatment that was put forward, however slim its chances for success. And, however insidious cancer was, Connie's will to fight it seemed to grow. He had never intended to give up without a fight. His unyielding nature was his best medicine and his strongest ally.

Connie's stay in the hospital was brightened whenever Pat could find the time to visit. At the sight of Dr. Neligan coming through the door Connie's lethargy would disappear. By Dr. Whitmore's orders, Pat had access to Connie's charts, and usually some member of Whitmore's team could be summoned to bring Pat up-to-date on Connie's progress. I welcomed those visits as much as Connie. Pat could tell me how Connie was and what was being done for him. Connie rarely told me anything and the hospital's doctors told me absolutely nothing. Through Pat's visits I could learn the seriousness of Connie's condition and his reactions and tolerances to the treatment he was given. What I had learned was seldom encouraging, but it enabled me to plan ahead, something the hospital doctors seemed to deem unimportant. How the family copes was not their business. They were engrossed only in getting the patient well enough, if possible, to go back home where, presumably at the snap of a finger, all things would fall into place. Pat's attitude was vastly different. He knew our household and was almost as concerned as Connie and I about the importance we placed on finishing *Bridge*.

Connie, who refused to take medication when working, disliked it equally at other times, no matter how necessary it seemed to be. Sedated, he often forgot that he had had a host of visitors and would look bewildered at some mention of their stay. Marilyn Evins daily sent fresh orange juice to him, which he often forgot to drink. David Evins, Ben Wright, and Paul Gitlin were constant visitors, and often Ted and Jean Safford, Suzie Gleaves, Abe and Betty Ajay, John Tower, and others came in to see him. With them all Connie carried on animated conversations which, after their departure, he could not recall. One day, after learning from hospital personnel that he seemed confused and disoriented, Pat decided to test Connie for himself. In the midst of their conversation, Pat suddenly said, "CJ, how long have you been here anyway?"

Connie stared at him and thought. "I remember once during the war dining at the officers' mess in Wellington Barracks," he said. "One of the dining room orderlies was Irish. I asked him, 'How long have you been a dining room orderly?' The poor man raised his eyes appealingly toward heaven. 'Since the Last Supper,' he said." Connie looked at Pat. "That's how long I've been here, Neligan," he said solemnly. "Since the Last Supper."

Still, fatigue and lethargy began to characterize his days. His blood chemistries, particularly calcium, and acid and alkaline phosphatases, were not responding to treatment and anemia was a rather constant problem. On Monday, May 7, he received his second course of chemotherapy and two units of whole blood. The next day, Tuesday, he reacted as he had done the previous week. He slept almost constantly, awakening briefly to complain of pain in his back and legs. The same worries still occupied his mind. According to a nurse's note he:

asks questions concerning other patients' diagnoses. Seems to be comparing all aspects of cancer, trying to find answers.

Even as he looked for them, his health appeared to slip further.

On Wednesday, May 9, doctors' "Follow-up and Progress Notes" read:

Pain in chest and hips more severe. Patient still complains of lassitude following 5 F-U May 7. Acid p'tase 33*

Nurses' notes for that day read in part:

... Has pain in legs, hips and back ... Medicated for pain X 1 [once]. Appears to be a little unsteady on feet ... Still complains of fatigue. Sleeping in naps most of day. Feels depressed ... IV started this p.m. Transfusing well. Appetite poor. Remained in bed all evening. Seems weaker.

Indeed he was.

I arrived on Thursday just as visiting hours began. One look at Connie convinced me that something was going very wrong. I ran back to the nurses' station and asked that Dr. Whitmore be paged. I heard the first droning summons even as I headed back for Connie's room.

I was not alone in observing a great change in Connie. The 8:00 A.M. to 4:00 P.M. nurses' notes for that day state:

Patient complains of general malaise. Stated unable to walk about because of weakness in legs. Coughing up thick sputum at intervals ... Voiding quantity sufficient ... Tolerating food fairly ... IV patent [wide open] and running well. Episode of emesis [vomiting] early this a.m. Speech seems slurred at times. Seen by Dr. Kaiser today. Resting.

Dr. Kaiser's note reads:

Clinically seems to be deteriorating with elevated BUN (48) and calcium (15+ today). Main complaints include multi-focal bone pain, lethargy, slurred speech and episodes of confusion. Plan more

* This was a jump of 29 above the highest limit in the normal range.

334

vigorous treatment of hypercalcemia and repeats of IVP. ? [question] increase 5 F-U to 1 gm Monday.

A note of a different kind was also written on May 10. In the doctors' "Follow-up and Progress Notes" there is one final entry for that day. No time is given on the entry and I cannot be sure if it was written before or after my arrival at 2:00 P.M. In light of what occurred during the hours I was there, I am inclined to think the report was written after 8:00 P.M. It reads:

Endocrinology emergency note:

Calcium 15.6 mg . . . Patient with widespread bony metastases of prostatic cancer now on Chemotherapy with 5 F-U and Cytoxan. Agree with institution of prednisone and oral phosphates although latter will need close monitoring of renal function. Would increase Intake and Output to 4 liters/day and follow serum K+* as well as BUN, Calcium, Phosphorous.

There was no response to the page for Dr. Whitmore. I sat on Connie's bed, putting cold cloths on his forehead, talking to him, shouting at him to answer. He appeared to be in a coma. Desperately I shook him hard, afraid of hurting him but more afraid of getting no response at all. His eyes flew open and pain passed across his face. He closed his eyes again. He had not seemed to know me.

At the nurses' station the call for Dr. Whitmore continued. At 4:00 P.M. as the eight-to-four shift was going off duty, I asked one of the nurses to get *anybody*. I was frantic. The nurse apparently passed my message to the oncoming shift and in a moment a summons began again.

Hurrying back to Connie's room it seemed to me that he had deteriorated in the few minutes I had been at the nurses'

* Potassium count. It plays a role in the conduction of nerve impulses and some of Connie's symptoms were muscle weakness, dizziness, and mental confusion. Intake would have to be watched carefully to be certain the levels were adequate in intravenous feeding.

station. Again I shook him hard, massaged his hands, put cold cloths on his forehead. The futility of my efforts made me continue them more urgently. There was nothing else I could do.

Shortly after 7:00 P.M. a nurse came into the room. She appeared as worried as I was. She told me that the page had finally been answered. Dr. Whitmore had been out of touch, apparently in the operating theater all day. That still did not explain why *someone* had not come. The doctor who had, just minutes ago, answered the page was on the eighth floor. The nurse seemed embarrassed as she told me that the doctor had informed her that he was seeing patients floor by floor. When he finished on the floors above he would be down to ours. I stared at her.

"I don't believe it," I told her. "I *know* this is an emergency. My God, he'll die if somebody doesn't come to help him soon." But deep within himself, Connie was hanging on. Through all those hours, it is the only explanation I can think of that seems to fit.

It was nearly 8:00 P.M. when the doctor arrived. I screamed at him: "I've had a call out for almost six hours."

He started to say something, but I interrupted. "Get in here and look at him, for God's sake. Look!"

He bent over Connie for some minutes and suddenly raced past me and out into the corridor. Within seconds the floor came alive as people hurried into Connie's little room. Someone asked me to go outside. There was work to be done.*

Distraught, I could only pace the corridor. Suddenly I realized that I had forgotten all about Vicki, alone at the house. It would be well past midnight before I could get back home, if at all that night. I went to a telephone and told her only

---

* In the nurses' notes there is no report written up for the crucial four-to-twelve-hour shift on that Thursday evening. In the entire nursing records covering Connie's stay in Memorial during that admission, only two other entries—for the same time shift—are missing. Nowhere in any of the nurses' or doctors' records is there any mention that Connie had not been seen by a doctor, despite the constant page (also unrecorded), since 2:00 P.M. when I arrived in his room until close on 8:00 P.M. when hospital personnel began to rush to his bedside.

that I had been detained "visiting Daddy" and would be home eventually. I hung up before she could ask any questions. At the time I had no answers and not much hope to give her.

It was nearly 10:00 P.M. when one of the doctors came out of Connie's room and, taking my arm, led me to a bench near the elevators. My anger had long since evaporated, but with every hour my fears had grown. The doctor began to speak soothingly. Almost nothing he said made any sense to me until I clearly heard him say that Connie was coming around. There was no further need for alarm that night.

The relief after those long anxious hours made me suddenly weak. I realized how tense I had been. The doctor suggested that if I felt able to drive, I should go home and get some rest. I would find my husband much brighter when I came next day, he said. He apologized for the time I had waited for help. His acknowledgment was cold comfort and I ignored it. If, as he said, Connie was responding and would be better, I felt those positive signs could have been brought about hours earlier. The state in which I had found my husband at 2:00 P.M., I thought, need never have happened.

I asked the man to call Dr. Neligan because I could not remember what he had told me about Connie's setback. I was too tired to understand it and, even totally alert, my relief at hearing he was responding would have been too great to take in all the facts.

Before I started home I made an entry in my notebook at the little garage across from the hospital. It had never occurred to me to do that when the doctor was speaking to me. The note I wrote reads:

C rallying, doc says. Being cared for. Nothing more I can do tonight.

But there was much I could think about. I believed that Connie's kidney was in danger of failing. As the doctors well knew from Dr. Van Syckle's report some twenty-two months earlier, he had only one functioning kidney, the left, and

Memorial's own IVPs had disclosed "nonvisualization" of the right organ.

Although the levels of certain of Connie's blood chemistries and a manual abdominal exploration suggested liver involvement or enlargement, continued hypercalcemia combined with the high elevation of urea nitrogen (BUN) seemed to me to be highly suspicious signs of the onset of kidney failure, as did many of the symptoms Connie had begun to display: lassitude, confusion, restlessness, vomiting, and shock.

But, in truth, no one specific sign could be singled out for blame. The doctors were doing everything possible. Put quite simply, cancer had by then gained the upper hand.

For the first time I knew I must try to face the awful possibility that Connie might not win his battle.

$$\doteq 3 \doteq$$

ON FRIDAY, MAY 11, Pat drove me to the hospital. Connie was no longer in the tiny room he had occupied since Monday, April 23. We found him across the hall in 501, a large, airy room close by the nurses' station. A twenty-four-hour urine collection was in progress, an IV running. Earlier, he had been taken for an IVP. The film showed no evidence of obstructive uropathy to the left kidney. Yet his blood chemistries had not shown any significant improvement and, in some instances, were worse than before. His hemocrit and calcium counts were slightly better, but urea nitrogen (BUN) was, as before, extremely elevated at 48 and acid phosphatase had climbed again. On May 9, Wednesday, it had been 33. On Friday it was 37.4, 33 points above normal. The slurred speech that had been noted by Dr. Kaiser and by nurses on Thursday was still present. I had not heard it before. Connie had not spoken during the six hours I was in his room, anxiously awaiting a doctor.

"What's going on here, CJ?" Pat asked as soon as we walked in.

"Listen," Connie said. He was obviously finding it difficult to form words and syllables. He pointed to his mouth. "Thish is what's going on." His eyes were anxious. After several tries, he said, "Christ, Pat, did I have a stroke on top of everything else?"

Pat tried to reassure him. "I'll check your charts, but I would put that idea right out of my mind, if I were you. Your blood chemistries have been acting up a bit. Have you seen a neurologist?"

Connie shook his head. "Not recently. I haven't seen anybody," he said, speaking some words over until he got them right. He stretched out his hand to me and I sat down on the bed beside him. "Haven't even seen Katie," he said, looking at me.

There was little point in telling him about the day before. I had known he was unaware of my presence. I sat and talked with Connie as Pat disappeared to read his charts and talk with doctors. Unlike himself, Connie said very little. He appeared exhausted but he also seemed alert, taking in everything I said. Geoff's school year was over and he had written us before we had gone to Saint Martin that he would like to bring a girl home for a two-week visit. I had been too concerned to think about his homecoming or make any plans for it, but I thought he would be arriving very soon. That news made Connie happy, although he managed to ask, "Is he serious about this girl?" Only time, I told him, could give the answer to that question.

He was equally interested in the news that Victoria, who

had applied for an *au pair* summer job with a family in Paris in order to expand her French, had a position. Marie Schebeko, Connie's French agent, and one of the editors with Robert Laffont—our close friend and Connie's French publisher—had been to see the family. Both felt Vicki would be with pleasant people. She was to leave for Paris on Thursday, June 14. While he had encouraged the idea initially, Connie was not enthusiastic once he learned that the plans were finalized. "Be gone all summer," he said. "Should have checked out the family myself. Suppose it doesn't work?"

"Then Marie will help her find something else to do. You wanted her to keep her French and improve it."

Connie shook his head. "All summer without my little girl. Long time." He turned his head toward the window. I was afraid of what he might be thinking. I bent over and kissed his cheek.

"She'll be back before you know it," I told him.

"Hope so," he said softly, and seemed to doze a bit.

Shortly after Pat came back from his conference in the hall, we learned that Connie was to be given his third chemotherapy injection within a few minutes. Instead of the usual seven-day interval between treatments, this one would follow the second by only five days. Suddenly Connie became agitated. He begged us to stay with him. His alarm and fear were very evident.

"Don't leave me. You don't know what it's like," he said.

We were about to find out. Within minutes after the injection was given a look of horror passed across Connie's face. "Help me," he said. He held out his hands. On either side of the bed Pat and I grabbed hold. "Pull," Connie said. "Pull! I'm sinking down."

His grip on my hand was almost viselike. I looked across at Pat. He was watching Connie closely, his face compassionate and worried. Gently he began to speak to Connie, to reassure him. He strengthened his own grip. The soft words of encouragement and support continued. After a time Connie's grip on my hand relaxed. Reason and peace returned to his face. His body, which had become rigid during those moments of panic, relaxed. Weary but calm again, he lay looking up at us.

"It's like drowning," he said. "I can't fight my way back to the top. It's always like this."

His reaction to the injection had badly frightened me. Yet within minutes he appeared to have recovered. He still did not want us to leave, but Pat had to be at the hospital in Connecticut, and I assured him that I would be back the next day, Saturday, May 12. At the door we turned. His face was full of sorrow and loneliness. It was hard to leave him like that.

Pat was mostly silent on the drive home. Connie's slurred speech disturbed him as did the continuing elevation of certain of the blood chemistries. He seemed confident that everything possible was being done for Connie. Still, he did not tell me much that he had learned. Perhaps the remembrance of Connie's behavior after the 5 F-U injection nagged at him as it did me. I felt chilled and very, very frightened.

As Pat and I drove up to the house, Geoff ran down the steps to greet us followed by a very pretty girl. Before I could leave the car he threw his arms around me.

"How's Dad?" he asked.

I had no idea how to answer. Both Pat and I were saved the trouble. Geoff introduced the girl whose manners were as charming as she was attractive. Pat left us to drive on to the hospital and I went up the stairs between my tall son and the girl he had brought home to visit.

Prolonged illness makes it difficult for the healthy to try to maintain any semblance of normality. One is torn between an all-consuming desire to be with the loved one in the hospital and the practical knowledge that life at home must still go on without letting illness tinge every plan. Somehow we managed. Coping on various levels does not allow much time for morbidity. Besides, in spite of all that I had experienced and seen of Connie's condition since it had worsened in late March, I had to keep believing that he would survive his crises. That trust in him was my source of strength. It always had been in all the years of our marriage. One can accept intellectually the likelihood that cancer will win out, but emotionally one fights it again and again at the times and places it chooses, and tries to rest up between those bouts.

On Saturday, May 12, Geoff, his girl, and Vicki went into the city with me. I had telephoned Connie to let him know that Geoff and his friend were home. He had sounded alert and was anxious for us to arrive. Only two visitors were allowed in at a time. Vicki and I went up first. Connie had showered and put on his dressing gown. He was seated by the window, writing in his notebook. I could not believe the change in him. I think he was determined to pull out all stops for the children's visit. Geoff and his girl reported the same high spirits Vicki and I had noticed. Perhaps our children were his true therapy.

He continued to improve over the weekend. Nurses' notes record that he appeared to feel much better, depression had lifted, and he had no complaints. He had a host of visitors, so many that I was often forced to telephone his room and ask someone with a visiting card to come downstairs so that I could see him myself. Dick and Jean Deems had just arrived back from a trip to Australia and Connie was anxious to hear all their news. David and Marilyn Evins dropped by, as did Matthew, bearing another thermos of fresh juice which Connie all but finished in one sitting. Paul and Zelda Gitlin were in, as was the announcer Ben Grauer, a dear and longtime friend. It was the kind of weekend that did most for Connie's spirits. Outgoing and gregarious, he was always happiest with people around him. He even joked about his hesitant speech and spent some time urging Ben Grauer to imitate him in order to hear how he sounded to someone else.

On Monday, May 14, he was taken to the Neurology Department for further examination. In part, that report reads:

... In last 3–4 days patient noted to have ↑ (increased) slurred speech associated with ↑ (increased) calcium and recent renal decompensation. Also had ↑ (increased) nausea and vomiting and Rxed with Tigon. Back pain, bone pain much improved. Feels well, in good spirits. Speech hesitant and slurred at times. Appears he has difficulty moving tongue to R. He denies difficulty swallowing or breathing ...

After tests were carried out the doctors decided to do an electroencephalogram and skull X ray the following day, Tuesday. Connie did not get much sleep before the work-up. Dr. Whitmore had told him that he might be discharged on Wednesday, May 16. That news, as much as the care he was receiving, charged him up enormously. Nurses' reports indicate that he slept in the early evening on Monday but was awake during the 12 midnight to 8:00 A.M. shift on Tuesday "intensely working on a writing project." He had started in on future notes for *Bridge*. He was not even out of the hospital and he had had a serious setback, but he was back to work again.

He ate well, denied pain, was talkative and cheerful. His mind had already left the hospital and was somewhere with the Allied troops in Holland. On that 1944 battlefield his own pain and worry did not exist. Yet his condition was still of great concern to the doctors.

The Neurology report of the EEG and base-of-skull films reads:

Appears to have a Left XII nerve paresis [speech disturbance] of mild degree probably related to nerve involvement at base of skull. He thinks it may be improving and does not want to have a full work-up now. Agree he can be followed. Please give him office appointment to see me [after] discharge.   Shapiro."

Cancer appeared to have metastasized even to the cranial nerves.

Connie was once again too busy with his own plans to

think about the critical stage his body was in. I stayed home on Tuesday after learning he would be discharged the following day. It was just as well. The phone rang constantly with orders from him. Anne, who had been hospitalized herself and had been back to work for only a week, restoring some order to our lives, made an appointment for Connie's barber to visit him early Wednesday morning at the hospital. In high spirits, Connie decided that Dr. Whitmore needed a haircut as much as he himself, and told us later, obviously relishing his reversal of their roles, "Willet looks much better than he has in days. On examination, he is elegant again and is doing productive work."

So was Connie. Our good friend, Myles Eason, had volunteered to come in with me to pick up Connie. While Myles maneuvered our car around and around the block waiting for us to appear, I had gone first to collect the prescriptions Dr. Whitmore wanted Connie to have. Then, after a trip to the cashier, I went up to the floor where Connie had been for twenty-four long and anxious days. He had been given course #4 of his chemotherapy injection. The dosage had been raised from 750 mg to 1 gm and his reaction was recorded as "uneventful." Perhaps the thought of his homecoming had made that treatment easier to bear.

He was waiting for me, dressed in a light gray wool suit, impeccably groomed and barbered. His weight had dropped back to 175 pounds and, aside from an indoor pallor, he looked incredibly healthy. It was hard to believe that this was the same man whose life I had despaired of only six days earlier. A bevy of nurses were in the room and two of them accompanied us downstairs and to the car where Myles was patiently waiting.

Connie was delighted to see him and Myles was, I think, rather astonished at the buoyancy and optimism Connie exuded. My reports to close friends like the Easons of the gravity of Connie's illness must have seemed grossly exaggerated to anyone who saw him on that morning.

With nurses' help he eased himself into the back seat of the car and pushed away the pillows I had put there. To the nurses he said, "I love you all but I'm telling you one thing. I'm damned if I'm ever coming back to this place again."

As we drove off he turned to wave good-bye. He was out of the hospital. As far as he was concerned, he was out forever.

CORNELIUS

Sunday, June 10, 1973. It has been so long since I have used the tape recorder that I had to check it out to be sure it is still operating. I have a fixation about keeping cameras, recording equipment, and automobiles in good working order. Probably because I never had the money to have any of those things when I was young, I am fiercely protective of them now.

I have been leafing through my notebooks for the past couple of months. The scribbles look as though they had been made by someone just learning how to write. They are readable but disturbing. From April 22 until May 16 I was back in Memorial. I think I nearly died there, which may account for the peculiarities of the handwriting. Several daily entries are missing and I can only assume that I was either too ill or too frightened to make notes.

One entry, however, is quite clear. It is for Sunday, April 29. A friend of mine died that day. She had the room next to mine. I knew her scarcely a week and yet I knew her very well. Cancer patients have a bond that surpasses a healthy person's understanding. The presence of fear and the agony of pain are transmitted without words by one of us to another. I cannot say how this is done. I only know it happens. My young friend wanted to die. I wanted her to stay. But her reserves were gone. She was being crucified by pain she could no longer endure. Now she is one more statistic on the medical charts, filed under "Lung and Bronchus." She will become part of a curve on a logarithmic scale and no one will know her name. It is not important on cancer charts. Age, sex, treatment, are important. Nothing else. The individual is deftly excised and sluiced down the medical drain.

I've had a very bad time, both in hospital and since I came home. I thought I had suffered a minor stroke while there because I could not seem to form words. That problem is much better now. No one—not Neligan, Whitmore, or the neurologists—have given me an indication of what could have caused it. It could be the chemotherapy I am now on, some drastic change in the blood or lymphs, or quite possibly the cancer is simply spreading everywhere.

There is nothing more appalling than the state I am in at present. I thought I had experienced the full spectrum of humiliations. I was wrong. I am sitting in a wheelchair in the office because I cannot walk back and forth to my desk. Each day Kathryn helps me propel a walker down the few steps from our rooms to the foyer and then gets me into this chair and backs out the front door to start the walk that has become a journey. There are seventeen steps from the front door to the driveway, with one landing where Katie can rest. I don't know where she gets the reserves of strength to haul me around. She straps me into the chair so I won't fall out and raises the front wheels high in the air while she takes me down with the large back wheels, sliding them gently off each riser and down to the next. I try not to moan because she does do it gently and should not be doing it at all. At the bottom we rest for a moment on the driveway before Katie starts for the office. Our drive has a slight downward elevation and a couple of times she has not been able to hold the chair except by dragging her feet behind it. I have tried to help by attempting to slow the back wheels with my hands and although I've rubbed some skin off, it does impede the forward speed.

Nearing the office the driveway rises again and this is the hardest part for Katie. I can propel the wheels with my hands quite successfully now, which saves her from having to push all my weight up the incline. Then she turns me around again and we back into the office. I want to cry every trip we make because I would rather be gone for good than for her to have to do this kind of thing. I am hoping to get some young lad to come and do the pushing and pulling because I simply cannot have Katie exerting herself like this.

Other aspects of my present condition are far worse. I am incontinent. It is the most embarrassing, god-awful thing in the world. I have a car robe over my knees and a urinal bottle on the far side of my desk. I cannot get up and get to the bathroom, so I have to use the bottle and very often I have had to ask Annie to leave the room quickly in the middle of dictation or work on copy. I cannot tell when I have to use the urinal and the need is often upon me before I can prepare myself or Katie or Annie.

My wife refuses to leave the room, just as she insists on bringing trays of food up and down stairs for me, keeping boxes of moist towelettes at my side, putting thermos jugs of water down at whatever place I may be, and helping me to roll over and grab the walker at night when I have to be in the bathroom for long periods of time. She never seems to sleep herself and usually greets me back at the bed with a pot of hot tea, toast, and marmalade. It may be four in the morning, but she is always there. Lately we have been doing some of our best work on the book at night. I am very excited about it, and in spite of the appalling creature I have become, I am careful to let nothing of myself show through the work. If I did, Katie would spot it and edit it out.

On Thursday, May 31, according to Anne, we finished the 310th clean page of manuscript. Prior to that, while I was in hospital, Katie told me she was working on the pages but needed my complete outline to keep on going. I was so angry I think I got myself well enough to come home. We can only do this book together, not apart. Even if Katie is, as General Jim Gavin says, the most knowledgeable woman about military writing he has ever talked to, there are things that I can do in an instant that take her an hour to figure out. She was bogged down trying to explain the layout and structure of the Arnhem bridge in order to show the position of Johnny Frost's men when they reached it on the night of September 17, 1944.* I had her bring in the copy she had done and spent the best part of one night in hospital setting it straight. Once that was done she put the men into the story and wrote up the account of the first attack to capture the bridge that Frost carried out that night. But we have got to do it together. We work best that way.

The first thing I did when I got home from hospital was to call both Annie and Katie up to the bedroom and then, and only then, did I dictate the rest of the outline to Annie. It will stand up, I'm sure. I bet the girls that when the book is finished they will see that I have not had to deviate from the outline at all. Somehow it was very important for me to do that outline. First, I had to prove to myself that the drugs I'd been given in hospital had not affected my mind, as something seems to have affected my speech. Second, just in case I shouldn't make it to the end, Katie will know where to take the book.

It is my impression that a great many people think I won't be around much longer. In fact, I had the same thought myself shortly after arriving home. People called in and I didn't remember seeing them. Then one night—it could not have been more than a day or two after I came home—I felt very strange. I had no sensation of pain, no urgency to get to the bathroom, no recollection of past or present. It was quite peaceful to lie there like that, and yet I rather felt I should do something about it, because I felt a bit unnatural.

I must have dozed off because it was morning and Katie was bending over me, yelling something about waking up. I was too tired to open my eyes. I could feel her hands on my face, chest, and arms. She tried to move me but I didn't feel

---

* At Arnhem, Colonel (now General, retired) Frost's 2nd Battalion, British 1st Airborne, was the only one to reach the bridge almost intact.

like moving. I had come to like my condition and I was more comfortable than I can remember being in days. The next I knew, Neligan was there, and he poked around my body and, like Katie, talked to me. I could hear him perfectly well but I thought if I didn't answer he would just go away. Quite frankly I didn't care what he did as long as he left me alone. That was the precise time I thought I might be dying—and I didn't care.

But Katie did. She slapped me quite hard. I was so surprised I opened my eyes. We have never hurt each other, except with words. She slapped me again. I could not think why. Then she said, "CJ, you are not going to die. Do you hear me? I will not let you just lie there and die." She seemed very angry but she put her face against mine and my cheek was wet from her touching me. She was crying for me and fighting with me at the same time. I don't know where she got the strength but she suddenly pulled me to a sitting position. The pain I thought I was leaving behind shot all through my body and I was in agony for a minute or two. I asked her why in the hell she had done that and she began to laugh and cry simultaneously. The pain was a good strong reminder that I was not going to be permitted to sleep or float or anything else that was soothing and comfortable. My wife had seen to that.

Neligan came back around eleven. Apparently he and Katie both thought I had been in a coma and apparently my face had gone very pale. Pat was delighted to see it flushed again. I didn't tell him that my wife had beaten me up. He listened to my heart and fussed around with my drawerful of medicines and after that everything was fine, at least as far as he and Katie were concerned. They had me talking and in pain. The latter is certainly a sure sign that one is not dead.

But death does occupy my mind. In the early days of this cancer I was afraid of it. Now that emotion has totally evaporated. I only wonder how long I can keep it away because I must fight until the book is finished and for as long as possible after that. I shall try never to feel peaceful and pain-free again. These symptoms, I imagine, may be quite closely linked to death because I am neither at peace nor without pain when I am well.

That is a ridiculous turn of phrase, but I don't know any other way of putting it. Fast-paced mental activity and constant pain are now my criteria for being well. Their absence would mean that I was dead or dying. Still, a lot of people seem to think I am about to hand in my dinner pail.

It is amusing how one's friends react when they think there is no hope of survival. About ten days ago Ben Wright, Pete Kriendler, and Mike O'Neill drove out from New York to see me. They arrived about midmorning and came up to the bedroom. I am not accustomed to seeing them display exquisite manners on our fishing trips, so it was rather a surprise to see the decorum they displayed. I simply sat and watched them acting unnatural until I had finally had enough. I told them they were boring the hell out of me and if they had come to view the remains that I would send them an invitation in advance. That broke the ice and we had a good day's talk.

A conversation I had with Pat was a little more disturbing. It started innocuously enough with us discussing some local real-estate problems. How we got around to cemeteries I don't remember. Pat asked me if I had ever thought of where I wanted to be buried. He said he and Vera had discussed that themselves because if something unexpected ever occurred, they did not want their children confused as to what to do. Now Neligan can sometimes be as transparent as window glass. I asked him if he thought I was dying and he replied no, but that I should give some thoughts to these things. Frankly, it doesn't much matter to me. When you're gone, you're gone. I would have liked to be buried at Saint-Laurent with the men who made the Normandy invasion. That is my spiritual home, but I suspect burial there would prove impossible and so I told Pat that Ridgefield was fine with me or wherever Kathryn wanted. I don't really want to talk about those things because I would have no control over them, and besides they induce morbidity which might inject itself into the book. That I cannot allow. There is too much greatness in the people involved in Market-Garden for my emotions to mingle with theirs.

Last Tuesday was my birthday and I still hadn't made it out of the bedroom and down to the office. Instead, Annie and Katie had been working up there, which meant they carried mounds of material from the office to the house. But that day I was really not feeling well, and I was both touched and embarrassed by the attendance I received. Louise McKeon and Vera Neligan had each made me a cake. Paul and Zelda Gitlin sent out champagne. Our dear friend, Helene Merrick, who is one of the brightest, loveliest women I know, made the bedroom look like Christmas. She brought over flowers, a plant, some excellent gin which John Tower will surely help dispose of, some Jack Daniels, and a basketful of vegetables. The Neligan kids sent me a large rubber elephant with all their names on it and their wishes for a happy birthday. Myles and Kath Eason called, Dick and Jean Deems, John and Shirley Tower, David and Marilyn Evins, Dick and Helen Hoyt—all were on the phone at one time or another. I appreciated it very much but I hope it's not a harbinger of things to come. I intend to be around for a while yet. The real problem with having cancer is that people get tired of waiting for you to die of it. Perhaps I am too obstinate or just too mulish to go ahead and accommodate them. Besides if I tried, my fragile little wife would slap me out of it.

As I have been recording all of this I have been aware over the past half hour that the pain in my legs is increasing in intensity. It is impossible to do much exercising in a wheelchair but I don't want my leg muscles to atrophy. I have just tried standing. I find that by hanging onto the edge of my desk with both hands I can hold my body weight, but only for a second or two. I will have to use the walker much more and try to find some means of working standing up so that the legs will have something to do. The pain on standing has been so bad for weeks that it almost seems as though I cannot remember a time when it did not hurt.

I gather I was given a lot of narcotics in the hospital because when I first came home Pat was giving me Demerol injections. I must have no tolerance for pain-killers at all. They put me to sleep and my mind is confused when I wake up. Pat had one of the district nurses here show Kathryn how to give me injections of Demerol in the muscle. I don't think I was really aware of exactly what she was giving me until one day last week. Then it dawned on me. The drowsiness and lessening of pain are all right at night. I need the sleep, but I cannot have drugs like that going into my system during the day. When she got near enough to me I knocked the syringe out of her hand. I don't think I've been so angry in a long time. I'd be a zombie if I permitted this to go on. I can manage the pain with lesser drugs and still go on with my work. I told Katie I didn't give a damn what Pat or Willet wanted, I was not having any more Demerol. No one seems to realize that pain makes the mind sharper. I think I am writing better with cancer than I ever did without it. How odd that an illness like this should spur one on to better work. Perhaps it is only that I have learned to ignore my condition when I am working or maybe I have just become accustomed to this gnawing, growing thing inside me. Actually I suppose there is no rationale, but it would be ironic if my writing was improving just when I might not live to see if I can do even better. I would like to live to do many more things, but I don't think about them because *Bridge* must be finished first.

On Friday, Neligan took me to Norwalk Hospital for two units of whole blood. The procedure is much like that at Memorial. They have to type and crossmatch to be certain the blood to be transfused is compatible with mine. The process seems to take forever. I got a glimpse of Neligan's orders. Under "Brief History and Diagnosis" Pat had written, "Ca Prostate—Severe anemia."

I suppose that finding came from the Main Medical Laboratory in Danbury. A man named Joe Vecchiarino came to the house to take vials of my blood. Apparently this will be an ongoing thing. It is a little unsettling to have someone drawing one's blood early in the morning in one's own house. I associate that procedure entirely with hospitals. Joe, however, makes it as painless as possible and he is quite a fascinating man to talk with. I've got to start reading up on blood and chemical constituents so that I can discover for myself exactly how I'm doing. I had not thought I was anemic but apparently Joe's report to Pat must indicate that and certainly I feel a little less lethargic than I have been.

Yesterday, Jerry and Barbara Korn's daughters came to visit, along with their young men. While I see Jerry frequently when I am in the city, I hadn't seen the girls in years. They are quite beautiful young women. Maggie and Ellen are identical twins and Sue is, I think, the baby. I am a little confused because Katie and Barbara were both pregnant at a time when Jerry and I were working at *Collier's* and I honestly can't remember if the twins or Sue were born then. At any rate I thoroughly enjoyed seeing them. Geoff and Vicki were home and we spent a pleasant warm day on the terrace. Maggie had some thoughts of becoming a serious painter and it came out in the conversation that she had more or less given up her work. She was reticent about the reason. My own feeling is that she has not given her talent time enough to grow to know what its potential is. As with anything else in the arts, practice is the only way one has to improve. Unfortunately the young are in a hurry. If something doesn't work out immediately, they feel disillusioned and very often stall out. I hope Maggie won't, just as I hope this year at college has given Geoff a glimmer of just how far he can go. Thank God there is enough money in trust to see both Geoff and Vicki through their educations. If I did nothing else right in my life, at least I provided for their future by seeing to it that the monies were put aside in order to help give them a solid base of knowledge from which they can spring into careers. I don't care if they start at the bottom, it's still the best place to learn. But I am relieved to know that if anything should happen to me they will not be denied an education.

Katie will be down to get me soon. I should have been working instead of spending this past hour fiddling with the recorder and taping my thoughts. Still I believe this is good therapy. One seldom has a chance to put down the many things that cross one's mind. Writing demands strict discipline of thoughts but a tape machine is not so stringent. I can relax with it because I'm using it to free my mind of certain worries, and to assess out loud my chances for survival. They are very slim, but the fact that I can acknowledge that helps me to stop worrying about myself overly much. I must take care not to turn inward, even on tape. It would, I think, be an almost certain sign that subconsciously I was giving up. Even without hope, no one should give up. There is so much more to life than fear of death. Each day is like a gift to enjoy and savor. Oddly enough, in spite of earlier morbid moods, I wouldn't change places with any man.

KATHRYN

On Thursday, June 14, a reluctant Victoria left for France. Connie was back in bed. After every energetic rally, he would slip back into exhaustion. But he did not stop working. Propped up in bed, he continued to turn out handwritten pages at a speed he had never before achieved. He was working intensely on the day Victoria left.

As the time for our departure for the airport neared, Connie's mood darkened, only to be masked by cheerful joking whenever Vicki came in and out of the room. I was going to the airport with our daughter; Mary Luke, with characteristic generosity, had come to the house to be with Connie until I returned home.

Father and daughter said good-bye to each other privately.

I waited on the steps above the driveway with Jerry Lewis, who would drive us to the airport and bring me back again. Through the open bedroom window I could hear Connie's voice, strong and lighthearted as ever, promising Vicki he would be fine and with luck would have the book finished by the time she came back home.

"Of course," I heard him say teasingly, "you may not be able to read English by then. Just remember, baby, who and what you are. Get the most of this summer. Anything you need, Marie Schebeko or Bobby Laffont will help you with and so will all the people at the Paris *Reader's Digest*. Whenever you get lonesome, call."

After a few minutes Vicki came down the steps to where Jerry and I waited. Her eyes were full of tears. "I just want to tell you that if anything happens to Daddy while I'm gone, I'll never forgive you," she said.

"Nothing will happen. He's going to be all right."

"Mom, you don't know that and neither do the doctors. Oh, hell," she said, not unlike her father, "I don't want to go. Please."

"It will be all right," I told her. "If anything should go wrong I promise I'll get you back here quickly."

She was silent all the way to the airport in spite of Jerry's attempts to cheer her and my optimistic remarks about how good the summer would be for her.

Matthew Evins met us at the airport. Connie had given Vicki a Nikon to take with her and Matt had dashed out to buy a case for it. Connie had mislaid his own. On research trips his cameras were each carried in aluminum cases, nestled in heavy foam cutouts, along with the various lenses he used. Matt just made the departure gate in time, swinging the Nikon case over his head. He kissed Vicki on the cheek and then she flung her arms around me. "I don't want to go. I can't tell you why. Please don't make me go."

I suddenly felt that it must seem to Vicki as though we were pushing her out for the summer, to spare her the pain of Connie's ordeal. "You'll have a marvelous time," I told her. "I promise I'd never let you stay over there if I thought Daddy was in any danger."

She was the last passenger to board. The camera case dangling by its straps in her hand, her face streaming with tears, she turned back once to look at Matt and me, and in that moment I had a wild urge to rush up, take her by the hand, and bring her home. Then she disappeared from sight.

Matt and I stood watching until the plane pulled out and started for its runway. I had much to think about. She was only sixteen and in the three years of Connie's illness, with the worries about money and the book, and the presence of cancer which seemed to have been with us always, I had not given her the thought and time she needed. I had never talked with her frankly about her father's health and my preoccupation with him had caused me to forget her needs, her everyday life. Now I was sending away a little girl who badly needed us and the reassurance of our love. In the three years since cancer had come to stay, Vicki had matured, with all the attendant worries teenage girls are given to. Because of my preoccupation, she had been forced to turn to others for companionship, to solve her own problems at school, to hide her fears and withhold her confidences because at home there was no mother-in-residence who really listened.

The people who had become her friends and confidants I did not know or knew only slightly. Not since she and Geoff had left home that rainy night in 1971 had I really been totally involved with them as people. Now Vicki was gone, taking her problems and worries with her.

I, not Connie, had built the wall of seeming disinterest, shutting her away from all she really loved. And so her angers, frustrations, and longings were all visited on others at school and elsewhere. She took her punishment for occasional misbehaviors at school, never blaming their origins on the fact that at home she had no one to talk over problems with. Her confidences, likewise, as I was to learn, were given to others who preyed upon her vulnerability under the guise of giving help and love—but were, themselves, ruthless and far more emotionally disturbed than was Victoria.

With young Matt beside me watching the plane taxi off, I felt a sudden fear. She didn't even know for sure how much I loved her.

⹀ 4 ⹀

KATHRYN

By Saturday, June 16, Connie was back at work in the office. Vicki had telephoned us from Paris on Friday and hearing her young voice and her assurances that all would be well had seemingly revitalized him once more. Additionally, we had gained another helper. One of Jerry and Barbara Korn's daughters had found us a young man who wanted a summer job and who was strong and capable of taking Connie back and forth to the office. His name was Jody, and he was also bright and eager to help in other ways around the office. He came to live with us from late Sundays to Fridays, going home on weekends. Geoff had acquired a summer job with a builder and was often up early in the mornings and out late in the evenings, so that Jody's presence was doubly helpful.

During the early part of the month correspondence had begun to pile up, as it did every year close to Connie's birthday and the anniversary of the Normandy invasion, a day apart. Ben Grauer had once suggested that Ike had always intended to start the invasion on June 5, Connie's birthday, and had regretted the delay ever since.

Longtime friends, World War II veterans, French men and women, and correspondents had, ever since the publication of *The Longest Day,* used June 5 and 6 as the time to write to Connie. In 1973 the volume of mail in June was heavier than it had ever been. The word of Connie's illness had made the rounds among his oldest friends. They were bent on cheering him as they had always done—by insults affectionately written and by atrocious gifts. Joe Ryle had settled on a mirror with *Time* magazine's logo and border around it and Man of the Year emblazoned across the top. Mary Hemingway had sent a handsome pencil with a note that read: *"Now* will you get on with *it?"*; and Walter Cronkite had handed over his "most prized possession"—a stained piece of marble fastened to a wall plaque emblazoned with bronze letters which read: Hitler Stood Here. Walter claimed to have hacked the marble out of the bathroom at Hitler's old headquarters in Rastenburg, East Prussia.

Connie had been too ill earlier in the month to enjoy or even see the mementos and letters. With Jody, Anne, and me in attendance, he settled down to sorting the mail and gifts. Joe Willicombe had sent him an old column written by Frank Conniff, who had been one of Connie's closest friends, about the twentieth anniversary D-Day trip reporters and columnists had made to the Normandy beaches in 1964.

In part Frank's column read:

One of the kicks of re-fighting the Normandy campaign has been the daily companionship of Cornelius Ryan, author of the largest nonfiction best-seller in France's history, "Le Jour le Plus Long," or, as roughly rendered stateside, "The Longest Day."

Mr. Ryan is a large, explosive Dublin-born extrovert who became an American citizen after the war and settled down amidst the bucolic beauty of Ridgefield, Conn. He flaunts spacious sports jackets and rakish caps as his identifying regalia. Some say America

358

obtained him from Ireland in a straight player deal for John Huston, but Mr. Ryan is mum on this speculation.

. . . It is when you enter Ste. Mere-Eglise, target of our first parachute drop on D-Day, that the full impact of Mr. Ryan on Normandy becomes apparent . . . [His] appearance on the streets is the signal for civil celebration. Mothers hold children up to be photographed with him, books are produced for autographs—in the small town of 700 souls, over 5,000 copies of his book were sold in one store—the Calvados and wine suddenly appear, and mon cher amis, it is great to be along.

"This never happened to John Huston," gurgled Mr. Ryan happily in his only comment on the Huston-Ryan trade reports.

. . . It couldn't happen to a nicer export from Dublin; and what's John Huston done for Ireland lately?*

A letter of a different kind arrived from Jack Thompson of the *Chicago Tribune,* whom Connie had described as "a shaggy poet." As Mary Hemingway's note and gift had intended, Jack, too, was attempting to cheer Connie and to goad him into action. He wrote:

Dear Dr. Ryan: On the eve of your day, my thoughts turn toward the old Ridgefield road runner . . . My agents tell me you've been having a rough time of it . . . They tell me this chemotherapy jazz can change a person's personality. And that, of course, could be a plus, eh, old boy?

Seriously, tho, why do you let a few aches and pains retard your completion of the "new" book, a manuscript my elitist eastern correspondents assure me is the best thing you have ever done . . . That "new" book, as we all well know, has been under gestation far longer than any elephant's miseries; indeed, it bears more resemblance to the 17-year cicada's pregnancy. Why, I can recall way back at the 25th anniversary of D-Day reading some of the mss. in your office and listening to your interminable tales of Market-Garden as we laboriously fought over the Dutch sandtables.

* Copyright Hearst Corporation. Frank Conniff died on May 25, 1971. A renowned columnist, a steadfast friend, he never learned of Connie's illness.

. . . I don't mean to lean on you, merely to irritate your risibles into getting off your ass and getting to work.

Best love. The Beard.

Connie's answer to Jack was far different from the notes he had written to his friend in the past.

Things have not been too well and this chemotherapy jazz can indeed change a person's personality. Who can tell, that beard of yours might look presentable now, for the first time.

I usually write to you in a lighter frame of mind but just this once I have to turn serious. . . . The last three years since I contracted this unfortunate ailment have been very tough. I am nearly broke and to date medical costs have run close to $68,000. I have had the best of attention and I'm only alive because of it. But our savings are being whittled down. Thankfully I've set up trust funds for the kids so they can get through college.

. . . I've no idea whether I am good for 6 months or 6 years because chemotherapy is a real hit-and-miss affair. . . . Summing it all up, Jack, I've always had the guts to fight back and I'm continuing to do so, but between you and me your old pal is scared shitless.

. . . I wanted you to know the truth.

Connie

And to Herb Caen in San Francisco, he wrote:

. . . I don't know whether I shall die before the book comes out or not. . . . My affairs are in relatively good order and if anything should happen you'll be duly notified and invited to the best Irish wake that's been seen around in a long time.

Jack Thompson, Ben Wright and the D-Day clan know the full story but, in general, the public knows nothing at all about the cancer situation so don't you mention it . . . the truth is that I ain't getting ready to step into the old pine box just yet.

Connie

Indeed he was not. Even as Jody was daily wheeling him to work and Anne and I were sharing his discomfiture at the urgent and frequent incontinence that interrupted his work and often reduced him to tears of embarrassment, Connie received the first subtle hint that an award signifying the highest recognition of his life and work yet made was soon to be given him. The president of France, Georges Pompidou, had decided to honor him with France's most distinguished decoration, the Legion of Honor.

We were incredulous. Within hours telegrams and letters began pouring in from Paris and from Washington. It was impossible to learn how the distinctive honor had come about. I believe that many French and American friends had played a role in putting forward Connie's name.

According to M. Xavier Marchetti, adviser to the then French president, the decision was made immediately at the Élysée Palace as soon as President Pompidou, reading through the proposed honors list, saw Connie's name. Beside it, the French president swiftly wrote the single word, "oui."

On Saturday, June 30, we learned that the Legion of Honor would be presented to Connie at our house on Sunday, July 8, by the French ambassador to the United States, Jacques Kosciusko-Morizet. He and Madame Kosciusko-Morizet, along with members of the French diplomatic corps in Washington, would fly to New York where the consul general of France in New York, M. Gerard Gaussen and Mme. Gaussen, would meet them. The entire diplomatic party would travel by limousines to Ridgefield. Their route would be monitored by New York State Police and, at the entrance to Ridgefield which abounds New York's state line, Ridgefield Police Department cars would take over the motorcade and escort the official party to our house where other Ridgefield police would be waiting, car radios tuned to alert us of the exact moment the cavalcade appeared at the top of our long driveway.

Connie could think of little else all week. The honor represented to him international recognition of his life's work. In Europe he had long been recognized and respected as a historian of the first rank. In the United States, his adopted country, he had once been described by Henry Steele Commager as "one of the great amateur historians. That doesn't mean he's not professional in his skills and techniques. [He is] amateur in the sense that he has not been taken in by the academy"—(that is, by the academic community). The last sentence had hurt deeply. For years Connie had longed to be invited to join The Society of American Historians, which had been founded in 1939 by Allan Nevins and others to promote distinction in historical writing. Many of the fellows of the society were men and women with whom Connie maintained correspondence and to whom, from time to time, he freely gave access to historical papers and documents he alone had been able to find. He had never been asked to become a member. As he labored toward the finish of *A Bridge Too Far*, the news of the honor to be paid him by France assuaged that oversight.

It did nothing to soothe me. Delighted as I was for Connie, I was in a state of panic. His illness, our intense work on *Bridge*, the constant care that Connie now required, had left me no time for outdoor work. The gardener we had once employed had moved on to a better-paying job. The flower beds, rock gardens, lawns, and hedges had not been tended in more than a year. The forest and accompanying underbrush had almost marched to the terrace, and the terrace itself, of black slate, had not been cleaned in months. My outdoor furniture was badly in need of new cushions and upholstery. My only thought as I viewed the house and grounds was that they were both disasters. There was no way that we could be ready for such illustrious guests in the space of a single week.

Once again I had forgotten the power of friends. Upon learning of the decoration to be given Connie, many of our Ridgefield friends practically took up residence to work in the house and on the grounds. Myles and Kathleen Eason labored from sunup to sunset on the rock gardens and among the flower beds. Roses were dug up from friends' houses and moved to ours. Kathleen Eason and Dolores Connor shopped for foam cushions and fabrics, and within five days Dolly Connor had made the outdoor furniture look like new. Mike Sedor, a veteran of the Normandy landings, trimmed the hedges and formal flower beds, and Betty Ajay filled the centers of each formal bed with masses of white petunias.

Young Neil Casey, still in high school, worked daily on the huge terrace, scrubbing every slate by hand. Margery Thompson and Shirley Tower cleaned our office from top to bottom, roping off in red ribbon only our two desks, which were cluttered with current work. Polly Forcelli and her task force of ladies set to work on my menu, abetted by Marilyn Evins's cook in New York. Our friend Gino Bob Polverari rounded up others to help pour the wines. In New York young Peter Morrell, whose family owns a wine shop and who had been a fan of Connie's since the publication of *The Longest Day*, worked out a list of wines for each course and a Laurent-Perrier Cuvée Grand Siècle 1961 for the toasts following the investiture.

The house was humming with activity as Margery Thompson ironed tablecloths, Jean Safford and Wynn Aldrich worked out flower arrangements, and Ann Crammond gathered great hanging baskets of flowering plants for the terrace. The ambassador's party was to arrive at 12:30 P.M. on Sunday, July 8. There would be thirty-six for luncheon at six tables. Not only would my up-to-then ample dining room be crowded, but I found I sadly lacked enough linens, service plates, wineglasses, and flatware for such a special occasion. Vera Neligan came to my aid. She and Pat carried in box after box of their own beautiful silver, china, and glass to supplement my own. Dick and Jean Deems, who could not be with us, obtained tall standards and French and American flags and had them driven out from New York to flutter near the formal gardens off the terrace.

Larry Aldrich brought us bronzes and paintings by such masters as Viera da Silva, Maurice Esteve, Bazaine, Masson, Picasso, Beaudin, and Cesar and supervised their placement in our living room.

Louise McKeon hunted down special herbs for the cold cream of leek soup we had planned as a first course, and Dan McKeon gave Connie some valuable references for his acceptance speech. Jean and Jimmy Gavin flew in from Boston and Jean supervised the seating at the tables, arranging my place cards according to diplomatic protocol.

On early Saturday evening before what we had come to call "Fete Day"—the pronunciation varied according to fatigue of the volunteers—we wheeled Connie to the terrace. Preoccupied that week with his acceptance speech and still at work on *Bridge,* he had been scarcely aware of the work being done around him. He could not believe the transformation.

Even as he sat in the sweltering summer heat (we had been promised more of the same for the following day), the Easons were fingerpicking the last blades of grass from the rock garden. Jean Safford was dry-mopping the terrace, Neil Casey was gently hosing down peat moss and mulch around the borrowed roses, and Wynn Aldrich was giving the flowers and tables a final inspection. Connie was under instruction from Margery Thompson and Shirley Tower not to go near the office until the festivities the next day were over. They had polished all the ashtrays, and both knew Connie's penchant for putting an ash in each clean tray. "He feels they look neglected if he hasn't got a cigarette going in each one,"

Shirley complained. Since the dining room could barely accommodate the thirty-six dignitaries, most of our friends who had done so much work would not be seated at the luncheon. It was arranged that guests invited only to the official ceremony would meet in the office, where the Thompsons and Towers would act as hosts and where wine and hors d'oeuvres would be on hand. When the luncheon was over, they would all come up to the terrace for the investiture.

In spite of the excitement Connie slept soundly that night. I did not. I had been trotting from house to office daily, getting in the way of my friends, who had the organization of our household well in hand. I was exhausted but mentally I kept running over last-minute details. I could not think what to wear, and I was worried about how Connie would be able to get through the day.

At 7:00 A.M. on "Fete Day" I awoke to see Myles Eason on the lawn, picking up leaves that had dared to drop during the night. Neil Casey was attaching miniature French and American flags to our mailbox, and Louise McKeon had provided still more to be used among the centerpieces on the tables. By 8:00 A.M., the temperature stood at 91. Ted Safford arrived with large floor fans which he positioned beneath the piano. We had never had occasion to wish for central air conditioning before. The eighty-four windows and sliding glass doors in our house had always provided us with cross breezes even in the warmest weather. But on Sunday, July 8, no breeze stirred.

At 8:30 A.M. Pat Neligan arrived to examine Connie and to stay with him for an hour before going home to dress. "Katie, Pat, I want to tell you something," Connie said.

Anxious, Pat and I sat down on Connie's bed. My husband's face was solemn.

"What is it, CJ?" Pat asked.

"Just this." Connie paused, his voice trembling. "This is the greatest accolade that has ever been given me in my life. I'm damned if I'll accept the Legion of Honor from a wheelchair and I'm damned if I'll strap on a rubber bag for this incontinency. I'm not going to use either of them ever again. I intend to greet the ambassador of France at my doorstep on my feet and I sure as hell am not going to allow any problems in the lower regions to occur." He looked at us. "That's it," he said. "I just wanted you both to know."

"Connie, you can't stand," I told him. "Your legs aren't strong enough."

"I've got Jeff Seitz's cane. I intend to use it," Connie said.*

I started to protest again but Connie interrupted. "Damn it, Pat," he said to Dr. Neligan, "you get me on my feet. I'll do the rest."

Pat looked at me. "That's it, then, Katie. But," he went on, turning back to Connie, "I warn you, I'll be right behind you all the time."

"No." Connie shook his head. "I have to stand alone."

At 12:10 P.M. a Ridgefield policeman came sprinting to the house. "They're just turning into your road now," he said. "They'll be here any second."

Pat had returned an hour earlier to help Connie get ready. They came out of his dressing room. I looked across at my husband, standing erect in a neat pin-striped suit, white shirt, and dark blue silk tie. Pat's eyes were full of tears and so were mine. Leaning on General Seitz's stout cane Connie took his first careful steps into the room. Then he stopped and looked at me. "Are you ready, Henrietta?" he asked.

We reached the threshold of our door just as the ambassador stepped from his limousine. The diplomats and their

---

* General Seitz had suffered a stroke and was in a hospital outside Washington. As the strength in Connie's legs had ebbed after his first operation in 1970, Jeff had lent him a beautiful hardwood cane with a silver inset. It had been presented to the general by officers at one of the posts he had commanded, and Connie had used it frequently until he had become unable to walk. The wheelchair he was using belonged to another friend, Harold Merrick, whose wife Helene, had brought it over for Connie.

wives came up the steps. Tall and elegant my husband greeted them each by name, and we welcomed them into our home.

I had never seen it look so lovely, and the terrace and formal gardens beyond were a mass of blooms and color. The works of art and bronze which Larry Aldrich had arranged with such care looked as if they had always been there. The place sparkled.

The exquisite manners and friendliness of the ambassador's party put us all at ease, and the help of Jean Gavin and Austine Hearst were invaluable to me in hostessing and chatting with small groups of diplomats and other dignitaries. Just as elegant as Jean and Austine, managing somehow to maintain an appearance of coolness in the stifling heat, were Marilyn Evins and Vera Neligan who arrived in from the kitchen, where they had gone over last-minute details with Polly. And down in the office, the only air-conditioned place on our grounds, the Towers and Thompsons were looking after a host of friends whose cars were adroitly parked by off-duty Ridgefield policemen as soon as guests stepped from them.

The luncheon went beautifully. The ambassador and the consul general were at my table, their wives at Connie's just across from me. There were many compliments on the food and especially on the wines Peter Morrell had selected. The rush baskets full of daisies had been arranged by Jean and Wynn with such artistry that they looked casually "country" against the fruitwood and painted French chests in the lime-and-blue-papered dining room.

I kept stealing glances at my husband. He was chatting with the members of his table as though he had never known a word called "pain." Yet, at the end of the luncheon as guests trooped to various rooms to freshen up before the ceremony, I saw Pat make his way quickly to Connie's side. The ambassador joined them and suggested that Connie rest for a few minutes. It was a gracious gesture and an understanding one. The three men walked slowly to the stairs leading to our bedroom where Connie and Pat continued on alone. I stayed with the ambassador and our guests, ready to summon those in the office by intercom when the ceremonies would begin. As we walked about, chatting, I saw with amazement that New York, Connecticut, and French television crews had arrived, along with a commentator from Radio Luxembourg.

Then suddenly the moment itself had come. The terrace began to fill with people. The ambassador, Madame Kosciusko-Morizet, and I waited at the bottom of the steps as Connie, dressed in another suit, shirt, and tie, came slowly down the stairs with Pat.* Connie was paying a price for his determination to walk instead of being an invalid. It was a price he would pay to the end of his life. Never again, except at airports, did he allow himself to be wheeled anywhere. France's great medal had already begun to work a minor miracle in our lives.

On the terrace, flanked by the flags of the United States and the Republic of France, and with Madame Kosciusko-Morizet and me in attendance, the ambassador began his address:†

"My distinguished friends, we are here today to honor a great American, a great Irish-American, with the greatest distinction awarded by the French Government . . . [Turning to Connie, he continued:] When *The Longest Day* was published, General de Gaulle wrote you personally and thanked you for telling the entire story of D Day and for making a very detailed and accurate reference to the French Resistance . . . I well know your dedication to our country. I know also that you consider Normandy . . . as your second homeland.

"Let me tell you that, for us . . . you demonstrated that it was

---

* Pat told me later that the heat and pain had actually drenched Connie's clothes. He had showered again and, with Pat's help, dressed in fresh clothes from the skin out.
† The ambassador's speech says so much about Connie and how he is viewed in France that I felt I should include it almost in full.

perhaps rare but possible nonetheless to be a journalist, writer and historian all at the same time.

"Some time ago, a literary poll was taken in France to see who were the best-read authors in our country. The five best-read were: Victor Hugo, Alexandre Dumas, Margaret Mitchell, Cornelius Ryan, and Emily Bronte.

". . . The date chosen for this ceremony—today—is highly significant, for it takes place between the Fourth of July and the Fourteenth of July, between the commemoration of the Independence of the United States and the celebration of France's National Day . . . today is certainly the most appropriate moment . . . to remember as you did so well in your books all the American and all the French men who have fought side by side in the war until victory.

"I shall not betray any secret by telling you that it is the personal wish of Mr. Georges Pompidou that you be honored at this moment, and that he signed a special Executive Order to do so.

"As his Representative in this country, as Ambassador of France, as a Frenchman, as a member of the Resistance, it is my privilege to present you with the Cross of the Legion of Honor."

It was brought forward on a royal purple pillow, its colors glinting in the hot sun. As the ambassador pinned the decoration, I saw Connie's hand begin to tremble and I moved forward, afraid that he would fall. But it was emotion that had caused the tremor, not illness.

Connie began his acceptance speech in French. Then he said, "It would be wrong, I think, for me to continue in my faltering French. There are other things I must say today on this occasion which I believe are best said in the language in which I write."

Switching to English he spoke briefly of his background and of his good fortune in knowing the peoples on both sides of the Atlantic. He spoke also of his books and said:

"My writing has not been about war; instead it concerns the human spirit, the courage, the loyalty, and the despair of people caught up in war. All these form the essence of my twenty-five years of research and labor. The people of France have obviously understood my books very well . . .

"This decoration, the highest that France bestows, I accept in memory of many others . . . the members of the French Resistance, Commander Philippe Kieffer who led his French commandoes ashore on D Day, Admiral Jaujard on the cruiser *Montcalm* . . . the men of my own profession, the Allied soldiers and brave French men and women who fell that day. In gratitude to the French people I accept this decoration in memory of all these others . . . Engraved on one of the crosses overlooking the Normandy beaches are the words: 'Into the great mosaic of victory, these priceless jewels were set.' On behalf of them all I thank you, Mr. Ambassador, representing President Pompidou, as I thank the people of France."

He stood in the sun, erect and proud, the Legion of Honor pinned to his lapel. I do not think he heard the applause that rolled across the terrace. Gino Bob brought champagne on a silver tray to the four of us, and silent toasts were made. Then the ambassador came swiftly to Connie's side. "My dear friend," he said, "let us go inside to sit and talk." Jimmy Gavin moved quickly to Connie's other side, someone threw back the sliding screens, and the three men walked indoors to a sofa. Television crews and reporters with microphones followed them, trailing equipment. Guests trooped inside away from the merciless sun. I caught a glimpse of Pat and saw both pride and worry on his face.

Soon the ambassador and his party rose to take their leave. Connie insisted on seeing them to the door. As their limousines rounded the curved driveway in front of the house, the diplomats waved and blew kisses from the windows of their cars.

Only when they had cleared the driveway and disappeared from view did Connie turn from the doorway. "Well, Docs," he said to Pat and Ted, "You're looking at a new man."

"Go up and rest, you idiot," Pat said. "I swear I don't know how you did it."

"I do," Connie said. "God gave me back my legs. The French gave me the Legion of Honor, and my friends—" He stopped abruptly. Carefully, he started for the bedroom stairs. I reached out to offer him support.

"Don't need it, Katie," Connie said. "I'm going up to rest up and think about today. Tomorrow I go back on the *Bridge*. It's got to be my thanks to everyone who ever helped or read my work. It's got to be as splendid as today has been." He slowly turned on the stairs and looked down at Pat. "You know something, Neligan? I think the Man Upstairs is going to let me finish it."

$$\doteq 5 \doteq$$

FOLLOW-UP AND PROGRESS NOTES (Brought Forward)

7-25-73 Appetite and digestion excellent . . . Has continued to require percodan and levodromeran . . . during the day. The sole definable pain is in his right thigh medially and is aggravated by standing . . . Denies other bone pain but admits that this could be concealed by his narcotic usage. Of interest is the fact that the pain does not awaken him at night* . . . has abandoned the use of urinal . . . Had last 5 Fu 3 weeks ago and last cytoxan 1 wk. ago. WBC . . . reported as 3200 . . . Taking deltasone [a cortisone compound] 6x daily . . . Since cytoxan was discontinued one week ago he states that he feels better, is eating better, energy has increased and pain, if anything, is less.

---

* Connie was not exactly truthful with Dr. Whitmore. Since he had refused the Demerol injections in early June, Pat had ordered other pain-killers—Percodan and Levo-Dromoran. Connie did not take them during the day. Dr. Whitmore has remarked that pain did not awaken him at night. It did not because it was then that he took the narcotics.

Complexion . . . somewhat sallow and he has puffiness of the face and neck of Cushing Syndrome. Neck—no adenopathy. Breasts— no significant changes. Abdomen—negative. Groins negative . . . although testes are probably smaller than before endocrine therapy, they are by no means clinically atrophic. Pubic and axillary hair remain within normal limits. Rectal—elastic, somewhat firm prostate but digital rectal findings, if anything, suggest some local softening of the gland . . . Recent SMA 12 [complete blood profile] shows no hypercalcemia and BUN is mildly elevated.

. . . Patient certainly has had some measure of improvement on the regimen of corticoids, 5 FU and cytoxan although it is impossible to say which agent or agents have been instrumental in achieving this response.

Accordingly, it is recommended that he continue on the same regimen of steroids and chemotherapy, withholding 5 FU for the present but reintroducing the cytoxan in one week if the WBC has started to rise*. In addition, it is suggested that he reinstitute DES 1 mg daily on the basis of the possibility that it may have been having a favorable suppressive effect on the estrogen sensitive component of his tumor. Although it seems likely that lumbar plexus involvement rather than bone metastasis per se may be responsible for his right leg symptoms and atrophy, a repeat x-ray of the lumbar spine and pelvis is suggested along with the possibility that radiation therapy to the lumbar spine and right hemipelvis . . . would probably prove palliative in either event.

Dr. Whitmore.

CORNELIUS

This is Thursday, July 26, 1973.

Yesterday I saw Willet Whitmore who seems to think that the chemotherapy is working. However, I am to go back on

---

* The white blood count, at 3200 or 3.2, was very low. Chemotherapy cannot be given when the count falls below normal ranges. Thus, Dr. Whitmore's recommendation to withhold 5 F-U and Cytoxan until the count was again within tolerable levels.

the estrogen hormone again, and perhaps Cytoxan, depending on my blood counts.

In the hospital I was put on a different kind of hormone. I've been reading up on its derivation in the medical dictionary. It is a cortisone or cortical hormone and its effect on the body—at the level of medication I'm on—is far more apparent than that of the female hormones. Given in excess, cortisol hormones, produced from the outer layer of the adrenal gland, change the body's appearance drastically, even as they work internally to restore and regulate cancer's interference with metabolism.

The external signs of the hormone's actions are called Cushing's syndrome. I looked him up too: Dr. Harvey Williams Cushing, a neurosurgeon famous—among other things—for his investigation of the misbehavior of the pituitary and adrenal cortex glands. Their hyperactivity produces physical symptoms that are appalling and these symptoms are known as Cushing's syndrome. Now medicine is using that very hyperactivity to fight cancer.

Some of the changes are already apparent. In less than a month my weight has gone up nearly eight pounds. However, this obesity is caused by the female hormones, I think. The corticoids produce far worse effects. As one continues to take high dosages of them, startling alterations in appearance occur. The face in my mirror is no longer mine. A moonlike fatness has obliterated my features and enlarged my neck. A 15½ collar no longer fits. I am wearing 16½ and that size, too, is getting tight. As time goes on, a slight bulge between the shoulders, like a very small humpback, will appear, along with additional chins as the neck continues to enlarge. I will become a fat man with a hump on my back and eyes that peer out from mounds of flesh. I'm going to end up a damned freak.

It is monstrous for Kathryn and the children to have to live with this. How the sight of me must appall them! It will be worse for Vicki. I was still myself when she went to France.

I prayed that I would not become an invalid, but it happened. Still, I managed to get over that and a cane is now my sole support. But to be an eyesore is disgusting. I had not realized I was so vain. It makes me sick at heart to look at myself. I am reminded of some lines I learned years ago: "Look into my face. My name is Used-to-Was. I am also called Played-out and Done-to-Death, and It-Will-Wash-No-More."

The plague of prolonged illness is the constant tendency one has toward self-pity. It is an affliction that I try harder to reject than the physical pains which, in spite of everything, daily intensify. While I believe that 90 percent of the battle resides in one's positive state of mind and a strong determination to win, willpower and mood are constantly undermined by cancer. It erodes not only the body but dignity and self-respect. The most difficult art to perfect is the art of being ill gracefully.

I have been deluged with telegrams, phone calls, and mail ever since I was given the Legion of Honor. A friend of mine, Olaf Olsen, gave me a memento— a film of the ceremonies. I noticed in running it through that I looked far different then, just two and a half weeks ago.

Among the letters I've had in regard to the decoration was one from young Matthew Evins and I will keep it the rest of my life. Sometimes friends tell you what they think you want to hear, but when young people bother to write, their sentiments come from the heart. The same is true of the veterans I have written about. Their letters indicate pride that this honor was given to me and, almost to a man, they have sent me best wishes for the success of the new book and expressed their hopes that we can meet soon again.

The friends in my profession take care to avoid any niceties in writing to a colleague. The same question has been posed in nearly all their letters: had the French decorated the wrong man? To this I replied that Napoleon had had a lot of Irishmen fighting for him and I thought payoff time had come. I added that since my associates themselves had never earned so much as a Good Conduct medal, I could understand their shyness in writing to an immortal.

Now I have got to return to the true immortals—the men and women of *Bridge*. The story and the material seem more compelling day by day. But the canvas is so large that I must constantly keep the reasons for the assault in the forefront of my consciousness. For example: Montgomery's concern about getting across the Rhine and into the Ruhr was matched only by his arrogance in believing he was the sole man who could accomplish the job. The ambitions and jealousies of generals are not very different from those of other men, except that when a general's plan goes wrong, thousands of people pay for his mistake.

To the general the cost of so many soldiers and civilians can be written off by a single sentence of dismissal. As Montgomery put it in his own book, "We did not, as everyone knows, capture that final bridgehead north of Arnhem."*

How little attention he gave to the men who had succeeded in their part of his plan—the U.S. 101st and 82nd Airborne Divisions—who captured and held their bridges, particularly the vital crossings at Son, Grave, and Nijmegen. And how characteristic of Montgomery to describe the massacre of the British 1st Airborne Division at Arnhem and its environs by writing, "there can be few episodes more glorious than the epic of Arnhem."

What is glorious about seventeen thousand military casualties or the horrors and penalties suffered and paid by innocent Dutch civilians? They and those who survived Montgo-

* *The Memoirs of Field Marshal Montgomery* (London: Collins, 1958).

mery's ill-fated plan cannot be dismissed in a sentence. Only their stories bring history alive, give it meaning, and teach us lessons which, sadly, we soon forget.

The little quote from Walt Whitman which I have had pinned on my wall for years becomes more important to me daily. "Underneath all," he wrote, "I swear nothing is good to me now that ignores individuals."

In a general's summation or a cancer statistic, the lone human being, frightened and suffering, is left out of the picture. I have spent my professional life trying to put him back in. There can be no understanding of war or disease without knowledge of what the individuals involved endured.

I have not mentioned on these tapes before that I have been so weak at times I have acquired the habit of resting on the office couch several times during the day. I outline a section, or several sections, and write as much as I can. But fatigue is continuous now and I find I can sit at my desk for only an hour or two at a time. Then I must lie down. Katie and Annie keep on working. Katie has so many interviews around her desk that it looks like moving day at the Ryans'. Still, she knows exactly what she wants at any given time and pulls two or three folders from as many piles. Then she inserts anecdotes from them into the general outline material; and when I get up from the sofa, we edit and pare until each interview is in the right place to strengthen and bring alive the basic story line. Annie seems to be everywhere at once. She has to repaginate and retype constantly because Katie or I have rewritten. I often wonder how she keeps everything straight.

I like resting in the office. This building is where I really live. When I stretch out on the sofa to rest, the muted softness of workaday sounds is soothing. I am in the midst of life, yet not of it in those moments. Eventually, as weakness passes, I get up. It is then, in the space of a single second, that the pain hits its hardest. I try not to hobble back to my desk. At times I feel too ill to work and I have to give myself a silent little pep talk. Always, after a few minutes, I can return my mind to 1944. I believe we are going at a faster clip now than with any other book we have done.

Just today I realized that we are rapidly coming up on the Nijmegen bridge crossing. There is so much good material about the street fighting and the river crossing by the 82nd that I would like to use it all. Of course, that is impossible. Each sector of Market-Garden could be a book in itself, and the difficulty is to keep one's eyes fixed firmly on the historical line, paint in the picture as fully as possible, and get on to the next event. Someday I would like to do a book of untold stories of World War II. The file drawers are full of material I haven't used because it could not be substantiated. But it would make fascinating reading—a book that was rather like a giant footnote to history.

Maybe someday Katie will do that book. I don't think I have got the time.

Sunday, September 23, 1973.

I have not used the tape recorder recently. The book is racing and I am giving it every particle of energy I've got. I cannot wait for the ending and yet I want to prolong it. I am afraid to come to the final page. For all I know, *Bridge* is keeping me alive.

Lately, after a hard day in the office, I have asked Katie to call Helene Merrick to join us for a little while in the early evening. She is one of the people with whom I especially like to talk. We are often on opposite sides of the fence politically. I think Helene believes that Watergate is a Democratic conspiracy, although from the moment Butterfield testified before the Senate committee about the existence of the

White House taping system, she has given in a little. I would find Watergate appalling no matter who was in the White House. It is a sorry story for this great nation. Americans are, by and large, a naive people. They cannot adjust to distortions of truth and honor in high places. They like to believe their own folk history and they like to believe that their presidents are elected by the will of the people and are, therefore, above reproach. Given a legend, they tend to make it a fact.

When they realize they have been duped and manipulated, Americans become disturbed, alarmed, outraged. But—and here is where I believe that naiveté has its purpose—Americans do not stop believing. They have a strength they are seldom aware of. They fall down and climb back up. Despite everything, they tend to survive.

More and more people seem convinced that I am not long for this world. That opinion always provokes me to a determination to hang around a little longer just to prove I can do it. Still, I was very touched by a recent tribute. On August 21, The Correspondents Fund of America, of which I am a trustee, presented me with an illuminated script, a testimonial to my years with the fund and to my journalistic standing. At a time when every form of the media is under attack, to be recognized by one's peers in the journalism fraternity tends to bring on a rather strong attack of humility, a most un-Irish trait and one that few people would believe I possess.

I treasure this accolade. Still, as it was read out, I felt as if I was standing at my own graveside listening to the good things people were saying about me. Right words. Wrong funeral. If they like the book, then I'll feel I deserved the tribute.

Late in August Vicki arrived back from France. Katie had gone in with Jerry Lewis to meet her at the airport and John Tower and I were wasting a little time, chatting in the office. Suddenly I heard the car horn and almost the next minute the outer door burst open and Vicki rushed into my office. I got up and held out my arms. She seemed to hesitate and then she threw herself against me so hard that my unreliable legs almost gave way. I know why she paused. She was not prepared for the sight of a strange fat man, trying so hard to show her the father underneath.

Her French is tremendously improved. That day it poured out in torrents. But in the serious aspects of her life she had come home battered in mind and bruised in spirit. She had gone to France deeply troubled—I was too ill to know it then. She had not talked out her fears or worries before she left in early summer because, as it was to turn out, she felt we had enough of our own already. The reasons for her anguish were mostly here at home. Fearing for my life and unwilling to take her mother's time, she had been treading dangerous water trying to keep from slipping down in sorrow. But she had. Now, bit by bit, Katie and I are pulling her up to the surface. She has already shown us the depths. I am struck by the bad advice she's had, by the sharks who would have preyed on her distress. My memory is very long. I will not forget the people who added to her pain and confusion, just as I shall thank the friends who tried to give her real help and assistance. But Vicki's torment has shown me how wrapped up in myself and my worries I had become. It will not happen again.

Over the days since her arrival home, Vicki, Katie, and I have had the best talks of our lives. There is a small prelude to them. In the evenings, settled in bed and reading for the next day's work, I hear the piano. Vicki usually begins with lighthearted show tunes and progresses to little pieces from Bach. The organist played "Jesu, Joy of Man's Desiring" when her mother and I were married, and Vicki is attempting to master even that. I have told Katie that I want it played at my funeral—the last time she and I are together at the altar of a church.

When I am finished reading Vicki comes upstairs to sit with us. Through these talks and confessions, questions and probings, I have come to know my daughter better than I ever did before. I would give my life for her but it is more important that I use the rest of it to listen and to love. She is much easier in her mind now. She has found that Katie and I can be her audience, that we are available, and that we care.

One of Vicki's habits is leaving notes for her mother or me to find at some later time. Just the other day this little note turned up among the papers on my desk:

Love goes from bliss to sorrow. Our family has shed tears because of love or loss. Sometimes the tears brought us closer together. Sometimes not. I think if we tried to have more happy, joyful experiences, we could knock out sorrow. Where love is shown by the embrace of a parent's arms around a child or by the glances between parents who love each other, that house is blessed. I know now that ours has always been, and that it shelters Geoff and me.

Daddy, past, present, and future—always—I love you.

Vicki

My own growing up now seems so uncomplicated compared to that of my children; my dreams and ambitions were crystallized rather early. Theirs are not. I have not understood my children as well as I might—a fault of most parents today. We work for them and tell them so frequently. But we are working for ourselves and our ambitions as well. We give gifts out of love but they are almost too overwhelming and the gift and not the love is what is remembered. Now Vicki is remembering love.

This has been a summer of accolades. They have both touched and troubled me. Not until *Bridge* comes out can I be persuaded that the body of work I have done over the years merits long-lasting recognition. I put the rest of my eggs in *Bridge*'s basket only because I will not have time to write the other two volumes I had planned. *The Longest Day* and *The Last Battle* were to be the beginning and end of a five-volume history on the European theater in World War II. *Bridge* was the middle book in my long-range thinking. I had planned a volume on either side of it. I won't live to write five volumes. The spirit is willing but the flesh has called a halt.

I have recently received one gift that I treasure because it is not for any achievement of mine. It is a testament to the courage and talent of the donor.

I have mentioned before that Jerry and Barbara Korn's daughters came to visit this summer. I had not seen Maggie, Ellen and Sue in years and their grown-up beauty astounded me as much as their childish good looks had once done. Maggie, I mentioned, had hoped to become a painter, only to give up her dream. She had, she said, no reason to paint, no motivation to go on. It was undoubtedly presumptuous of me to try to tell her that she must paint for herself and that only by doing so will the reason for painting at all come clear.

Well, Maggie has done a sketch, her first in some time, and sent it to me. It is a profile of a young woman, very like Maggie herself. There is a mysterious, haunting quality about the work that causes me to ponder it again and again. I have had it framed and Katie has hung it in the bedroom, always within my sight when I'm there. How many hours I have shared with Maggie's drawing! How often it has stayed with me through bad nights of pain! The girl in the sketch appears to contemplate pain both physical and spiritual—and accepts it. I have come to accept pain, too, but not to reconcile myself to it, and I hope Maggie never will. Still, the real Maggie and the Maggie of the picture have made some long nights easier to bear.

Geoff did not go back to college. I wish I knew the reasons why. One of them, I think, concerns the girl who came out here this summer. Young love has a way of dying out in letters, and I think he was deeply hurt when hers did. Still, when the money's been sent for tuition and the car is serviced and packed, the eve of departure is hardly the time to spring the news that the trip is off.

Katie and I had taken him out to dinner. We talked about everything, including the upcoming school year and then, over coffee, he said, "I'm not going back."

He had apparently been thinking it over all summer. He'd done all his packing and loaded the car. It was sitting in our driveway with a full tank of gas, ready for the long trip to the university. His explanations leave much to be desired. He believes college is no longer necessary for most people and he wants to "find himself" away from ivy-covered halls.

"Well, you're going *some*place, aren't you? You're all packed," Katie said.

He had some plans. He has moved in with some other fellows, sharing a small house in the next town. The subject of exactly how he lives does not seem to concern him very much. His summer job, at which he worked very hard, is over. He has some tentative thoughts about house painting, some thoughts of working to help disturbed kids. He wants to try to write, to experiment further with photography, to learn more about the stage and movies. All these he could have learned about at school. Those who have to teach themselves must have very strict codes of self-discipline and Geoff has not developed those as yet. I can make no sense of this at all. If the tools to learn are handed to you, use them. Geoff prefers to forge his own.

Well, he turned twenty last month. It's his life and he's got to live it as he sees best. Still, I wish he had told us what was on his mind earlier. But we have seen little of him this summer. He slept here and went to work and saw his friends. Home was a way station—a place to shower and change and go out from again. And yet, I know he loves us and he knows that we love him. We just can't seem to get it together, as he would say.

I remember when he was a little boy and I was working on *The Longest Day* screenplay in France, Katie took him to see *Camelot* in New York. She wrote me that she had arranged with friends to take him backstage to meet Richard Burton. Always the squirmiest little lad in his group, she said he sat right through intermission, staring at the curtain. After the play he didn't want to go meet Burton. He walked home with Kathryn to the apartment we had then in Turtle Bay, holding her hand, absolutely silent. That night he took the tape recorder I had taught him how to use and sang snatches of songs from *Camelot* to send to me. The whole family was coming over to Paris to join me in about a month, but Geoff sent off his little tape immediately. By the time Katie and the kids arrived, I had found a big apartment for us and, with the help of my friend Avery Fisher, who was in Paris on a business trip, we had rigged up our Fisher radio and a record player. I wore out that little disc Geoff made before the family ever got to France. Something in his voice made me cry every damn time I heard it. I guess I was homesick for him. I think I still am. It's been a long time since I've really known my son.

KATHRYN

Even as his own strength wasted away, Connie's mother's health was failing. For more than a year Emily's letters had revealed an increasing depression, yet her belief that Connie was on the mend never faltered. Her love, her incredible faith, her prayers for us all filled every page of her letters, but there were strong undercurrents of her own fears and obvious loneliness.

Shortly after Connie's return from Memorial in May, I had apprised his brothers of his condition, contrary to his wishes. Only Joe, in Washington, D.C., was in rather constant contact with us and therefore up-to-date. But I felt that Gerard, David, and John in Ireland should know that their brother's health was deteriorating, and I was worried about Emily as well.

Their response was immediate. All three brothers telephoned several times to inquire about Connie.* Usually their calls came when he was sleeping fitfully, in intense pain, or unable to summon the strength after a day's hard work to talk with anyone. Only with Joe in Washington did he speak often and then only for short periods. I believe that as the eldest he wanted always to be at his best in talking with the Irish family; when Connie did not feel firm and confident he did not wish to speak with his brothers. I gave them as much news as I could and from them I learned that their mother's condition was indeed unsettling.

After a particularly worrisome letter from Emily in which she detailed many of her problems, I had written to David, who appeared to be in and out of the family house most frequently, giving him the names and addresses of specialists Pat knew well in Ireland. I wanted Emily in the best possible medical hands. The appointments were never made. Emily wrote in a faltering hand that David did not entirely agree with Pat's recommendations and that she felt too ill to proceed on her own. Consequently she was never to see the men Pat felt could best help her. Connie, when he learned of this, was bitterly angry. Within a few weeks I learned from David and John in separate communications that Emily had

---

* It was a particularly difficult time for Gerard. His wife, Vera, had been discovered to have cancer of the breast. Not until he telephoned me late one evening did I learn of her condition. I do not think Connie ever knew of it.

become so depressed and physically weak that she had been put in a nursing home.

On Sunday, September 30, a gloomy fall day, Connie and I were working in the office when the phone rang.

Connie swiveled his desk chair around to pick it up.

"David," he said. "How are you?" There was silence and then, "What the hell do you mean, I should be glad my mother's dead?"

I stared at my husband. Connie's face was ashen but he was also angry.

He listened for a minute, said, "I'll come," listened again, tears gathering in his eyes. He put down the telephone and turned to me.

"Do you know what David said?" Connie asked. "His first words were, 'You'll be glad to know your mother's dead.' Christ!" He stopped and covered his face with his hands. He swiveled his chair to face the wall, his back to me. I started across the room and then slipped back to my own chair. I did not know what to do.

"Then," Connie continued, still facing the wall, "he said, 'What I meant was, you'll be glad to know Mother is no longer suffering.' He said there was no need for me to come over. He would take care of everything. My God! Who the hell—?" He turned to me. "Katie, you'll have to pack. I'll call Annie to get us plane reservations."

Instead, I called Pat. With Connie's low energy, the chemotherapy and blood transfusions he needed almost every two weeks, Pat, who knew the family, was adamant. Connie was not well enough to go. As David had said, there was no longer any need. I felt that I should fly over, but the question was, how could I leave Connie? Pat said that I could not.

We were at an impasse but not for long. In the end it was Connie who decided not to go. No words from Ireland or from Pat and me would have stopped him. As he had done when Kathleen died, as he had done throughout his life when dramatic and tragic events occurred, he closed an emotional door and kept his feelings locked away. He had longed to see his mother but had not wanted her to see him as he looked. Now, the time of reunion had passed.

To Geoff and Vicki, Connie gently explained that Grandmother Ryan had died. He did not talk about his mother again. In my family Bible, in which he had always faithfully recorded the marriages, births, and deaths of the Catholic Ryans alongside those of the Protestant Morgans, he made no entry, nor did he in his diary.

In August 1973, he had sent money to his mother as he had done in the then twenty-three years of our marriage and for many years before. He wrote three more checks—one a florist's bill—that pertained to Ireland. Then, he went back to the book his mother knew would "flow from his pen." Only to an old school friend who wrote him a letter of sympathy, did he reveal his feelings:

Yes, I loved my mother very much. It will be hard to go on with the knowledge that she is not there. I have been ill myself and did not have full information as to the critical state she was in. Had I not been sick I would have handled it, as I have always done. Now, although I would like to see you and the old crowd, I have no desire to visit Dublin. I am growing old. I am trying to do it gracefully and with dignity.

Doggedly, Connie went on with the book, shutting out grief. By Friday, October 5, we were closing in on the final tragic pages. The piles of interviews which had stretched the entire width of the glass wall of our office had dwindled steadily as we finished with them and I put them back in the files. Whole regiments had been put to rest. Only the valiant few left in the British sector and the Dutch civilians residing in the little village of Driel remained; their stories would be the finale to the long years of research and writing.

He seemed to draw the paratroopers' tenacious endurance

into himself. In those long hours he did not seem tired. The days of resting on the sofa were gone as we neared the end of *Bridge*. He took his corticoid and estrogen hormones faithfully and as unobtrusively as possible. If I asked how he felt, his standard reply was "Fine." I think he meant it.

During those last weeks of work I had been too engrossed in keeping up with him to look at my cork bulletin board where reminders and snippets of copy were kept. We had long since used each relevant note on my little board. I had ticked them off one by one in the months of writing.

"Have you checked your board lately?" Connie asked one afternoon.

I was struggling with a dangling participle. Dangling, it made the sentence read better, I thought, but it would never pass Jerry Korn's nit-picking eye.

"No," I answered absentmindedly and went on with my work. So did Connie.

Later, after I had taken the reworked pages to Anne, I looked at my cork board. There, alongside paragraphs from an interview with General Eisenhower, were two small newspaper headlines, one pinned below the other. They read:

Ryan's Time Running Out

and

Liberals Nominate
Mrs. Ryan to Run
In Husband's Spot*

I stared at Connie. "Why did you do that?" I asked.

"Another man's headline seems to be the only way to get my own message across," he said. "There are some things, Katie, you have always got to keep in mind." Without a pause

---

* We had both followed the story of William Fitts Ryan's battle against Bella Abzug in the primary contest for New York's 20th District in 1972. Mr. Ryan had won the primary. Before the general election he died of cancer. His wife, Priscilla, running on the Liberal ticket, lost the Congressional seat to Mrs. Abzug.

he continued, "Have you got the interview on Major Cain? I think I want to use something from it again." And he went back to work, leaving me to stare at the sad and chilling implications of those words.

On Saturday, October 27, *A Bridge Too Far* was finished. About 4:00 P.M. that afternoon Connie brought me three pages. I changed only the last paragraph by cutting off four lines. I showed it to him. He nodded. Then he stood up and hugged me. "God has been so good to us," he said. "To me."

One member of our family had been following events far more closely than we realized. On Sunday afternoon, October 28, I was putting the last of the file folders in their proper places. The office looked almost too neat. Gazing around it I felt both sadness and relief that *Bridge* was finished. Connie, too, had a forlorn, lost look. Our depression was not to last for long. The outer office door burst open and Geoff came in, eyes gleaming.

"You finished," he said proudly. "I knew it. I could feel it coming closer every time I stopped in." He stood and looked at us. "Hey, you guys, I'm so proud of you." He produced a paper sack and slowly drew out a bottle of champagne. "I bought it last night," he told us, going to the little office kitchen for three glasses. "It's not the best but I hope it tastes O.K."

Carefully he opened the bottle and poured the champagne. He brought us each a glass. Standing between our desks he said, "I don't think anybody in the world ever had more guts than you two." He raised his glass. Connie stood up.

"There's one," he said to Geoff. "You."

It was one of the best moments in months. In spite of the many assaults against it, our family bridge had held secure.

$$\overset{\mathrm{II}}{\underset{\mathrm{II}}{=}} \; 6 \; \overset{\mathrm{II}}{\underset{\mathrm{II}}{=}}$$

CORNELIUS

This is Saturday, November 10,1973.

I find it hard to believe that the book is finished. There have been so many dark days when I did not believe I could summon one more ounce of energy. I don't think I ever realized what a strain it was keeping cancer a secret from publishers and far-flung friends. Now the necessity for silence is over. We have not let anyone down, my contracts are fulfilled, and the manuscript is as good as I would ever be able to make it and perhaps even better than previous works.

Looking back through my notebooks I see that it was mid-August of 1970 when I tried to get the first sentences of *Bridge* down on paper. From then until May 31, 1973, we were able to complete only 310 pages. On October 27, just two weeks ago, we came to the end—a total of 666 pages. It took thirty-four months to write the first 310 pages and just five months to write the last 356.

I have much to be thankful for. I am alive, as well as I will ever be again, and "in remission." There is a specialness about *Bridge* that cancer made possible. When I set about writing *The Longest Day* and *The Last Battle*, I was fascinated by the oddities, the curiosa, memorabilia, myths, and the strengths and weaknesses of the average person caught up in battle. My object was to find out what people thought and felt. In the new book I had the opportunity of looking into the darkness of the abyss and I gained a greater insight into the emotions of my subjects than I ever had before. I hope the book reflects the inner courage I discovered in men and women and that I keep on finding day by day. I think *Bridge is* a better book than the last two. Strange to say, there is a virtue in having cancer. It makes one more sensitive to others.

This is noticeably true in my relationship with my family. I now see Geoff and Vicki mentally and physically healthy, taking up their lives with purpose. The old angers and antagonisms are gone. We are friends and, like true friends, we sometimes disagree. I wanted Geoff to go through college. The degree was important to me, not him. In his reading and on his job he is learning daily. He is discovering his own philosophy of life. He is honorable and honest. The finest education in the world cannot guarantee integrity and so I have come to terms with what I wanted for him and what he is making of himself. And in human value the end result is the same.

Victoria is quite definite about going to college next year. She is becoming more and more caught up in music and theater. Among the professions these are as hard and demanding as any I know. She will have to learn to accept disappointments, rejections, and setbacks, but if she believes in her abilities she will find a way to make others aware of them, too.

With the book finished it would be easy to sit back and rest. It would also be dangerous for my morale. Somehow I feel that inactivity and leisure time would give cancer an edge. I'd think more about it and probably tend to pamper myself. I want to keep on working. It is not enough to have written *Bridge.* I've still got a lot of ongoing doctors' bills and, while I'm depending on the book to lift some of the financial burdens, I am also very eager to see it properly launched. I think, too, that there are a few projects Katie and I can do together that will keep my mind off cancer and challenge my writing abilities. I am still striving for perfection and the best way to approach it is to keep on working. And so I will.

In spite of Neligan's grumblings that I should take life a little easier, I have no intention of complying. I am trying to postpone something that Goodman Ace wrote about in the *Saturday Review* a few years ago. He recounted his experiences in arranging a funeral for a member of his family. "What it amounts to," he said, "is we go into a funeral shop to buy a man something that he wouldn't get for himself and that he has never had before."

He should have added, "and what he did not want."

KATHRYN

In the late fall of 1973 the bleak struggle between medicine and cancer seemed deadlocked. The scattershot invasion of malignant cells throughout Connie's body appeared to have been halted in some areas of bone and tissue. On November 12 Dr. Van Syckle found "significant interval improvement in the appearance of the skull," compared to a previous scan on August 8.

Five days later on November 16, Dr. Whitmore wrote:

> ... Ambulates with a slight limp due to some discomfort and weakness ... but he does not use a cane. Gets along with surprising agility and evidence of his mental acuity is supported by the fact that he recently completed another volume of his World War II history.

But the erratic hit-and-run nature of the cancer cells produced disquieting news as well. Tamed in one place, they held fast in others. Dr. Van Syckle had found widespread metastatic involvement of the ribs in August. In November that situation was neither better nor worse. But the thigh bones—the strongest bones in the skeleton—had been weakened further. Not only was cancer entrenched in Connie's shoulder and hip bones but there was evidence of new spread, this time to the right knee.

To combat the deadly cells the specialists had put Connie back on a high daily dosage of Cytoxan—the chemotherapeutic agent 5 F-U had not been given since June—along with DES and the cortisone derivative Prednisone. Additionally, he was taking Zyloprim, a drug given to inhibit the rise in uric acid levels that chemotherapy can cause. The dilemma—finding the right combination of medicines without producing severe toxic reactions in the patient—seemed resolved for the time. Dr. Whitmore concluded:

... he is doing remarkably well on the present regimen and we would be reluctant to make any changes therein.

But no single formula was ever to work for long in the silent battle in which cancer strove for total mastery over Connie's life.

With something approaching his whirlwind energy of the past, Connie had delivered his manuscript, worked on photographic layouts, rechecked the meticulous maps that Raphael Palacios had drawn, and closeted himself with Paul for a discussion of foreign contracts for the book.

The long struggle to finish *Bridge* was over. Concern about bills, our family's future, Connie's determination to keep active and to keep writing, were by no means resolved. For Connie, it was not enough to have written *Bridge*. He was determined to see it through publication and beyond. Then, and only then, could he feel peace of mind, he said.

In mid-November, taking Vicki and me with him, he barnstormed across Europe, seeing publishers, agents, principals in the book. In health and appearance he was greatly changed from the man his European acquaintances had known. He wanted to face them and get the initial shock over with. He had written the stories of his "kings" as he had come to call the men and women in his books. Having done so, he could see them all with a clear conscience. He had fulfilled his obligation to himself to tell of their ordeals.

The fast-paced journey—through Holland, France, and England—gave him little opportunity to rest and relax. Yet he did find time to play a prank with his daughter. Their practical joke would become a memory he would recall happily in a few months, only hours before his death.

We were in Brussels after a day of meetings and conferences in Amsterdam about *Bridge.* We had arrived there in the early evening. We would stay overnight and, to show Vicki some countryside, would take an early morning train to Paris. After a leisurely dinner at one of Connie's favorite restaurants, we three strolled down the corridor of our hotel floor. At one door a menu card—marked for the morning breakfast and hung on the outside knob for room service pickup—caught Connie's attention.

He read it. "Not really enough to eat," he said, and taking out his gold pencil he ticked off more items on the menu.

I protested but to no avail. Victoria promptly agreed with her father that most breakfast orders were, indeed, far too sparse. Mischievously they tiptoed down the hall together, conferring in whispers about particular orders before adding an item or two. They were careful to pass up those menus with delivery times as early as our own would be.

Back in our rooms Connie made out our breakfast orders. "Our getaway meal," he told Vicki with a grin. "I don't think I want to be around here when breakfast is delivered to some of these rooms in the morning."

"I shouldn't think so," I told him. "That was childish behavior and you should both be ashamed."

"We're just trying to make sure they eat well," Vicki countered.

Connie agreed. "We have attempted to further the cause of good nutrition. We've either succeeded or we've set it back for good."

In January 1974, Connie received the honorary degree of Doctor of Humane Letters from Ohio University. It was a high point in his life, the only tribute of its kind he had ever received from an American university. In a hasty two-day trip we flew to the Athens, Ohio, campus where Connie was given his honorary hood. He made a speech to the students at the College of Communications and went through numerous student interviews and questions regarding his work methods, particularly those he had used in writing *Bridge*.

Then, only weeks later, he was granted a recognition he had believed was forever beyond his attainment.

In April 1974 he was notified that the executive board of The Society of American Historians had elected him a Fellow. The annual awards banquet was to be held on April 24 at The Colony Restaurant in New York, where the new Fellows would be introduced. He was as taken aback as he had been on learning the previous year that he was to receive the Legion of Honor. He read aloud to me the second sentence of the society's letter, his voice breaking at the words:

Such recognition is conferred only upon those authors who have done substantial work of literary and scholarly distinction.

I left my desk and threw my arms around him. He was trembling. "No man in his lifetime, Katie, ever received all the honors he ever dreamed of," he said. "What more could any one ask?"

"Well, there's the Pulitzer," I said, "and if you start writing novels instead of histories maybe you'll get a shot at the Nobel Prize."

He shook his head. "I don't think *Bridge* will get the Pulitzer—although," he smiled at me, "one does always hope. And if I wrote novels for the next fifty years I'd never be able to match even the acceptance speech Faulkner gave in Stockholm." William Faulkner's address in accepting the Nobel Prize for letters in 1950 was among yellowing clippings pinned to Connie's wall. Long before cancer struck, he had underlined these words:

I believe that man will not merely endure: he will prevail. He is immortal . . . he has a soul, a spirit capable of compassion and sacrifice and endurance. The . . . writer's duty is to write about these things. It is his privilege to help man endure by lifting his heart, by reminding him of the courage and honor and hope and pride and compassion and pity and sacrifice which have been the glory of his past.

He had memorized those words. They had been the philosophical heart of all his World War II histories. And over the past crucial months they had been the words he himself had struggled to live by. His efforts had not been in vain. The recognition by the body of academic historians, their acceptance of his work, had come at last.

Connie was in a flurry of excitement before the society's dinner in New York. Like Pat, I was concerned by the way he pushed himself and I knew, despite his protestations to the contrary, that his energy was very low. He had seen Dr. Whitmore only once in 1974 and had come home from that examination to assure the children and me that he was totally fit. Dr. Whitmore's notes of that visit, on February 13, tell a different story. In part, they read:

States stiffness in his joints has increased although he remains active and ambulatory. He states that he feels he is deteriorating in the sense that he is getting weaker . . . He has had transfusions each of two units of blood on three occasions in the past four months, the last a few days ago . . . Recent skeletal survey . . . was reviewed . . . Again one sees some films which appear to show some evidence of healing and other films where changes can be interpreted as progression. He has mixed osteolytic and osteoblastic disease extensively involving bones but especially the pelvis and vertebrae . . .

The findings in the final sentence were to play an ominous role—robbing Connie of the elation of his new honor and plunging him back into excruciating pain from which he would never again recover.

Wednesday, April 24, 1974, the day of The Society of American Historians' dinner was breezy and cool. As the day progressed a damp chill permeated the air. I drove Connie into New York. As always he was impeccably dressed but his medication had worked still more significant changes on his body. His collar size was now 18½, a source of extreme mortification to him. The Cushingoid appearance of his face had intensified, as had his abdominal girth. Still, although he refused to believe it himself, his dignity, carriage, and mannerisms were as impressive as ever.

He wore a light wool black overcoat and carried General Seitz's cane. He had not recently needed it, but in crowds he found it a useful protection. I parked at an underground garage not far from The Colony, letting Connie off on the sidewalk before I drove down to park. Neither of us had noticed a black iron bicycle rack bolted to the sidewalk near the garage. When I came up to ground level after handing the car over to an attendant, Connie was nowhere to be seen, but a crowd of people had gathered at the edge of the walk. Hurriedly I joined them and, pushing my way through, saw Connie lying on the cold concrete.

I knelt beside him, frantic.

"Connie!" His eyes were closed. "Connie," I said again, "Can you hear me? What happened?"

He tried to speak but his breath came only in gasps.

A man beside me said, "I saw it happen. He caught his cane between the racks of the bicycle stand and just seemed to twist around. Then he lost his balance and fell."

Two young men, dressed in jeans and frayed jackets stood near Connie's head. Alone at night, I would have been frightened by them. Now, along with the man who had explained to me what happened, they became a source of comfort and strength. One of them leaned down to Connie. I half expected him to rob my husband there in the street. Instead he gently pulled Connie's coat closer about his ears and neck and, as I watched dazedly, took off his own tattered jacket, rolled it into a ball, and gently eased it under Connie's head. "I don't want to raise him, but I don't think his head should be lying on the pavement," he explained.

The first man touched my arm. "I'm going for the police and an ambulance," he said and started to make his way through the crowd.

"No," Connie said in such a strong voice that we were all startled. He was very pale and his breath came in small gasps but he was also determined. The man rejoined me.

"You're from Ireland," Connie said.

The man nodded.

"From Mayo, I expect," Connie said between short breaths.

"How did you know?" our benefactor asked. "I haven't lived there in over twenty years."

A faint smile played over Connie's face. "I know the county accents," he said in that same breathy way. "Even though I'm a Dublin man myself."

"I never would have guessed. Please let me get an ambulance."

Connie shook his head. He looked at the two young men standing near where I knelt beside him, trying to massage warmth back into his hands. "Do you boys think you can get me on my feet?"

Both nodded. "But take it easy for a few minutes longer, sir," one said.

"Let's do it now," Connie told him. "I feel like I'm stiffening up inside. If we wait I might not be able to get up."

Gently the boys caught Connie from either side. Our new Irish friend politely asked the other onlookers to move away and one by one they did. Bracing Connie's neck and shoulders with their arms the boys slowly got him upright. He cried out once and bit his lips but made no other sound. With his hands on the bicycle rail, the Mayo man on one side of him and I on the other, Connie swayed but did not faint or slip. The boy who had put his own thin jacket under Connie's head picked it up and, finding a fairly clean part of the lining, gently brushed off Connie's coat and trousers. He even rubbed his coat across my husband's shoes. Connie asked for Jeff Seitz's cane and I gave it to him.

"What's the time?" he asked faintly.

"Almost seven," one of the boys answered.

"Katie, we've got to go. We'll be late."

I stared at him. "It's impossible. We don't know what you've done to yourself. Let's go to Memorial right now."

There was a little silence. The men with us exchanged glances. They knew Memorial's fame. "Maybe you'd better, sir," one of the boys said.

"All I need is a taxi." He was still breathing in short gasps but his words were firm.

The man from Ireland stepped out into the street and within a minute a taxi rolled up before us. The boys opened the door. "Get in, Katie," Connie said. "I don't think I can slide across."

Once settled he stopped the three men from closing the door. "Please let me pay you for your help," he said. All three looked aghast.

"Absolutely not," said the man from Ireland.

"Pay us for what, sir?" one of the boys asked.

"O.K.," Connie said. "Has somebody got a pencil and paper? I don't think I can reach in to get mine. I want your names and addresses."

"No money," our Irish benefactor said.

"No. Books," Connie told him. "I write them. I'll send you all books."

One of the three produced pencil and paper and each wrote his name and address. The paper was handed in to Connie and I took it from his nerveless fingers and put it inside my handbag.

"God bless you," Connie told the three.

"And may He look after you, dear man," said our Irish friend.

The three of them stood in the pavement watching our taxi pull away. The unsung angels who had rescued us made an odd combination but they were bound together by compassion and kindness.*

Connie was unable to lean back in the taxi seat and each bounce of the taxi made him stifle a groan. He refused to entertain my repeated pleas that we get him to the hospital.

"I've waited too long. I will not miss this evening," he said.

We arrived at The Colony, I almost holding Connie up, to find that most of the guests were already at their tables. It took me anxious, arduous moments to remove Connie's coat; then he laboriously followed a waiter, with me close behind, to a small table where, we found, we were to be seated with old friends, Emmet John Hughes and Orville Prescott. They chided him for making an entrance but almost immediately Emmet, sitting across from Connie, stopped the banter and got a waiter. The cocktail hour was long over but Emmet said

---

* It was two weeks before I got around to sending the books. I received a letter from the Irishman's wife. Her husband had died the preceding week in a car crash. The other books came back, stamped "Return to Sender. No such address." The kindness that we had been given was never to be repaid.

399

quietly, "We all need a drink here. Connie, what will you have?" My husband shook his head. "Bourbon," I told Emmet. "Some ice, a little water." Emmet gave the rest of our orders and asked quietly that they be brought quickly. Seated between Orville and Connie, I saw that Connie's hands were trembling in his lap. Orville gently congratulated him on finishing the new book and he and I talked about a memorable dinner the Prescotts and the Ryans had spent with our poet friend Phyllis McGinley and her husband Bill Hayden. Connie was silent and Emmet eyed him with concern.

The drinks arrived promptly but Connie did not pick his up. "Sip the bourbon," I whispered to him. "Maybe it will help a little."

"I can't," he said so softly I could hardly hear him. "I don't think I can hold the glass in just one hand."

Slowly he dragged his right hand to the table. After a moment or two he inched it toward the glass. He was breathing through his mouth and trying very hard to keep the sound from being noticeable. Emmet and Orville began talking rather loudly to each other. Both kept their eyes from Connie. I reached out to pick up his glass.

"No," he said almost angrily. "No!"

He willed himself to pick it up, and his entire arm appeared to tremble as he got the glass to his mouth and took a swallow. Quickly, as if the effort had taken all his control, he set it down with a small thud, splashing the liquor. He could not hold it any longer.

Emmet and Orville drew him into their conversation. It did not require his response and Connie sat and listened. The dinner was served but neither of us could eat. Connie was unable to use his knife and fork and I was too frightened even to contemplate food.

The speeches began on the brightly lit podium, the tables dim around it in muted darkness of candlelight. Just as the names of new Fellows were being read, Connie turned to me. His face was beaded with perspiration. "Katie, get me out of here. I've got to get home."

Emmet rose quickly and pulled out the table. Connie put both hands on it and hauled himself up. I handed him his cane. Then hobbling agonizingly, making his way past the little tables where startled faces stared up at us, Connie walked out of the dining area. He could not move his arms enough for me to pull his coat on. I draped it over his shoulders to give him what little protection from the wind it would afford.

We found another taxi and Connie endured a second painful ride to the garage where I'd parked. There I found two attendants on duty and asked one to go up and stand by my husband while the other located our car and drove it up the ramp.

Inside the car I took off my own coat and wrapped it completely around his chest and waist before strapping on his seat belt. The ride to Ridgefield was as terrible for him as the taxi trips. He became nauseous. I pulled off the shoulder twice during the trip home, helped him out, supporting him as sickness overwhelmed him.

Just before we reached Ridgefield Connie said faintly, "Katie, it feels like I've broken every bone in my body, but I know for sure I've broken my ribs."

At the house I somehow got him up the stairs, and leaving him in a bedroom chair, dashed for the phone to call Pat. Fortunately he was in. He came immediately.

Together Pat and I undressed him. Throughout the ordeal Connie's lips were tightly sealed but his face was racked with pain. Tenderly Pat's expert fingers went over him as he listened to my story of what had happened. He opened his case and brought out rolls of elastic bandage. It was too late to get wide bandages or even an elastic corset. Drugstores had long since closed.

"You're right, CJ," Pat told Connie quietly, "you've broken your ribs. Tomorrow early we'll get you proper bandages.

Now I've got to tell you something I don't much like saying. You're going to have to try to sleep in the chair. I don't want you to lie down at all, understand?" Eyes on Pat, Connie nodded his head. "I'll give you something for the pain, but it won't help much tonight. Still, try to sleep a little." Connie closed his eyes. Tears gathered and ran down his face. He could not raise his arms to brush them away. Pat pulled out his own handkerchief and gently wiped my husband's face.

With Connie settled and apparently drowsy I walked down to the door with Pat. "His ribs—in fact just about all the bones in his body—are like matchsticks," Pat said. "I have to keep him upright. The one thing we don't need is a floating rib splinter traveling around."

"How long will he have to try to sleep like that?"

"Ten days, maybe longer. Maybe several weeks." Pat paused. "I've got a big reclining chair. It's a brute but I'll get my boys to bring it over tomorrow. He'll be more comfortable."

"Dear God," I said, "hasn't he suffered enough?"

"Yes. He has," Pat answered. "How did the dinner go?"

"I don't know," I told him. "He fell before we ever got there and he was determined that nothing was going to keep him from it." I began to cry for the first time that night. Connie had wanted to be invited to become a Fellow of The Society of American Historians for years. Finally it had happened and he did not even get to hear his name read out.

= 7 =

CONNIE'S ENFORCED RETIREMENT from active life lasted a scant week. Although he continued to sleep upright in the reclining chair Pat's sons had hauled up to the bedroom for him, he refused to spend any time there except at night. The elastic corset Pat got for him was almost as painful as the damage to his ribs. It bit into his flesh and ugly red lines encircled his body. Baby oil and Vaseline soothed the cuts a little, but it was agony for him to have me try to move the corset up or down to free him from the constant abrasion.

On Wednesday, June 5, her father's birthday, Victoria graduated from private school. Connie, still encased in the elastic corset, stood with other proud fathers, taking numerous pictures of his daughter in her graduation dress.

Just six days later he and I were back in Europe where Connie held meeting after meeting with Dutch officials to explore the feasibility of gathering principals and press in Holland for the thirtieth anniversary—September 17, 1974—of the battles described in *Bridge*.

It was clear that he was not well. His nerves were frayed, his fractures not yet mended, and he was on his feet or in conferences far longer than he should have been. Yet he refused to rest. We moved on to London for conferences and lunch with British publisher Hamish Hamilton and his staff, making plans for *Bridge*'s London publication.

On Tuesday, June 25, we were in Paris. That day Connie was too weak to continue his grueling schedule. Dr. Jacques Fouré, whose wife Kiki is my oldest friend, arranged for Connie to have a complete blood test at The American Hospital. Only to Kiki did Jacques confide the news that the results of the tests were extremely erratic and abnormal. In turn, she suggested to me that I try to persuade Connie to return home as soon as possible.

My attempts were fruitless. After only a day's rest Connie saw his French publisher, Robert Laffont, and then went on to wind up his final conferences in the Netherlands. But he was paying a terrible price for his efforts. The cost was becoming more than his body could meet.

While we had been traveling in Europe, Vicki had been attending casting calls for the Ridgefield Workshop's summer production, *Finian's Rainbow*. She sent us an exuberant telegram: "Guess who got the lead? I did." Her father sent back an immediate reply: "Guess who's not surprised? Mom and I."

She was already deep into rehearsals when we arrived home on Saturday, July 6, and, as usual, she asked for her father's help. With the gracious permission of the Ridgefield Workshop officers and staff (not, I suspect, that it would have made much difference), Connie immediately plunged into rehearsals even as he worked at the finishing touches on the plans for the thirtieth anniversary of Operation Market-Garden, with the aid of Jack Thompson and Ben Wright in the United States and the helpful services of Dutch officials. Between Market-Garden plans and rehearsals for *Finian's Rainbow* Connie was by then putting in an eighteen-hour day. He had even gone so far as to find the pianist who had played in the orchestra when the play opened years before on Broadway, and a handwritten note attests to his determination to make the music live up to the actors and vice versa. He wrote:

One violin, 1 viola, 1 flute/piccolo, 1 clarinet, 1 piano, 2 trumpets, 1 string bass, 1 drums . . . Orchestral interludes . . . Overture.

On Sunday, July 28, our friend George Newell died in his sleep. We had seen George and Billie almost every week when we or they were home, and George, one of Vicki's staunchest fans, had ordered yellow roses, only a day before his death, to be delivered to Victoria after the first night's performance on Friday, August 9.

Connie drove immediately to see Billie. He stayed a short while, came home, and went to the record player. The overture of *Finian's Rainbow* drifted sweetly through the house.

Connie listened for some minutes in silence. Then he said, "I'm conducting the orchestra the first night. I want to make that evening a special tribute to George. Damn it," he said, close to tears, "why did he have to go and die on me?"

On Monday, July 29, not his usual day for a visit, Connie drove in to see Dr. Whitmore. As always when I did not accompany him, he told me nothing of his examination, except the laconic "Fine. Good report," to which I had become accustomed. As usual, too, he had not apprised Dr. Whitmore of his hectic schedule, or, I assume, of his weakness and the battery of tests which had been made in Paris. He seemed determined to tell the doctor as little as possible. Perhaps he feared that a true accounting of his activities would have caused Whitmore to caution him or slow him down. Pat's urgings had come to nothing, and, upon hearing that immediately after the play on opening night Connie intended to go off for two days fishing in Canada with Ben, Pat, no fisherman, announced that he was going too. If Connie could not be deterred—and he could not—Pat intended to be there in case of trouble.

The opening night of the play was a mixture of joy and sorrow. We had invited a large group of friends in to dinner, although the host and his daughter made only the briefest of appearances. Billie Newell, looking frail but determinedly cheerful, was in our group. Geoff and I acted as hosts for the dinner and afterward we drove to the auditorium for the play.

The lights dimmed and I saw Connie walk slowly out to a high seat in front of the orchestra. It had been arranged there because he would be unable to stand during the entire performance. He had bought a baton for the occasion. He used it that night and presented it later to young Phillip Van Lidth De Jeude, a talented musician, who would conduct the orchestra during the rest of the play's run.

As the opening strains of the overture began I felt my eyes smart, and I began to tremble. Helene Merrick, sitting by me, reached out and held my hands. I knew I would never again sit through a play in which father and daughter had worked together. Listening to the complicated, lovely, lilting tunes I thought of all the nights Connie had come home from rehearsals at midnight or later and remembered something he had said. "These kids hate me, Katie," he told me one evening as he sat down carefully in Pat's big chair. "I work their tails off. We did three run-throughs and I told them no one was going home until everybody got it right," and then, in a burst of pride, he said, "Lord, those kids are good!"

"Then why don't you tell them so, and then they won't hate you?"

"For Pete's sake, why would I do that? I don't give a damn what they think about me. If I get soft, they'll think they've got it made and put in less effort. I want to keep it just the way it is. The tougher I am on them the better they perform."

His attitude must have carried not only to the orchestra but to the cast as well. All the young people brought the show glowingly alive. I watched my young daughter singing "Look to the Rainbow," her voice true and tinged with a bit of Irish pronunciation that neither Vera Neligan nor Connie, both Dubliners, had been able to teach her. She had picked it up by listening to the cast record of the original production. She stood on the stage and sang to her father, watching every movement of his baton as he wove the music around her. No one in our row of seats was dry-eyed.

When the last scene had been played and the curtain had come down, the applause and calls of "Bravo" were deafening. As the curtain rose for the actors' first call, Vicki stepped forward and blew a kiss to her father. The entire cast and orchestra applauded. Connie raised his baton to signal the orchestra to rise, and again the applause swelled. Then he turned slowly, one hand on the high stool to steady himself, and bowed slowly to the crowded hall. Geoff, seated behind me, whispered in my ear, "Mom, I never knew how good Vicki was and Dad—" His voice broke and he leaned over to kiss me. "You've got quite a husband, lady," he said.

"I've got quite a family," I managed to get out.

The curtain calls were still being taken, and flowers were brought onstage for the actors. George Newell's yellow roses were vivid against Vicki's dress. Geoff and I had sent her flowers, as had many of our friends. They spread like a garden at her feet but it was George's bouquet she held.

After the performance families and friends stood about in small groups. Pat and Ben were backstage with Connie and someone sent word that Geoff was needed. I started after him but he cautioned me away. "Don't worry," he said. "I'll be right back if anything's wrong."

He returned quickly, carrying his father's evening clothes on a hanger. Because Ben, Pat, and Connie were to leave immediately for the airport after the performance, Connie had brought a change of clothes, his fishing gear, and river apparel to the auditorium. Geoff held out the suit to me. "Feel it, Mom," he said. Everything, including Connie's tie, was as damp as if it had all been removed that instant from a washer. I was reminded of the Legion of Honor ceremonies. Then, too, Connie had needed to change clothes completely. Weakness and pain had drenched his clothing as it had done before.

Vicki and most of the cast and orchestra came out the stage door and walked around to us. Again, they received the plaudits of bystanders. The door opened again and Connie, followed by Ben and Pat, emerged. Connie was dressed in casual flannels, a soft, open-necked shirt, and a blazer. He was riding on a wave of enthusiasm. He made straight for Billie Newell, kissed her, and the two of them talked quietly for a minute. Vicki handed me her bouquets and joined them, her arms circling Billie's and Connie's waists. Then, the three of them walked over to us.

"Well, Katie," Connie said, loud enough for the cast and musicians to hear, "what did I tell you? They did a fair job, didn't they?"

There were exaggerated groans all around. "I don't envy

407

young Phillip his job conducting that lot." Connie motioned to the orchestra personnel. "He's too young to scowl as well as I do."

"Thank God!" somebody said fervently.

Connie took my hand and we walked toward the car that would take the men to the airport. Vicki and Geoff—still carrying Connie's damp clothes—followed close behind. At the car, almost all our guests turned up to wish the fishermen luck. Connie got painfully into the front passenger side. I leaned in and kissed him.

"Catch some big ones," I told him.

"I may not have time," Connie said. "Ben and I will probably spend all of two days untangling Neligan from his line." Pat started the car and it began to move off slowly. As it disappeared around the bend and headed toward New York, clusters of people were still in the parking lot waving goodbye. I stood with Geoff watching until we could see the taillights no longer.

On August 19, after he had had rather disappointing fishing in Canada, Connie and I flew to Chicago for his taped appearance on Bob Cromie's "Book Beat." Old war buddies, the two men had kept their friendship thriving throughout the years. Their stories and jokes before airtime were, to my mind, far more fascinating than the actual interview but, as both explained, they couldn't tell those stories on the air; "We would have been bleeped out."

Upon our return Connie plunged again into the work for Operation Market-Garden. American, British, and Polish generals—as well as the press of many countries—were going to Holland for Market-Garden's thirtieth anniversary and the many ceremonies commemorating it.

In September we flew to Europe once again for those events. Barely into the trip Connie was exhausted, stretched almost to the limit of his endurance. He continued to waste his fragile strength still more. I could do little but stand by and watch, ticking off the days until we could get home again. Connie, it seemed to me, was daily losing ground. He was losing it faster than either of us knew.

On Monday, Septemper 23, we arrived back in New York. There, we were met by further demands on Connie's time. *Bridge* had come out in the bookstores in the United States while we were in Europe and sales were moving very fast. Many press, radio, and TV shows had been lined up awaiting his arrival. There was a great deal for Connie still to do. Too much. I noticed that his legs had become very swollen and his limp was pronounced.

Prior to our spring departure for Europe we had talked about spending the winter of 1974 in New York. Geoff was on his own and by September Vicki was in college; from her letters and phone calls she was enjoying her new life. The interview and speech schedules that had been arranged for Connie would take him all over the country. If we had an apartment in the city the trips to and from airports to home could be shortened considerably. Additionally, Connie had begun to voice aloud his fear that some new medical treatment would be required. If so, he wanted to be close to Memorial. We found an apartment at the Sherry-Netherland and I made a series of trips to Ridgefield, bringing back clothes, typewriters, and personal mementos to make the place seem more like home. Weekends, if Connie's schedule allowed, we planned to be in Ridgefield to enjoy the autumn, but we would go back into the city each Sunday. We had acquired a caretaker and now there was no need for us to worry about the house or the animals.

On October 9, 1974, Connie saw Dr. Whitmore for the first time since July. Following our return from Europe in September he had been interviewed on the "Today" show, attended a Book-of-the-Month Club luncheon in his honor, taped several radio shows, been interviewed by magazine and newspaper writers. Additionally, he had given a speech at the Dutch Society dinner, another at the Dutch Treat Club, and together we had spent two days at Fort Bragg, North Carolina. There, Connie was honored at a colorful ceremony highlighted by the presentation to him of a baton which members of the 82nd All-American Parachute Team had exchanged in midair before opening their steerable chutes and landing precisely on colored circles in front of the reviewing stand.

The frenetic activity of the past months had sapped Connie's vitality. It was almost as painful to watch him walk as it must have been for him to do so. Still, he made no real complaints. He spoke of weakness and tiredness, but he resisted all my attempts to get him to omit portions of his heavy schedule. He was suffering greatly, however much he still tried to hide it. Obstinately he refused to rest. I was puzzled by his attitude. I did not know that he feared a slowdown of activities would bring on morbidity and depression and cause him to lower his guard. I did not know that he had come to regard cancer as a tangible murderer, stalking his every move.

On that October Wednesday when he saw Dr. Whitmore, my husband was apparently somewhat more candid about his health and his activities than he had been in all that year. Dr. Whitmore wrote:

Has been more or less stable until the last week or two during which time the pace of his social responsibilities has increased as a consequence of the success of his most recent book. . . . Bowel function has been poor with alternating constipation and "pure water." In the past 24 hours he has had increased right hip pain so that he is taking percodan with levodromeran 4x daily and sometimes doubling up on the percodan. In addition, during this same interval, he has had some discomfort in the right chest with ambulation. No peripheral edema but the pain in his right hip radiated down as far as the ankle although primarily in the right thigh. He is taking Elavil t.i.d., prednisone t.i.d. Xyloprim q.i.d. and cytoxan 100 mg. daily but has had no 5 FU for several months.

On examination he clearly does not look as well as when I last saw him, there being a slightly cyanotic tinge to his entire outlook and more evidence of pain in the way he ambulates and moves. . . . There is certainly rib tenderness in the right costal arch area. Abdominal examination reveals no significant positive findings. Genitalia atrophic. Rectal—small, rather fibrous inconspicuous prostate with a probably palpable seed overlying the right side.

Blood count and chemistries drawn prior to examination and x-rays obtained of the lumbar spine and pelvis and right hip area.

Dr. Batata saw the patient in consultation and plans made for initiation of radiation therapy to the area of his maximum pain. If there is any abnormality in his blood chemistries of critical nature, hospitalization may be advised, but otherwise will try to maintain him on OPT [outpatient] basis.

Clearly, cancer was again gaining the upper hand.

$$\doteq 8 \doteq$$

CORNELIUS

Today is Saturday, October 12, 1974. I have been out most of the day at book autographing parties in this part of Connecticut. Geoff drove me from one to the other. I did not think I would get through the day.

Tomorrow we will be leaving for New York to stay in the apartment and on Monday, the fourteenth, I am to begin radiation therapy to the right hip. The pain in that leg has become excruciating. There is no longer any way to talk myself out of awareness of its constancy. I think I am going to have to take pain relievers on a steady basis, but even then I don't think they will help very much. I began to increase dosages several days ago and have noticed little if any relief. Oddly enough, I don't think these drugs are affecting my mind or distorting my mental outlook. I have been very much afraid that narcotics would unhinge my reasoning powers but now the pain is stronger than the drugs' abilities to override it.

In Holland in September I met a lady at the airport as we were waiting for our flight home to be called. She was very large, almost too big for the wheelchair in which she was sitting. I became aware that she had been staring at me. Finally she asked, "Are you on cortisone?"

I admitted I was. "Don't take it anymore," she said. "It won't help your cancer."

I must have registered surprise.

She explained that she, too, had cancer. From my appearance and her own treatment in the past, she assumed that the massiveness of my face and neck were due to corticoids. "When they start giving you such large doses the game's up anyway, isn't it?" she asked. "Just stop taking them. I've reached the end of my line and I suspect you think you've got yours in sight. Go out looking the way you want to look. That cortisone isn't doing anything anymore." She smiled. "You'll feel better because when you look in the mirror you'll see yourself and not what cortisone has made of you."

Katie was very angry and tried to move us away, but I understood that the woman's views were expressed with the kind of forthright honesty cancer patients use in conversation with one another. And her view may be valid. I do know that I hurt in so many places and so constantly that chemotherapy and other treatments are just not doing the job. Except for the radiation therapy which might help at the site of my greatest pain, the right hip, I would doubt that there is much more to be done. I think I have used up the therapies the medical profession can command to bring against cancer. I still wonder, as I have done for a long time, if events might have taken a different turn had I gone to Palo Alto and put myself into Malcolm Bagshaw's hands. But the move was impractical from every aspect, and *Bridge* would certainly have been far longer delayed than it was. At least my mind is at peace about the book. It is selling very well and the reviews from everywhere have been gratifying.

I have been trying to get a little further on future writing plans, but pain and tiredness make it difficult to think about new projects. I cannot seem any longer to immerse myself in ideas and forget everything else.

Each morning for the past two or three years when I have wakened the first words I've said are, "Thank you, God, for this fine day." It has not mattered if the weather was bad or good. What has been important is that God had seen me through the night and given me another day to work and to be with my family. I continue to thank Him. He has allowed me to do what was important.

I have received more than my share of blessings. I have been able to cram so much into my life that it has been brimful of happiness. The most rewarding moments, the best writing I think I've ever done, the love I'd had from my wife and children and the joy I've taken in their accomplishments— all have been realized in the years I've had cancer. But I will still continue to fight it. I don't have time to die.

Part Five
THE LAST MONTH
October–November 1974

KATHRYN

At 8:30 A.M. on Tuesday, October 15, 1974, Connie limped
out of the apartment at the Sherry-Netherland and got a cab
to Memorial. There he took the first of five radiation therapy
treatments to his right hip. According to Patient's Appointment tickets he brought back with him, each with a counter-
foil and carbons for the accounting department, he was to
receive radiation daily, excepting weekends, through October 28. He was also given a plastic card like a charge plate,
with his name, home address, and case number on it above
the hospital insignia—an arrow pointing skyward, its shaft
crossed by three bars, and the words "Memorial Center Outpatient Department" at the right.

He showed them all to me, then folded the sheath of appointments around the card and put them in the breast pocket
of his jacket. He seemed strangely reluctant to talk about the
morning. He stretched out in the bedroom and rested for
about an hour, then got up to go to a luncheon conference
with Paul Gitlin.

On Wednesday, the sixteenth, an overcast morning, it was
more difficult for him to get up. He felt ill and could not eat
any breakfast. "I wouldn't keep it down," he said. I watched
him from the apartment door as he dragged himself down the
corridor, a raincoat thrown over his shoulders. At 12:30 that

same day he was to make a speech at the Four Seasons restaurant to *Reader's Digest* advertisers. From the hospital he
had called David Evins and asked him to meet us at the
restaurant. By then it was raining hard, and Paul Gitlin telephoned to say he had ordered a car to pick up Connie at the
hospital. Then the driver would call for me, deliver us to the
luncheon meeting, and return us to the hotel.

Connie was pale but exuding the kind of nervous energy
that I associated with most of his public appearances. His
face looked far thinner than it had in months. I wondered if
he was taking his corticoids. Ever since I had attempted to
give him a Demerol injection in June of 1973 after his second
hospitalization and he had resisted so fiercely, he had carried
all his medications in a small leather bag from which, at given
times, he privately selected the pills he wanted.

Arriving at the restaurant we were met by Fulton Oursler,
Jr.—a *Digest* editor with whom Connie had often worked—
and escorted to an upstairs room where David Evins, Peter
Schwed of Simon & Schuster, and the men to whom he
would speak were having cocktails. Connie declined one.
Somebody asked to take his picture. Motioning Peter and
David to him, he put his arm around me and laid his cane on
a chair out of sight. I could feel the trembling of his body but
his face was devoid of pain, totally calm. Afterward, he sat
down at a small corner table and spoke animatedly with
everyone who approached him.

We were seated alongside a podium with two small steps
leading to it. Connie made no attempt to eat when luncheon
was served. Soon after the main course, Fulton mounted the
platform to introduce the speaker. He touched briefly on
Connie's background, on his World War II histories, and on
his achievement in writing *Bridge* while he was so ill. Fulton
told the audience that they were indeed fortunate to have
Connie among them; he had come to the luncheon from a
session of radiation therapy at Memorial.

"Christ!" Connie muttered to me. Under polite and sympathetic applause he negotiated the steps to the podium. "Gentlemen," he began, "I suffer from a terminal case . . ." He paused and the room was completely silent. Connie leaned over the podium, smiled widely, and said, ". . . of *greed!*" The room erupted with laughter and relief. For over forty minutes he held his audience spellbound with stories and anecdotes about the writing of *Bridge*. I know that's what he talked about but I don't remember anything he said after that first incredible sentence. He finished to a standing ovation, stepped carefully off the platform, and sat down heavily in his chair. Men crowded around to shake his hand and wish him well. He laughed and joked with them. At one point he turned aside to me and murmured, "Find out where the car is, Katie. I've got to lie down as soon as possible." We left as quickly as I could get his coat and mine.

The rest of that week Connie forced himself to dress and go to the hospital, but he came home immediately after each appointment and went to bed. We had dinner with Hamish Hamilton, over from London, but Connie canceled all other engagements. On Friday he was too ill to go to the country, and Jerry Lewis drove in on Saturday, October 19, to pick us up. The date was important.

That evening we went to a function that had long been planned. To celebrate the publication of *Bridge*, Vera and Pat Neligan were giving a dinner party for nearly seventy guests in Connie's honor. As time to go drew near he was too tired to dress and I helped him into his clothes and dinner jacket, leaving Vicki, home for a few days from college, to deal with the problem of his evening tie. He, who had always prided himself on independence, could not manage the effort involved that evening. Still, he had no intention of missing the party. Vera had consulted him weeks earlier to find a date in his busy schedule when she and Pat could plan the evening, and Connie's responsibilities as the guest of honor weighed far heavier on him than the agony he by now was clearly showing.

Somehow he got through the hours, chatting with guests, toasting his hostess, chiding his host, who he claimed "needed a haircut—as usual," and complimenting Vera on her serene and lovely room, lit by hundreds of candles, and rich with the scent of flowers. We left shortly after dinner. For many of his friends, that evening was to be the last time they would ever see him alive.

On Tuesday, October 22, 1974, I was awakened in our bedroom at the Sherry-Netherland by the sound of harsh sobs. Connie was sitting on the side of his bed, tears streaming down his face. Quickly I hurried to him and knelt beside him.

"Damn, Katie, I'm sorry," he said brokenly. "I can't get up to go to the hospital. You'll have to get me dressed and go with me."

I helped him with his bathroom chores and tried to soothe him. "I'm so ashamed," he kept saying. "So ashamed."

"Of what?"

"Of being helpless. Oh, Katie, when is it ever going to end?"

I had no answer. The radiation therapy had failed, it seemed to me. In the past few weeks my husband had gone steadily downhill. And his decline had seemed to worsen in the seven days since treatments to his right hip were begun. Eventually I got him dressed but he could not walk across the apartment to the door without help.

At the Outpatient entrance to Memorial an attendant came running as I tried to help Connie from the taxi. Quickly he got a wheelchair and we took Connie to the radiation therapy department.

Dr. Batata, who had supervised his therapy, came to meet us. Attendants put my husband on a stretcher. He turned his back to all of us and pulled his knees up, curving the upper part of his body into a fetal position.

"Admit me," Connie said, his voice to the wall. "I'm not going out of this hospital again until I can take care of myself like a man."

I started to say something but Connie cut me off. "Don't waste time, Katie. You can't take any more of this and I can't either. Let's get this thing settled once and for all."

The "settlement" took time. I wanted to reach Pat or Dr. Whitmore but was unable to get in touch with either man. Finally I gave up—and gave in. Connie's agony was too much for either of us. Connie was undressed and put into a hospital gown; his clothes were folded at the head of a rolling stretcher and we went to Emergency Admitting. He was not seen by anyone except nurses, kind but ignorant of his case, for some hours. I waited, separated from him by a curtain, growing angrier by the minute. He had had neither breakfast nor lunch. His pills in the leather bag had been removed. He was given nothing for his pain.

At some point a doctor came and I was asked to leave. I filled out the admittance forms and waited. At about 5:00 P.M. I was told to go to the fourteenth-floor visitors' waiting room; Connie would be brought to that section. The usual hunt for a bed had taken as long, it seemed, as the meticulous medical history, physical and neurological exams, and X rays.

I spent an anxious hour on the fourteenth floor waiting for Connie. Time and again I checked the corridors and elevator banks, terrified that I would miss him. No one at the nurses' station seemed to know that he was on his way. I asked one of them to get on to emergency admissions. "Why don't you people communicate with one another?" I asked frantically. "I was told to wait on fourteen. You say you have no record that my husband will be coming to this floor."

A little after 6:00 P.M. I saw an unattended stretcher alongside a wall. I found Connie on it, pale and exhausted. What little control I had left vanished. My husband had been in the hospital since 8:30 A.M. For close onto ten hours I had waited in one place or another for news of him. To come upon him alone in a corridor, unattended, touched off my anger and my fear. I shouted—literally—for someone to come. After some minutes a nurse and an attendant arrived.

By then Connie himself was aroused. My anger and his pain were not well received by the two employees. "If you don't be quiet, I may not take care of him at all," the woman said. I stared at her. I became quiet. Caring for Connie was all that mattered.

At the entrance to a two-bed room, I saw an empty bed and the dim figure of a man in the other. "Are you Bones?" he asked as Connie was being wheeled in. "This whole floor is Bones."

Connie didn't answer. I was equally silent. The nurse and the attendant paid no attention to the other patient's question as they moved Connie from the stretcher to the bed while I snatched up his clothes, still on the cart where they had been since early morning. At the door the attendant turned back to look at Connie and me. "My, my," he said, "we got ourselves a couple of tough cookies, have we?" The nurse paused too and smiled. "Not for long," she said. "They'll come around. Believe me." I walked toward them. "What's your name?" I asked the nurse. Usually there were name pins on the uniforms, but I had been too upset to think about that until then. She was half turned in the doorway and I could not see her pin. "It doesn't matter," she said, "I know yours."

Connie had seen many doctors, but even haunting the hospital as I was, I did not see one for two days. During that time, however, I learned both the nurse's and the attendant's name. The doctor I finally met, a pleasant man whom I was to see only that one time, listened to my story about Connie's entry to the fourteenth floor. "I'm afraid there isn't anything to be done," he said. "Why don't you just forget it?" In time my two antagonists became, amazingly, a source of occasional comfort and help to Connie, but their behavior on the day he was admitted was something I would never forget.

A GU Fellow Note for Tuesday, October 22, the day Connie was admitted to Memorial for the third time reads in part:

Fell. Ribs fx [fracture] subsequently healed. The R leg pain has increased sciatic like distribution. Local RT [radiation therapy] begun for ↑ [increased] pain and suggest ? [question] pubis path. Fx. Pain seemed to increase and assoc. bowel frequency with lack of control. Enters for eval. No voiding Sx. [symptoms].

Neurology notes read as follows:

54-year-old R handed male with Bx [biopsied] adeno ca prostate. Rx'd with Ch Rx [chemotherapy treatment] and recently with RT. Patient has diffuse bony mets [metastases] including skull and pelvis. For past 18 months % [complains of] numbness in R buttock and medial R thigh and of pain recently (1–3 mos.) on walking. Patient had hx [history] of pain in R leg 18 mos. ago which was not radicular [related to a nerve or vein root] but says this is different. He can find no comfortable position and pain increases with movement: Also % progressive weakness in both legs . . . Has atrophy of both legs and R buttock. C/o numbness across anus. Pelvic films 10/9 show fx R. Pelvic ramus.

Impression: CA prostate with diffuse bony metastases. Appears to have, in addition to R pubis FX, involvement of lower motor neurons . . . Whether this represents compression of cauda [terminal of spinal cord] or of nerve roots outside sacrum remains a ?.

To determine the answer to the question, a myelogram was done on Wednesday, October 23. It disclosed blockage in three, possibly more, regions over or on the outer membrane covering Connie's spinal cord. The neurological opinion was less than encouraging:

Myelogram shows definite blockage—possibly tumor—can't operate.

Consulting doctors then agreed to start Connie on radiation therapy the following day, Thursday, October 24. With technicians using a Cobalt 60 machine, he would receive a total of 3000 rads to the lumbosacral spine from October 24 until Wednesday, November 6.*

It seemed that the treatment, medications, and watchful care of doctors and nurses were working once again. Connie, after the first few days, was again cheerful, optimistic (at least with me), and looked more rested than he had in days. He read the newspapers carefully each day, took pleasure in his visitors, and, according to nurses' notes, offered few complaints. He took an interest in his roommate and they were soon on a first-name basis. Always unable to refrain from an interview if a subject was at hand, he discovered that "Harold," his roommate, had no immediate family, had been a carpenter in New Jersey, and "wouldn't have come here no way if I had had my say." Connie gave Harold numerous pep talks and shared his newspapers and magazines with him; often I would come into the room to find the two of them in a high-spirited character analysis of some of the hospital staff.

From their beds they were able to look out into the corridor and view ambulatory patients and visitors. Often complete strangers would stop in the doorway to chat with them. And Connie's friends were a constant source of interest and amazement to Harold. When Hamish Hamilton visited, prior to leaving for London, Harold remarked, "You're the first Limey I've seen up close," and when Ben Grauer arrived,

---

* Memorial records indicate some discrepancy in dates. I have depended on Dr. Whitmore's final report for this time period.

Harold was in a state of awe. Each New Year's Eve, he informed Ben, he listened to Ben's on-the-spot description of the Times Square celebration, "but it never occurred to me you was real," he said enigmatically.

One patient on the floor was a constant source of amusement to Harold. He walked completely around the corridor of the huge floor on an average of three or four times a day, pushing before him a rolling standard to which his IV was attached. Each day, he appeared to go a little faster, his face determined, his bare legs churning down the aisles. Harold was both mystified and puzzled by such exercise. Connie told him the story of Diogenes and his daylight search with a lantern "for a man." Harold was delighted by the story. He kept a small notebook by his bedside to record the patient's trips. "Hey, Connie," he'd say, "here comes ole Dodge again. This makes five times and he ain't found a man yet."

Within a few days Connie was transferred to a private room which had become available overlooking York Avenue. Harold watched the packing up, the clothing removed from Connie's closet, the shaving gear, toothbrush, and toiletries being taken from the bathroom. Connie was helped into a wheelchair. He was rolled across to say good-bye to Harold. They shook hands solemnly and Connie reached out and brushed back his roommate's hair.

"So long, old pal," Connie said. "If Dodge wins any footraces, let me know."

A nurse wheeled Connie out. I followed, carrying his clothes. At the door I turned and blew a kiss to Harold. He was staring blankly at the wall and crying.

The tests, medical histories, and charts went on intensively. Connie's medication was changed and nurses' notes indicate that he was upset about it. Still he seemed to be in less pain, although sphincter tone was lax and he was experiencing some fecal incontinence and diarrhea—probably from the results of radiation. His sleeping habits were erratic. Sometimes he dozed at intervals throughout the day. At night he was often given medication for pain at his own request.

On Wednesday, October 30, 1974 a medical oncology report which dated back to Connie's first hospitalization in 1970—listing findings, treatment, and results—indicated that once more cancer had eluded the chemical detectives sent to find and detain it. The report concluded:

On basis of above summary, it appears that DES/Cytoxan/Prednisone combination has run its course . . . At conclusion of R.T. and if no surgery planned we ought to try one of the combinations with Adriamycin which have been so effective in breast ca.*

My days became routine. Afternoons and early evenings were spent at the hospital from Monday through Friday. On Friday evening Jerry Lewis or Dick and Jean Deems would drive me to Ridgefield and I would return Sunday afternoon, going straight to the hospital. Although I was anxious, my mood was brighter than it had been in months. The source of Connie's continuing pain to the right leg had been found and the cobalt treatments appeared to give him no small measure of relief, in spite of recurrent diarrhea and nausea. Then, too, new therapy was being planned, and my hopes soared once again. No matter how wearing the constant battle I still believed, naively, a day would come when Connie could lead a productive, if limited, life once more. I had not seen or spoken with Dr. Whitmore since Connie had arrived at the hospital—nor did I ever see him until Monday, November 18, twenty-eight days after Connie was admitted—but I had made the acquaintance of two young men from his depart-

---

* Adriamycin is a cytotoxic antibiotic given intravenously in chemotherapy. It has been successful in the regression of not only breast cancer but in lymphoblastic and myeloblastic leukemia and in bone sarcomas.

ment, Drs. Katz and Crawford, who dropped in almost every evening when I was there.

Pleasant and cheerful, they spent a great deal of time with Connie and patiently answered all his questions. Yet I felt reluctant to leave Connie's room when they did for a private talk with them about his condition. He was, as usual, determined to hear all views and opinions about his health himself. And by then he had an additional health to worry about. Vicki had become ill at school and Dr. Safford had insisted that she come home to rest. Since I was in town throughout the week, she came to the Sherry-Netherland and was put to bed, where she more or less remained until Friday evenings when we went to the country. Connie was concerned about her although Ted assured him that mononucleosis, which appeared to have infected the entire school, could be best treated by removing her from the surroundings and enforcing rest.

For some days I had been aware of the fact that Connie, usually so vocal and interested in outside activities, was undergoing a slow but obvious change. During my visits he smiled, held my hand, inquired about Vicki, and discussed visits from Geoff, but at news of friends and future plans and activities he seemed to draw down a curtain. Often, coming into his room, I would find him staring at the ceiling, his thoughts far away. At such times I could do little but sit beside him, denied the sharing that had been one of the foundations of our marriage. He was less and less inclined to be helped to a big chair by the window where, earlier, he had liked to watch traffic rushing along the avenue. He seemed to feel at home only in his bed, and I would often come in to find that he, an avid reader, had not bothered to open the newspapers that were brought in each morning. He had begun to shut off everything outside the hospital and his room.

His blood chemistries were being constantly monitored and, depending on the findings, medications were decreased, increased, dropped, or added to as Memorial's vigilant staff of specialists sought to bring some balance and stability to his life. Meanwhile Connie was, I think, coming to terms with death. He had gambled with cancer and won from it the time to write his book, to watch his children reach near maturity. The time had come when a patch-up job and stopgap measures held no further interest for him, except as rather abstract curiosities. Indeed, he sometimes seemed amused at learning of new medical plans for his benefit and would discuss them with his doctors as if the three of them were talking about some other patient.

In late afternoon Monday, November 18, I was sitting on his bed when Dr. Whitmore and Dr. Katz came in. Almost immediately Connie needed to go to the bathroom, and Dr. Katz helped him there while Dr. Whitmore sat down on the bed beside me. He told me that he planned to release Connie soon. "He's suffering from hospitalitis," Dr. Whitmore said, "and I'd like to get him home again." That was the best news I'd heard. But no one had told me the bad news. On that same day Connie had been found to have a fecal impaction and his blood counts had fallen again. A new therapy was planned, using DES 5 mg daily and Schering Compound 13521.* He was never to start the new chemotherapy suggested by Memorial's Oncology Group. Even as Dr. Whitmore and I sat talking about plans for bringing Connie home, he had barely five days to live.

On Friday, November 22, I arrived later than my usual 2:00 P.M. appearance at the hospital. Jean Deems and I had been shopping and I had found a sweater; it was blue, a color that

---

* A medical compound followed by a number is usually an indication that the formula has been made to order for a specific department in a single hospital. Compound numbers are really codes, and information as to what the medication contains are kept secret. In spite of several attempts, I have been unable to learn, four years later, the components of this compound or what beneficial effects doctors thought it would have on Connie.

Connie particularly liked on me. Vicki was still resting at the Sherry-Netherland and I had stopped by there to leave off the sweater and check on her. She had become quite handy about ringing room service for her meals, even though I left food in the apartment refrigerator for her whenever I had to be out.

Jerry Lewis was coming to the hotel at 4:00 P.M. to drive Vicki and me to the country, and I hurriedly packed a small case and then caught a taxi to the hospital. There, I found Connie pale and quiet but he asked about Vicki. I told him her health was improving; she had ordered a rather enormous chef's salad for her lunch. Connie smiled and caught my hand. "Why not?" he said. "Remember when we added more to the menus in Brussels? At least she's only ordering for herself, not half a hotel floor." He paused. "Katie, you're a good little mother. You take care of us all. Say," he went on without a pause, "Diogenes has picked up speed. I clocked him today. He came past within four minutes in three separate laps." He smiled again. "Tell Harold, will you?"

I couldn't, but I didn't say that to Connie. Harold had died more than a week earlier. I had not wanted to bring it up, and that Friday was the first time Connie had mentioned Harold in weeks.

As we were talking, a technician wheeled a huge machine through the door. Dr. Crawford came in behind it. Immediately Connie's mood changed.

"Now what?" he asked Dr. Crawford irritably. "Why more X rays?"

Dr. Crawford smiled. "It will only take a minute."

Connie was positioned up in bed and the technician expertly and rapidly took the X rays and backed softly out. I stared up at Dr. Crawford. He was affable and smiling. I went over and kissed Connie.

"I've got to go," I told him. "It's after four now and Jerry Lewis will be waiting at the hotel. I'll see you Sunday. Be good."

Connie nodded. "Take care of Vicki," he said.

I waved good-bye and went out into the hall. Dr. Crawford followed me out and walked me out of sight of Connie's open door.

"Don't go to the country tonight," he said.

I stared at him. "Why not?"

His voice was hesitant. "It's a feeling I have."

"My God," I said, "what are you trying to tell me? Is Connie worse? I thought he was to come home in a few days."

Crawford was silent.

"Look, the driver has been waiting for me about half an hour now and I've got a sick young daughter. If you had any worries, couldn't you have gotten in touch with me earlier?"

For answer, he pulled a card out of his white jacket and wrote down a number. "Here's my home phone. I live in the apartment building right next to the hospital," he said, handing me the card. "You can call me anytime or I'll call you."

"Just tell me what's wrong."

He shook his head. "His lungs aren't too good."

"Is he in danger? My God! Why doesn't anybody tell me these things?"

"Look, maybe it will be all right. You take your daughter home. You've got my number and I've got yours. If you're worried or I think you should come back, I'll call."

I left Memorial like a sleepwalker. I could not think what to do: Send Jerry home with Vicki? Send Jerry home and put Vicki back in bed? Should I get in touch with Geoff (who was working on a movie documentary in and around the area but might be hard to contact)? Had anybody called Pat about Dr. Crawford's concern? Why hadn't Dr. Whitmore told me if anything was wrong? What was I to do with myself when I did get home?

Memorial's nurses' notes for Wednesday, November 20, two days before Dr. Crawford and I had our conversation read:

Appears sluggish mentally.

Had a glass of tea in bed. Not in pain. No nausea. Chilly sensations.

Patient assisted with a.m. care. Pt. appears weak and pale. C/o back pain. Med. X2 for pain with slight relief. Resting in bed all day.

OOB with help. Chest X-ray taken this p.m. Highly febrile, no diaphoresis [heavy sweating] so far. Med. given for pain X2. C & S done.* Fleets given—small effect.

On Thursday, November 21, Dr. Katz's note reads:

T—37° CXR [chest x-ray] [indicates] infiltrating mass-like density in the R mid-lung field; C/S* sent; on Schering 13521; % some constipation; WBC—3,100; Pl.—67,000; HCT—23.7.†

Nurses' notes for Thursday, November 21, are not very different from those written on Wednesday, except that Connie was slightly diaphoretic [perspiring], asked for a walker, and was out of bed once in a wheelchair. He was noted to be feverish, weak, and pale.

Dr. Crawford's notes for Friday, November 22, the day he spoke with me, are as follows:

T to 38° and afebrile now. Mod. bronchi [abnormal chest sound] R lung field. HCT today 22, WBC 2.5, platelets 75,000. No change in bowels, pain R hip although patient continues progressively ↑ [increased] weakness and shows some depression. At Dr. Whitmore's

* C & S or C/S stands for culture and sensitivity. Urine and sputum are two common examples of cultures tested in a liquid dilution of drugs. Such lab experiments determine the body's susceptibility to bacterial infection and to its tolerance or reaction to a particular medicine.
† The masslike density in the right midlung field could indicate the presence of a tumor or pneumonia. Dr. Katz's note indicates that Connie had been given the Schering Compound 13521. Dr. Whitmore's notes state only that the therapy "was planned."

suggestion I had a talk with Mrs. Ryan appraising her of Mr. Ryan's condition.

All I had ever learned of Connie's state of health was the gentle, quiet talk with Dr. Crawford in the hall. In the four days from Monday, November 18—when Dr. Whitmore told me of his hopes of sending Connie home soon—to Friday, November 22, when Dr. Crawford told me that Connie's lungs were involved, my husband had deteriorated rapidly, but I had been given no information about it at all. At the time Dr. Crawford was suggesting I stay in town, Connie had slightly more than twenty-four hours to live.

It was a silent, moody drive home to Connecticut that Friday. Vicki, wrapped in a blanket, dozed on the back seat. I sat in front with Jerry. "Not good?" he asked. I shook my head, staring out the side window. At one point I remember thinking hysterically: what am I doing going in the wrong direction? In point of fact I was as bewildered, ignorant, and confused as I had been during my brief conversation with Dr. Crawford. I badly needed somebody to make the decisions. Whenever crucial moves had been required, that somebody had always been Connie.

At home in Ridgefield I raced to the telephone and called Connie's room at Memorial. Paul Slade, our photographer friend, answered cheerfully. Paul had been one of the rather constant visitors at the hospital and always came on Friday evenings or Saturdays when I could not be there.

"How's Connie?" I asked Paul.

"Good. He's lying here giving me hell as usual."

"No, Paul. Listen to me. Is he—how does he seem? Just answer yes or no."

"That's a hard one," Paul said. "Sort of in between. Here, I'll let you talk to him. He's trying to take the phone from me anyway."

"Hi," Connie said. "Get home all right! How's Vicki?"

"Everything's fine. Oh, Connie, I'm sitting on your bed and looking at our beautiful house. The doctor said you could come home soon. I just know when you get here you'll feel all right. You'll be well again."

There was a pause. "Tell me what you're seeing," Connie said.

And I did. I told him about his favorite armchair, the bright brilliance of the November night filling the wide windows, Maggie Korn's picture facing his bed, the Baccarat glass monkey I had bought for him years before in France which was staring at me from the place where Connie kept it beside the phone. I told him about the dog, Alta, named for the fishing stream, who was lying beside his bed where she always slept, about the stacks of books that had come in for him to autograph, about some deep emotion between us that wasn't complete unless he was there to experience it with me.

He had remained totally silent throughout my recital.

He said, "I love you very much. God bless you always," and the phone went dead. In all the years I'd known him, that was the only time he had ever hung up on me. Slowly I replaced my own phone. I knelt beside his bed and said aloud, "Connie, listen to me. You've got to fight. Do you hear me? You can do it. Don't be tired. Don't think about being tired. Connie, listen. You have to fight."

I repeated those words at intervals all through the night, between calls to Pat and those to locate Geoff, which I finally managed to do. He wanted to come over immediately, but he had finished work late and had had no dinner.

"Just stay close to the phone," I told him. "We'll want to get in early tomorrow."

David Evins called. He had been to see Connie either before or after my talk with Connie and Paul. Connie had appeared to have some difficulty breathing, David said, and had coughed up some sputum into a tissue which he quickly balled up and threw in the wastebasket.

433

I called Dr. Crawford after David's call. It was then 1:30 A.M. Mrs. Crawford said he was out walking their dog and would call right back. In minutes he did. I told him what David had observed.

"I'll get right over there and find out what's going on. I'll call you back." He hung up immediately.

On our private line I called Pat Neligan again and then Paul Gitlin and then David. All were determined to be at the hospital early in the morning.

The listed phone rang. It was Dr. Crawford. He had thought from David's description that perhaps Connie had brought up blood, but if he had, no more had apparently been seen. Connie had had a small amount of stool incontinence and his appearance was poor, Crawford said. He had complained of pain, been medicated, and appeared to be resting, but his breathing was becoming audible and gasping. His blood pressure was 90/70, his pulse 100, his respiration 32.

"I'll call Dr. Neligan and tell him," Dr. Crawford said. "And I'll leave word at Reception that you, your children, and whoever else you want can go right up as soon as you arrive. You can't all be in his room at once, but at least you'll all be on the same floor."

"Thank you for your kindness," I said. "I wish there were more doctors around like you."

"Sorry I haven't helped you as much as I would have liked. I've come to admire Mr. Ryan very much. I don't imagine there's much point in asking you to try and get some sleep?" he said.

"It's after three and I've got to call our son. We'll try to leave here by seven."

"All right. I'll be at the hospital. Take care of yourself, Mrs. Ryan."

"You take care of Connie."

"Yes," he said. "I will. I'm trying."

Saturday, November 23, 1974. Even at 7:00 A.M. one could tell it was going to be a beautiful day. A warm weather front had moved in, making the day golden. Although it was warm, I put on the blue sweater I had bought the day before. We got into the car. Geoff sat up front with me, and Victoria, much improved but still fatigued, again took over the back seat. At that early morning hour the highways were nearly empty. The Saw Mill Parkway curved and dipped and climbed again, and for long stretches at a time ours was the only car.

Just after we crossed the Triborough Bridge we hit real traffic. Roadwork had forced a detour. Traffic was emptying slowly off the ramp and down onto 125 Street, bumper to bumper. I pulled out of line at the first street possible and we wended our way through neighborhoods I had never seen before. Children were playing on the doorsteps of dingy buildings and newspapers fluttered up and sailed on small breezes. I kept turning back toward the FDR Drive, only to find orange roadblocks barring every street I tried to take. Eventually—I don't remember where—I found my way to Second Avenue and headed downtown toward the tall, looming complexes of Memorial and New York hospitals.

We parked at the little garage across the street from Memorial and hurried to the hospital. The detour had caused us a good hour's delay. At the visitors' desk I gave my name.

"Yes, Mrs. Ryan. Dr. Crawford left word. You and your children go right up." This time we did not need the large, bright pasteboard visitors' cards permitting only two people at a time in the patient's room. Nor did we have to wait for an elevator. An operator I had come to know from many visits was waiting for us. Quickly we reached the fourteenth floor.

I ran down the familiar hallway to see Paul Gitlin and David Evins just turning the corner. Connie's room was just beyond that turning. I stared at them. "What are you doing here? Are we too late?"

"Late?" Paul said loudly. "You're a little early if you ask me. Your husband's been telling me off, as usual."

I raced around the corner, not waiting for Geoff and Vicki to catch up.

I stopped just inside the door to Connie's room. It seemed to be overflowing with equipment and with people in white. An attendant to the left of the bed watched over a white porcelain tray on which vials and bottles were neatly arranged on a white cloth. Blood pressure apparatus stood near the bed. On the other side, IV standards held bottles which dripped saline fluids and ampicillin, a synthetic penicillin, into Connie's arm. Oxygen equipment was in place and a nasal mask lay on the pillow. A nurse and another man in white stood near the foot of the bed.

But it was only the man in the bed I really saw. Thin of face now, the fine skin almost as pale as the pillows, the strong, long-fingered hands moving restlessly on the coverlet, Connie lay with his eyes closed, breathing in short, harsh breaths. I went directly to him.

"Connie," I said, and again, "Connie."

He opened his eyes and smiled. "Little Katie," he said with difficulty. "It's not Sunday. Why aren't you at home?"

I couldn't think of an answer immediately. "You've got your days mixed," I finally said. "It is Sunday."

"Saturday," Connie said.

I heard someone tell me that he must put the nasal mask back on. I positioned it. Almost immediately Connie tried to take it away.

"CJ, please. It's oxygen. Try to keep from talking for a little while and just breathe in through your nose and out your mouth."

"It hurts."

"It will help you. I think you've got a cold," I told him.

436

"Remember, I had a bad one last week. I shouldn't have kissed you. I think you caught my cold."

Connie shook his head. "Got pneumonia, I think," he said in pauses for breath. "Funny about cancers. Half the time you die of pneumonia."

"You're not going to die."

Someone told me not to encourage him to talk. The young attendant near me began to take Connie's blood pressure. Connie turned to watch the procedure. His eyes widened.

"Seventy-five/fifty-five," he said. "My God, Katie, no one can live with a blood pressure like that."

A nurse adjusted the nasal mask once again. I went to the bathroom and wrung out a cloth under the cold water faucet. I went back to the bed and laid it on his forehead and then gently began to pat his face. A peaceful look came over his features.

"Katie," he said, "nobody else knows how to do that right."

"Does it feel good?"

He nodded.

"Then I'll keep on doing it until you want me to stop."

The nurse crossed to where I was standing. She handed me two boxes of tissues. "Try to encourage him to cough. The more he can get up, the better. I'll also give you some soft towelettes to wipe his lips. They get very dry."

I nodded, and urged Connie to cough. He complied willingly.

"You see," I told him, "you're licking this cold. You're doing fine. The oxygen and antibiotics are clearing everything up. You've just got to keep on remembering to breathe in the oxygen and cough up as much as you can."

From the doorway I heard a small noise. I turned to see Geoff and Vicki standing there. I had totally forgotten them. "Can they come in?" I asked the nurse.

"Of course."

The children moved up to the end of the bed. Vicki's eyes

were full of tears, her color almost as ashen as Connie's. She stared at him, unbelieving.

He opened his eyes and saw his children and slowly reached up and pulled the oxygen mask away.

"What are you doing here, baby?" he asked Victoria. "You don't look well. Why did Mama let you come?"

"I'm fine," she said. Her voice broke. "I was lonesome for you. I'm all well now."

"Sure?" Connie asked.

She nodded and stared down at the floor, trying hard to control her tears.

"Dad?" Geoff said. He had caught his sister's hand and was squeezing it tightly.

"Hi, Big G." Connie made a small gesture around the room and its equipment. "Helluva thing, isn't it?"

"Not if it helps you get better," Geoff said.

Connie looked at them. "Take your sister to the apartment," he said, "then come back."

Vicki looked up tearfully. "Daddy?"

Her father watched her.

"I love you," she said, face wet with tears.

At Connie's side I quickly wiped tears from his own eyes.

"Go with your brother, like a good girl. Go now," he said as they both hesitated. Slowly they left the room, their eyes and Connie's holding on one another until the children were out of sight.

David Evins was still in the waiting room. Pat and Vera had not yet arrived. David called Marilyn, who immediately left her house to go to the Sherry-Netherland and await Victoria. Geoff stayed at the hospital, never far from Connie's room.

By noon Pat and Vera had arrived. Vera stayed in the waiting room for a time while Pat came in. As always, at the sight of him, Connie's spirits rose.

"What the hell are you doing, CJ?" Pat asked, his eyes moving steadily over the room, checking equipment and oxygen rate. "What'd you have, a party in here last night, hum?"

Connie looked at him. "Son-of-a-bitch Neligan," he said fondly.

Pat came around and took my place at Connie's side. He bent over the bed. "Now listen, CJ, stop the talk and start listening, hear? I want you to cough for me."

Connie complied and Pat adjusted the nasal mask once more.

"I want you to cough a lot. You're plain lazy, Ryan, you know that? You just want to lie here and go to sleep. Well, you're not going to sleep. You're going to cough up all that crap you've got inside."

Connie pulled down the mask and held onto it.

"I want a cigarette, Neligan," he said. "They're in the drawer someplace." He turned his head, searching for the bed table.

"Are you crazy?" Pat asked. "You want to blow us all to Kingdom Come? There's oxygen running in here and if you take off that mask one more time we're going to have a row."

He took the mask from Connie's hands, picked up swabs from the table, and cleaned it. He put it back in place.

Vera came in and Pat went through the same struggle again with Connie about the mask.

Still Connie attempted to talk, and had to be reminded constantly to cough. I caught a glimpse of Paul and Zelda in the hall and went out to them.

"You go sit down in the waiting room for a while," Zelda said. "I'll come in."

"Pat and Vera are here," I told her. "Geoff took Vicki to the hotel. I'd rather stay here."

Zelda was firm. "Geoff's in the waiting room. Marilyn Evins has gone to meet Vicki. She'll take care of her. David was here but he went home and will be back later. Now, scoot!" she told me.

In the waiting room the television was on. It was the day of the big college game between Michigan and Ohio State.

The sun was streaming in the windows and one could hardly see the screen. Someone made room for me and I sat down beside Geoff. He stared silently at nothing.

"Can he make it, Mom?" he asked.

"He's been in a lot of tight places before in his life. If there's a way to do it, he'll do it."

"Yeah, but is there a way?"

"I don't know. When Pat comes out we'll see what we can find out."

I walked back to Connie's room. Vera and Zelda were just coming out the door, followed by Paul. "We'll be in the waiting room," Vera said.

Inside the room I again got a cold cloth and gently applied it to Connie's forehead and face. I wiped his lips. I urged him to cough. I told him he was winning. I told him he had to win because—well, I couldn't imagine him any other way. I couldn't get a picture of myself in a world he did not inhabit. I did think of all the times in the past when he had tried to explain the business details and contracts of the books to me, when he had attempted to show me how the furnace worked and where the well was located and the position of underground wires. I had never listened because there would never be a need to know. Connie had always seen to those things. He always would.

I looked down at him in the bed. He was watching me.

"My poor little girl," he said. "My Katie."

I bent and kissed him and clung to his hand.

Close to 4:00 P.M. Pat held a conference with Dr. Katz in the hall while Vera and I listened. Dr. Katz had taken Dr. Crawford's place along about noon. The two men talked a medical jargon I could not follow. Pat asked a great many questions. Dr. Katz supplied answers. Finally Pat turned to me.

"They are taking all the positive measures they can, Kathy," he said. "Dr. Katz even discussed doing a tracheotomy earlier. Connie's been given digitoxin. There's one unit of packed cells in progress.* They're using oral suctioning equipment to try to clear his air passages."

"Are they doing everything they can?"

"Yes, they are," Pat said firmly.

"He's fought so hard for so long, Pat. I want him to have every chance."

"I'm telling you, these are very positive procedures." Pat hesitated a moment, then said, "But the poor fellow's suffering terribly. He's fighting but it's taking everything he's got." He looked at his watch. "I've got to see another of my patients here and then I've got to get back to Norwalk Hospital."

"Do you have to go?"

Vera put her arms around me. "I'll be at home."

"He's better when you're here, Pat."

"He's doing the very best he can," Pat said. "With or without me, God bless him."

Marilyn Evins came in soon after Pat and Vera left. Zelda, too, had gone home. Seeing Marilyn, Connie gasped, "I'd about given you up."

"Given me up?" Marilyn joked. "Don't you ever give me up, kiddo."

Her eyes were full of tears. She stayed only a short time, assuring me that Vicki was fine.

Ever since Pat's departure it seemed to me that Connie's condition had worsened. The breath sounds were now loud and very labored. I thought of Ann and the fight for life she had made in the room next to Connie's the year before. Connie's breathing was not unlike Ann's.

Nurses and attendants still came and went. I paid little

---

* A transfusion of red blood cells from which plasma has been removed. Packed cells help to reduce overloading of the circulatory system and work against dangerous bacteria in the blood.

attention to what they did except once when they tried to put the oral suction tube down Connie's mouth. His eyes flew open, he appeared in great distress, and then stubbornly he bit down on the tube so that it could neither go down or be removed. Only after much cajoling did the nurse get him to release it.

Around 6:00 P.M. David Evins returned with a small basket of sandwiches and a thermos of tea for Geoff and me. I was still at Connie's side, with my cold cloth. It was all I could do for him. Memorial's staff was fighting as hard for his life as he was himself. They let me stand beside him with the useless little cloth, endlessly patting his face.

Suddenly his eyes flew open. Directly opposite his bed was a picture of a fisherman casting into a river. "Geoff," Connie gasped.

Geoff came quickly to my side of the bed.

"The wrist," Connie whispered. "Remember to use the wrist."

At first we did not understand and then we followed his eyes to the picture. "I will, Dad," Geoff said. "You always tell me the success of the cast is in the wrist. I'll practice more."

Connie smiled. The harsh breath sounds seemed louder. We stood still beside this man who, in different ways, had given us life.

Suddenly Connie grabbed the sides of the bed and, with the great strength in his shoulders and arms, pulled himself upright. I put my arms around him to steady him. He reached up and put one hand on mine.

"Katie," he said, "I'm so damn tired."

He took two deep breaths and was gone.

The hospital staff thought it unusual that Geoff and I should insist on lowering him on the bed and taking from his little finger the heavy ring that bore his crest, but somehow we knew he would want only us to do those things, and close his eyes and brush his fair hair neatly back. With David Evins helping, we gathered his possessions. His heavy watch had stopped at 7:44 P.M. exactly. I wrapped it in tissue and put it in my handbag. We made necessary phone calls. I spoke with Dr. Katz a last time and with the priest who had been in and out. David, Geoff, and I walked slowly toward the elevators. Half the patients on the hospital floor, it seemed, had copies of *A Bridge Too Far* and the ones I knew I waved good-bye to. In that special kinship of victims and families, nobody had had to tell these patients that the battle in Room 1428 was over. Some of them cried as we walked by and some of them stared vacantly into space, accepting the fate that Connie had fought against up to the end.

We buried him not in Normandy among the men he wrote about and loved but in a little country cemetery near our home where French troops of Rochambeau's army had encamped 193 years earlier when they came to aid the cause of the American Revolution.

Veterans of the 82nd Airborne Division were Connie's honor guard, a score of friends his honorary pallbearers. The service was ecumenical because he was. A choir of boy sopranos sang "The Battle Hymn of the Republic" and a fine Irish tenor sang "The Minstrel Boy." The flags of Ireland, Great Britain, the Netherlands, and France flanked the altar, and representatives of those countries sat behind the family pews.

His casket was draped with the flag of his adopted country, and the Stars and Stripes was flown at half-mast at Ridgefield's town hall and at the fire department.

Church bells tolled as the processions lined up outside the church. Then an organist with a fine feeling for Bach played our wedding song, "Jesu, Joy of Man's Desiring," and we went up a church aisle together for the last time.

Walter Cronkite read two paragraphs from *The Longest*

Day and spoke of Connie in a tremulous voice he's never used on the CBS Evening News. A Protestant minister read Connie's favorite lines from Faulkner's Nobel Prize speech.

At gravesite, near Rochambeau's Frenchmen and American patriots, the men of the 82nd closed ranks around him. They folded the flag from his casket and brought it to General Jimmy Gavin, who presented it to me. A man who had jumped in North Africa, Sicily, and into the burning houses of Ste.-Mère-Église in France in 1944 read the 82nd's burial service for a comrade fallen in action and then put the division's shoulder patch on the casket.

Our cars pulled away, heading for home and the "bash" Connie had once—jokingly, I thought—made me promise to give "with no sad, lousy toasts, Katie. Just a bunch of the guys and our friends sitting around drinking and yakking about the war." As we left I looked back to see the 82nd veterans still drawn up by the grave. They stood by Connie until the casket was lowered into the ground and covered with earth. Only then did they return to the house to mingle with columnists and reporters and diplomats and their counterparts from the U.S. 101st Airborne, the U.S. First Army, the Third Army, the 4th Division—and with British, French, and Dutch people whose names are sprinkled through the pages of Connie's books and who took off, the minute the news of his death broke in Europe, to come to say good-bye.

In a letter Connie had written Victoria during the summer of 1973 when she had gone to work in France, he mentioned that the book was nearly finished and he was glad because he was tired. Then he wrote:

Vicki, if you ever have to, tell Mom that the only thing I want on my gravestone is just "Cornelius Ryan," then the dates of birth and death and, after that, just have her put the single word "reporter."

And I did.

ACKNOWLEDGMENTS

CONNIE'S TAPES, my records and Anne Bardenhagen's compose the heart of the book, but that heart depended, for total accuracy, upon a large body of medical records and statistics and on the cooperation of internists, surgeons, radiation therapists, laboratory technicians, and nurses.

It will become obvious that, next to my husband, the greatest debt of gratitude I owe is to that most compassionate, intelligent, and professional of women—Anne Bardenhagen. As she did with Connie, she goaded, prodded, threatened (yes, threatened in the kindest possible way) when my emotions were too dreary, my fear of failure too great to allow me to work. She has also the ability to laugh, to cry, to share with me the memories of the man we worked with. He is never far from our thoughts, nor will he ever be.

Dr. Patrick Neligan, that gentle man who hides behind his brusque professional exterior, has, I think, forgiven me my birthplace. I am not Irish, nor was I born in the Nile Delta as he once thought. I am Connie's wife, and Pat loved and cared for Connie almost daily from the onset of his illness to the last day of his life. Working long hours himself, Pat still finds time for me and the questions I have so often imposed upon him. My admiration for him and my thanks are insufficient for the job he has performed.

Without the belief of Dr. Willet Whitmore that I would

attempt to write this book as well as any layperson could, I might have experienced great difficulties in obtaining vital records which form the background to much of the book. Through his efforts and the cooperation of directors and administrators of Memorial Sloan-Kettering Cancer Center, in particular S. Jeffrey Bastable, Connie's medical records from the center were placed at my convenience. They date from Connie's first visit to Dr. Whitmore in August 1970, through his death in November 1974.

Dr. Joseph N. Ward sent me all the data he had collected of Connie's visit to him and helped me enormously by his encouraging words to me and his belief in this project.

Dr. Hugh J. Jewett of Brady Urological Institute, Johns Hopkins University Hospital, played a vital role in helping Connie and me toward the decision we would make regarding Connie's course of treatment to try to hold his cancer at bay. But Dr. Jewett did more. Not only did he, as well as all the other doctors, allow me access to his own letters and records, but he was an unfailing source of comfort and kindness. Like Pat Neligan, he often fitted me into his busy schedule, explaining medical background and history, reading and correcting various portions of the book as they pertained to him. His letters, filled with facts, encouragement, and deep interest, are among my prized possessions.

To the brilliant young professor and chairman of the Department of Radiology, Stanford University Medical Center, Dr. Malcolm A. Bagshaw, I owe a great debt as well. He made available to me his files and studies on Connie, as well as many articles and papers he has published in medical journals.

To Connie's journalist friends—Herb Caen, the late Bob Considine, Ben Wright, Jack Thompson, to name a few—who made letters and articles available to me, I can only thank them for accepting me almost as one of their own. To the Hearst Publications goes my appreciation for permitting me to use excerpts from columnists' articles. *The New York*

Times provided me with Jane E. Brody's fine articles pertaining to cancer, and the *New York Daily News* sent me the deep investigative pieces written by Kitty Hanson about people—victims, friends, and family—living their lives in the shadow of cancer and often turning those shadows into sunlight. *Time* magazine, *Reader's Digest, Newsweek, Saturday Review, Esquire,* and *W*—either through editors or publishers—brought to my attention a wealth of material relating to or directly focusing on the subject of cancer. These thoughtful, timely articles make it possible for hundreds of thousands of readers to be better prepared to face cancer if it does strike and to learn of techniques and treatments as quickly as the medical fraternity feels capable of publishing them.

The U.S. Department of Health, Education, and Welfare and the American Cancer Society made available pamphlets, articles, and books to help me in this work. Their vigilance in attempting to keep abreast of material is commendable when one considers the vast quantity of cancer facts and the rapidity with which they change as scientists and technicians reach ever-expanding goals. Such experts, who work alone and unknown against the racing clock of cancer, are the unsung heroes of cancer research.

Time will not allow me to record in this acknowledgment all of my many friends who deserve to be named here. Most of them are in the book, and I have cause to think they know my gratitude as I have cause to know their faith and understanding.

There are, however, friends who, like Annie, took the responsibility of making me work and believing that I could and should. They are: Paul Gitlin, lawyer and friend to all the Ryan family, courageous, loyal, and steadfast (old-fashioned words, perhaps, but applicable): Michael Korda, of Simon and Schuster, who never faltered in his belief that this book should be written just as he never faltered in his love and admiration for Cornelius Ryan.

And last and always first there is Jerry Korn, once Connie's "chief nitpicker" and lately the manager of "the bloody but unbowed fighter" he has forced me to be in order to write this book as well as I could. In the cold winter days immediately following Connie's death I said to Jerry, "We'll write a book about him, won't we, Jere?" He put his arms around me. "You will, kid. *You* will. I'll be close at hand to pick up the pieces." And I did, and he has.